THE
MALE HERBAL
Health Care
for
Men & Boys

James Green, Herbalist

The Crossing Press • Freedom, California 95019

Dedication

To the Elders and my first teachers—
Gypsy grandmother Charlotte Wilkins
and Pretty Grandma Faye Green;
Canadian medicine woman, Norma Myers;
Herbalist, Dr. John R. Christopher.
You fueled the passion of this male heart
with your healing warrior spirit.
To our trustful allies, our Plant and Animal Companions.

Note to the reader: Neither the author nor the publisher take responsibility for any effects which may be produced as a result of following any treatments or suggestions given in this book. Take good care of yourself, and good health to you.

Copyright © 1991 by James Green
Cover art and design by Janice Angelini
Botanical illustrations by Elizabeth Morales-Denny
Anatomical illustrations by Elizabeth Morales-Denny
Illustration of Apollo and Artemis by Ajana Green

7th Printing, 1997
Printed in the U. S. A.

Library of Congress Cataloging-in-Publication Data

Green, James, 1940-
     The male herbal: health care for men and boys / by James Green.
       p. cm.
     Includes index.
     ISBN 0-89594-459-6 (cloth) — ISBN 0-89594-458-8 (paper)
     1. Herbs—Theraputic use. 2. Men—Health and hygiene.
I. Title.
RM666.H33G73 1991
615' .321—dc20
                                         91-2024
                        CIP

With Deep Appreciation:
It takes the help of a lot of friends to write an herbal.
Thank you.

Mindy Green for your gentle love, your patience and your magical fragrances.

Jo Green for raising me with such spunk and humor.

John Fox for helping her.

Amanda McQuade Crawford for your laughter, your light, your kindred spirit and for pointing out my errors.

Mark Crawford for your warm friendship.

David Hoffmann for your British humour, your teaching and for constantly reminding me that "None of this is true."

Diana De Luca for the passion of your dance.

Gina Banghart for your Earth prayers and your Earth science.

Lawrence Banghart for your bilingual wit.

Tim Blakley for teaching us to play in the garden.

Richard Vogel, PhD. scorpio brother, musician and timeless friend.

Daniel Pinney for first asking me to study and share male health-care.

Rosemary Gladstar for inspiring me to begin this written work and the following one.

Cascade Anderson-Geller for your healing wisdom and for introducing men and women to the concepts necessary for practicing male/female mutual health-care.

Christopher Hobbs for your peaceful immune enhancing herbalism.

Beth Baugh for your gracious hospitality and quiet nourishment.

Ed Smith & Sara Smith for your integrity, your learning and all the help you've given me.

Ryan Drum for the astute observations you share with me and for your great herbal brews.

Roy Upton for your bright enthusiasm nourishing our herbal sciences and the TCM connection.

Kathi Keville for your knowledge shared with great heart and for the AHA.

Svevo Brooks for speaking with us in fluent Nettle tongue.

Feather Jones for your leadership and your herbal medicine.

Carol McGrath for your songs of life.

Bob Brucia for your integrity and playful wit, like a smiling eagle.

Michael Moore for your pioneering work reviving the concept and practice of the local medicine maker.

Forest Shomer for your seeds of Earth consciousness.

Don Ollsin for your healing journey.

Joy Gardner for years of friendship and the bridge to Crossing.

William LeSassier for building the foundation for so many healers and for reminding us that "we are what we don't excrete."

Daniel Kenner for your intelligent enthusiasm and attentive help.

Kurt Schnaubelt for the fragrance you brought into our lives.

Ken Collins for helping us all stay free.

Jane Bothwell for your heartfelt dedication to the plant community.

Michael Tierra for your Eastern Medicine translation and for helping me get Dr. C out of jail back in '74.

V. J. Keating III for taking care of the companion animals, wherever you are.

David Winston for the pipe ceremonies and your Earth stories.

Brigitte Mars for promoting the heart of your herbal peers.

Jeannine Parvati Baker for your mother courage and for The Woman's Herbal.

Rico Baker for the power of your male insights.

Nan Koehler for your beautiful family and your Artemisian healing.

Silena Heron because I like to see you smile.

Jeanne Rose for breathing fresh air into American herbalism.

Paul Lee for your garden and for putting academic wisdom into its proper herbal perspective.

Steven Foster for keeping the experts ever alert.

Rob Menzies for manning the forests.

Joel Alter, D.O. for helping me get back up when I was down and confused.

Paul Bergquist, M.D. for working with me to build a foot path between our healing arts.

Mark Blumenthal for your vision.

Rob McCaleb for tirelessly building bridges between the sciences.

Marcia Starck my Earth peer and Sky sister.

The California School of Herbal Studies for being there and for patiently tending the spring garden of today's Herbal Renaissance, and Herbie our wily feline ally for closely observing us all.

Each of you, your knowledge, your Spirit, your humor and companionship are my references for this herbal. You are the visionaries and troubadours of the science that I believe. You are the singers and musicians in the hottest dance in town.

Contents

Prologue   vii

1   Where is the Male Medicine of Folk Wisdom?
     Or, Why can't I Call a Guynecologist?   1

2   Recycling our Heritage: An Introduction   8
     to Herbalism & Related Topics

3   The Male Community   28

4   Female–Male Herbal Heritage   34

5   Green's Hypotheses   38

6   A Technology of Independence   52

7   Picking the Right Herb   59

8   Specific Male Problems   82

9   General Health Care   154

10 Materia Medica   187

11 The Male Herbal   193

12 And We Wonder Where the Seeds of
     Male Maturity Fall?   247

Bibliography   250
Resources   253
Glossary   261
Index   268

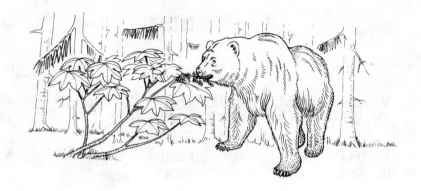

Grizzly bears were seen to eat the Devil's Club berries, and soothe their battle wounds by wallowing in the roots. The leaves and berries of the Devil's Club are shown below.

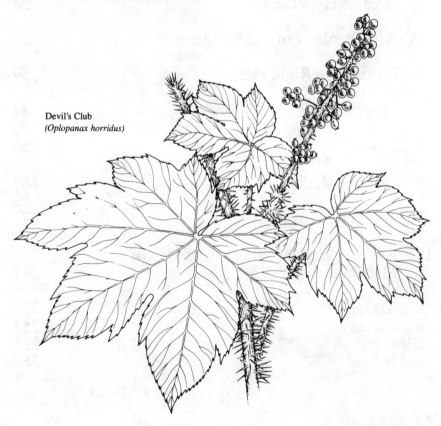

Devil's Club
(Oplopanax horridus)

Prologue

It is a mystery to me why we men have not sooner written a male herbal, so looking into the eyes of mystery, I offer this work as a beginning.

When I was a kid, running around in my little boy body, usually barefooted, wearing sloppy sweatshirts tucked into baggy corduroy pants hiked up to my armpits, I liked to see myself equally splendid as a giant grizzly bear. Of course I knew I stacked up as only a very small grizzly, but that didn't matter. I felt that human beings had the potential to be as magnificent and free as the grizzly, with equal heart and courage and independence. The grizzly could do anything. He could play, be mad, eat wild plants, roll around, sleep as long as he wanted to, roar, lick his own wounds and make them better. He (bears were always boys to me then, so were dogs; cats were girls and so were horses) was totally self-sufficient within his vast surroundings. I loved that. When my friends and I played cowboys and Indians, I would always be my favorite Indian warrior, Broken Arrow, but whenever I got killed, I'd change into a grizzly bear. Indians used wild plants to make themselves better too, and I thought that was great.

I looked with deep admiration to the man and the woman who could fix things. Individuals who could take care of themselves and help others; who had the wit, the common sense and the simple skills to live their lives independently. They knew how to build fires, how to grow vegetables, how to preserve food, and how to help their animals when they were hurt or sick. These folks, with knowledge and skill, tended their families using local medicinal plants. They rested when they were sick and knew when to advise someone else to do the same. They could moan out loud or even cry when in pain; why not, it seemed like the natural thing to do, though Broken Arrow wouldn't have.

I sense a profound loss of that sort of wise independence in human beings these days, the loss of our folk-wisdom and folk-skills, and I feel with terrible sadness the horrible loss of the great grizzly bear from the shrinking wilderness of our planet. I believe there is a connection in the parallel disappearance of the majestic grizzly bear and humankind's sense of self-reliance.

I want to do something to preserve and enhance both of these priceless treasures. This book is one of my efforts to help preserve endangered plant and animal species and the equally endangered health-care independence of my human peers. The energy that returns to me from this endeavor will, likewise, go toward preserving and protecting Earth's wildlife and wilderness lands, natural home of the grizzly, wild medicinal plants and the wise human being.

By profession, I am a wholistically oriented herbalist; a generalist, not a specialist. Specialization requires one to forget too much. I use predominantly the language and health-care models employed by the relatively conservative empirical sciences and systems of clinical investigation evolved by traditional western herbalism. For reasons I discuss in a following chapter, I do not search and reference reductionist literature that pertains to current herbal research. The herbal information I share with you is drawn primarily from the empirically explored, western uses of whole plants. I draw from information which is evolving through the experience and insights of modern wholistic practitioners and herbal clinicians who are continuing to work directly with human beings dealing with the health and disease conditions prevalent in today's societies.

To my heart and mind men, women and families are most alive when they are self-empowered by the independence of their self-reliance. A keen sense of self and the knowledge and skills of caring for one's own health are fundamental for living a truly effective life in this world. Herbalism is a basic human art and science. It holds the knowledge of how to use wild and cultivated plants for maintaining personal independence and self-reliance. The plant materials and essences used for personal health-care and environmental esthetics are ecologically sound. If harvested wisely, they come free with residence on this planet; medicinal herbs come with the territory. Herbs are integral, planet-provided food and medicine for all inhabitants. Herbal medicine is everywhere. It is in every forest, jungle, seashore, "vacant" lot and in almost every family's yard, if we know how to use it, if cultural amnesia does not remain so chronic and disempowering that the individual continues to see himself/herself merely as a victim of injury and "disease," unable to heal and sustain health without the external expertise of some elite authority. Someone once wisely noted, "Healing is a basic human function; it is neither a medical touch nor a supernatural power." Healing is a natural process of each person's evolution, as is disease. Healing belongs to each of us who dwells in a living body; it comes with the carnal real estate. But let us not allow ourselves to be deceived; neither the power to heal oneself nor the efficient use of herbal medicine relies on the existence of magic fix-it-quick chemical or herbal bullets. No brand of medicine or technology can deliver the goods that will fulfill that prized illusion, though many try hard to convince us that they can. Healing is far more profound and intimate than merely buying some corporate herbal or chemical health gimmick. There is a dignity inherent in the ability to tend to one's own condition; to live a knowing relationship with natural surroundings, possessing a personal independence with the skills to provide one's self with natural remedies and self-help; a dignity that I think is particularly fitting to the male nature and the male psyche.

Ah yes, the male psyche, clear images of you must dwell on the shadow side of the moon, a labyrinth even more mysterious than the female psyche. This book is about that mystery. This book is the progeny of shared personal experiences, opinions and hypotheses regarding the male spirit and male health-care in the United States and Canada, the two cultures that I know. It is written neither about men nor at them. It is written by a man talking with the other individuals of his gender. I offer these ideas and techniques in wholistic herbal health-care as concepts for males of all ages, all races, all countries and cultures to consider, to work with and to share. It is a beginning.

Before journeying into the mysterious and intriguing panorama of issues that specifically affect male health-care, maybe lining up a few soap boxes to stand on en route, I'd like to establish some ground rules and requests for the reader and this writer.

When an individual goes public, publishing a book discussing his experiences, beliefs and opinions, especially in the realms of health and personal power, it is important to give the reader a self-disclosure of one's bias. Currently, in this western culture of ours, the fact that I have written this book which has been published tends to display me as an authority. In light of this strange cultural phenomenon, I wish to supply the discriminating reader and herbal learner with appropriately insightful information to help him and her question this authority. Nothing that I say is presented by me as Truth (only Broken Arrow spoke Truth). Through your eyes, the printed voice of this book will share my knowledge, observations and opinions based on my experiences, punctuated by what wisdom I have gathered. Every individual has a share of wisdom to pass around. As your mind travels through the landscape of ideas I design and construct for you in this herbal, please do not slip into a passive state of observation. In the light of your experiences, question my opinion. I accept the risk of being proven wrong. I know I have attachments that my mind has cleverly camouflaged as reality which my heart has not yet enlightened with compassionate understanding and peace. I assure you that I care deeply about us human beings, about our planet and all the other incredible beings, grizzly and non-grizzly, that share this planet with us . . . . and I definitely have strong personal opinions about the issues that presently affect us all. If the fervor of my expression of these opinions ascends a street orator's platform for a brief moment, allow me the social blunder; it's just an idiosyncrasy of my particular humanness, probably related to my anatomical shortness. Do not fault me for my passion. Rather, make notes of your disagreements, get back to me and point out the possible error of my conclusions. This way we can interact and communicate as co-seekers and as co-members of a species that obviously has a lot to discover within itself. We are a transformative species that has a present need to share experiences and ideas where it comes to cohabiting a small planet, preventing disease and living our individual lives in a healthy ecological balance. I can live with the fact that some people will always think of authors as "experts" as long as it is noted that the only universal characteristic of experts is that they always disagree with one another. I personally don't give the label much credence. I rather prefer the term artist, or maybe wiz.

1

Where is the Male Medicine of Folkloric Wisdom?
or
Why Can't I Call a Guynecologist?

There is relatively little specific information concerning herbs and folk wisdom for male health-care presently available in the literature of our western cultures. I draw from the experiences of the small number of men who come to me for herbal consultation and the considerably larger number of women seeking help for their sons, male partner or other male relatives. It is difficult, however, to gather a diversity of direct wholistic information on male health-care, for relatively few men consult me or any other herbalist to discuss their health problems and the possible contributing factors. Personally, I'm no different. I seldom seek help. I probably wouldn't call a *guynecologist* if such a specialist in male medicine did exist. I must say, a major reason that I usually don't seek outside help is because I believe that a well nourished and adequately exercised body will take care of most problems if just given time and a lack of outside interference. However, I must also admit that I don't seek advice or therapy because I am a male, and for some reason many of us tend to keep our health problems to ourselves. This is due possibly to pride, fear, embarrassment, or a reluctance to admit illness and expose vulnerability. I don't fully understand the dynamics of this male trait, but it is there to some degree inside most of us.

In order to manifest more knowledge and wholistic understanding about specific male health-care, we have to listen, observe carefully, make accurate notes and share our experiences with each other.

Living and teaching at the California School of Herbal Studies, my home nesting within the school's fecund and prolific herb garden, the green light district of our acreage, I view our culture through a plant person's eyes, evolving a relatively unique male perspective. I am deeply concerned about our culture's health. I'm not concerned with the issue of whose or what kind

1

of medicine and system of health-care is "best." I think all sincere health-care sciences are remarkable, necessary and of equal value. I am concerned about the availability of quality health-care education for individuals, creating a society that supports a wide spectrum of legally available health-care choices; allowing and encouraging people to learn disease prevention first and, when necessary, to insightfully and freely choose their healers and their best medicine from a diverse field of health-care practitioners.

Having explored and studied a variety of fascinating health-care systems, I have found herbalism the most healing for me. I believe the wisdom and unique power of modern herbalism is dispensed and received through the nurturing relationship that plants help humans re-develop with Earth. It is important to work with herbs, especially one's locally growing herbs. Touch them, smell them, taste them, grow and carefully harvest them. It goes far beyond merely marketing and consuming them. This is a relationship that works to return the life style of a human being to a more compassionate, wise and humble perspective with the other companion species of this planet, teaching each of us in turn to "move over a bit" and share the planet's space and natural resources with our siblings, all the other equally essential beings. Through this relationship herbal healing touches us most profoundly. This, I believe, is the primary healing that herbs have to give to males. Nine out of ten students in our herb school are women. I suspect that the general male population does not find it as easy or convenient to observe and learn from plants as does the female, but when he does receive plant communication it comes home with great power, and his receptivity to plant medicine is considerably altered. From this point of comprehension and acceptance the energy, the pharmacological actions and the organic nutritional components of herbal preparations are more readily received by male body tissues.

I understand the skeptical caution of those individuals who doubt that so called "scientifically unproven" plant medicines heal the human being. I feel a balanced discriminating skepticism is healthy and wise, but, at the same time, I enthusiastically and in good nature challenge you to get in touch with me at the Herb School where I can teach you how to harvest, prepare, and use your own plant medicines. Then we can discuss with each other our experiences of the healing power of herbal science's remedies. I feel strongly that a medical profession or any group of healers surrenders a vital portion of its healing power and insight when the individual practitioners completely disconnect themselves from the making of their medicines by relinquishing this art and skill to another individual or group to perform for them. Contributing to the making of one's own medicine is a powerful human action and a major part of the human art of simpling. Simpling is the traditional art and timeless knowledge of using common, local, medicinal plants or "simples" for nutrition and healing. Plant medicines have always been there for us. They are simple to prepare and simple to use, and their use is an easily relearned wisdom. (Please see the chapter titled, "Technology of Independence" for methods of preparing herbal medicines.)

As mentioned previously, my search for a rich body of western herbal folkloric knowledge regarding prevention and treatment of chronic disease of the male organs and systems has uncovered a relatively small amount of written information, whereas, certainly, an extensive body of knowledge and empirical lore concerning female health-care exists and flourishes as common knowledge to anyone involved in the study of herbal therapy and wholistic care. Why haven't the males of our culture manifested an equivalent cornucopia of technique and natural wisdom regarding their own specific health-care and treatment? This is a question I ponder as I pursue natural health-care information for my gender. Is it that men appear to lack the degree of complexity of anatomical structure and function of their reproductive system; that they have no obvious reproductive organ cycle that requires them to routinely focus on their physical body, a cycle which alerts them to internal processes and changes? Is this the reason men haven't developed over the centuries an overtly conscious interest in their health and their bodies as women have? Or do males have an innate trust in their body's natural healing power that they rely on more completely than does the female? It is a common experience reported by most physicians that men in the age group 25 to 40 are seldom seen in their offices except with broken bones or some other acute injury. Whatever the reasons, in light of the obvious lack of traditional male health-care lore, it appears that western males have not collectively concerned themselves about personal health-care for many centuries past.

Initiating seminars about male health, I often begin with the questions asked in the previous paragraph, triggering lively discussion and animated opinions from both male and female participants. From the multitude of ideas expressed in these group discussions, it has dawned on me that possibly men are just now creating their gender's specific system of medicine and medical-care techniques. The impact of crisis "war" medicine is and was much more profound on the male than on the female simply by the male's exposure to its value on the battlefield, forsaking traditional supportive means of health-care as being totally inapplicable and lost to them. Maybe today's western, allopathic, technological, crisis medicine is the male's folkloric medicine in the making. The male of our species has, generally speaking, had technical, tactical and cerebral facility promoted and has not been pulled into body consciousness so much by cyclic, lunar, hormonal tides, but more by immediate situational need. He prefers to have control; historically, he creates and avidly pursues competition, reckless-ness, war and crises, and maybe these preferences are the manifest expres-sions of *his* particular hormonal tides.

Possibly the male, in general, requires and prefers medicine that is suitable for his more swashbuckling attitude about life. He requires medi-cine that is heroic in nature, not one that is nutritional. He seeks a medicine that is designed to be efficient in acute crises, not necessarily one that is preventive in nature. He prefers a medicine that will assist him to carry on his "driven-ness," one that gets him back up and back out on the field of whatever it is that he is unrelentingly endeavoring to accomplish. "Stop the bleeding! Quickly, kill the pain and suppress the symptoms so they won't get in my way and interfere with progress! I'm busy. Don't slow me down or attempt to change my direction. Do what needs to be done, but do it quickly and don't talk to me about who I am or about changing my life patterns." Allopathic medicine (chemotherapy, surgery and radiation therapy) specializes in these services and does it more efficiently than any other western system to date. It is a brilliant crisis, accident & wartime medicine. Herbs and natural wholistic health systems don't fill this requirement nearly as efficiently. And that's fine; certainly we all benefit from the availability of a diversity of healing and body-care modalities.

Unfortunately, in the last 70 years in the U.S. and Canada, the merchants and practitioners of this heroic crisis-oriented medicine have established a functional monopoly which has rendered most other systems of healing "unorthodox" and illegal. This in turn has limited personal choice of health-care systems (of which there exists a wonderful diversity) and has nearly eliminated open, exploratory education in homes and schools about alternative health-care, rendering most of the people in our culture unaware of how to care for themselves and how to prevent most chronic and acute health crises. Certainly much recognition and credit must be given to the family doctor. This dedicated family M.D. spends a large amount of time teaching and providing preventive health-care. He and she are definitely a breed apart from the innumerable medical specialists who often lose sight of the primary function of the doctor, which is to teach. The term "doctor" comes directly from the Latin word *doctor* = a teacher. Doctor was the highest degree in medicine, law or theology given by the medieval universities. It still is the highest degree, and today the doctor of medicine must continue to teach the ways of health to his and her patients, including the still healthy. Likewise, the term "physician" is derived from the ancient Latin word *physicus* = physical philosopher. The problem family doctors face daily, however, is that not many individuals are willing to comply with the insights and advice he and she give to them, e.g. stop smoking and drinking, eat an improved diet, get more exercise, etc. The individuals of our western culture in most part have chosen to become dependent on the drugs, surgery and radiation therapy of the allopathic system to treat and suppress the symptoms of their self-depleting living habits and, out of ignorance and media propaganda, believe this is the only valid medical care in existence. As a culture we have ignored and are losing the rich heritage which was handed to us by our culture's ancestral teachers and healers. Consequently, we who cherish our personal independence and favor the alternatives, who choose not to rely, solely, on the allopathic system, frequently find it difficult to draw to ourselves the traditional (currently referred to as unorthodox) alternate arts of healing.

By using the term "alternative" healing arts, I am referring to medicines and techniques that are based on empirical knowledge, i.e. that, based on centuries of observation, they have been repeatedly used with success. These are healing techniques which are not necessarily based upon the use of medicines according to their known physiological, chemical or biological action upon definitely known pathological conditions or perverted functions and which do not rely strictly on white powders, clear liquids, radiation and the scalpel. I'm referring to those medicines that work more slowly and systemically, that regularly incorporate time as an ally for healing. These are the traditional systems that use plants and other nature-designed Earth resources to nourish and rebuild body tissue; that attempt to support and enhance the body's natural immune system rather than suppress and replace it with the actions of serums and chemicals; that rely on the body's wisdom and methods of tending to its own health and repair rather than suppressing and manipulating the body's spontaneous healing energies. The alternative healing arts tend to educate the individual rather than assume responsibility for the individual's health, and they focus on promoting life style habits that help prevent chronic and acute health emergencies.

These "allopathic" and "alternative" medicines and systems of health-care are based on different economies, but therapeutically they are not necessarily mutually exclusive. They are sometimes complementary and, I believe, should be used in combination as needed. When corrective surgery is appropriate or when emergencies occur in times of true accident-emergency and natural disaster, or when the use of natural, non-heroic modalities require the assistance of allopathic medicine in spite of preventive habits, one should draw unhesitatingly on the specific technology of allopathic crisis intervention.

Attitudes are changing, and old inappropriate barriers are crumbling. We are witnessing the beginning of an inspirational time as male individuals express more desire and willingness to explore alternatives and pursue a variety of health-care sciences and wholistic insight; a time when the traditional uses of plant medicines can be re-embraced, focused on male conditions and teamed with allopathic technology to help take better care of the male population, both child and adult.

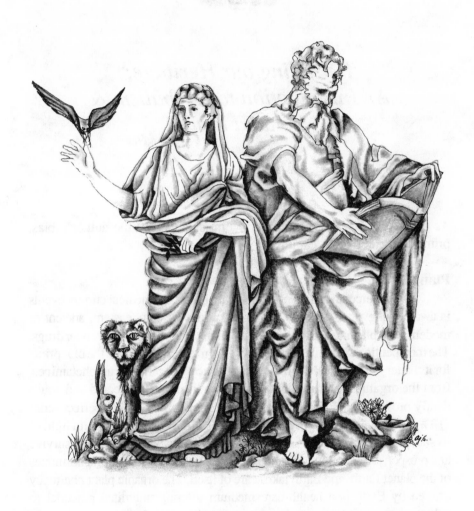

Apollo and Artemis — twin patrons of healing.
Assisted by two midwives, the beautiful and immortal Leto delivered a daughter Artemis who immediately assisted in the birth of her brother, Apollo. Apollo and Artemis develop into the twin patrons of healing; each healing in their own way, Artemis the artful herbalist and midwife, Apollo becoming the father of Asclepius the archetypal medical doctor of present day.

❧2❧

Recycling our Heritage: An Introduction to Herbalism & Related Issues

As promised, the following introduction should bare the author's bias, prime bent and salient leanings.

Plants

The perceptive student of medical history and medical current events is aware that every system of health-care, be it western, eastern, ancient or modern, uses plants as the basis of their potions, pills, balms and wonder drugs. The therapeutic power of mainstream western medicine derives the blueprints for its battery of chemical pharmaceuticals, such as aspirin and amphetamines, from the organic molecular models that are ingeniously created and abundantly provided by Earth's organic plant kingdom. It makes perfect sense that a self-contained planet such as ours, as it circles within the warm light of its star, provides absolutely everything its native inhabitants require to survive and prosper, an evolution of abundance. We are the flesh, bones and hormones of the planet Earth, and Earth takes care of itself. The organic plant pharmacy created by Earth is a health-care medium offering unlimited potential to enhance humankind's arts and sciences of healing, but plants have far more to offer than merely their healing chemistry; they offer us companionship and silent wonder. They feel things we feel; they give birth; they move around; they live in families, and they die. No companion creates more beauty, gives nourishment more freely, or lives and dies more gracefully than a plant.

> Silence is the language of the leaves
> and great teachers . . .
> Silent sensual wonder,
> flower speaks, bee hears.
> T. Elder Sachs

Herbalism

Intuitively employing Earth's cornucopia of plant foods and medicines, humans have devised over the centuries numerous and diverse systems and schools of healing. Traditional herbal health-care systems, some of which are native to our country, remain active outside our nation's relatively closed and narrow medical borders.

Herbal medicine is a "people's medicine." It is the oldest branch of planetary medicine, suggesting itself to all animals instinctively. Herbalism is the property and heritage of all cultures and Earth species, embracing far more than merely harvesting plants and taking teas or capsules to counter disease symptoms. Certainly it does provide us an unlimited variety of naturally occurring medicinal remedies, but it also supplies nourishing foods, esthetically sensual and medicinal aromatic oils, beauty aids, delicious (and sometimes not so delicious) herb teas, clothing, shelter and deeply enlivening, wild and peaceful environments.

In the wake of civilization's current ecological dilemma, the practice of modern herbalism asks something of us at the same time that it gives to us. It asks us to reintegrate with our planet, Earth, and to reconnect compassionately with all of Earth's companion species; to take responsibility, responsibility for one's self, one's relationships and one's surroundings. It asks us to relate to herbs not merely as material medicines, but as allied planetary connections, vital parts of the whole of our lives that can help us revive a balanced relationship with a planet that we need to put back into order, thereby preventing most of our afflictions. It promises greater health, effectiveness and abundance in return.

The herbalist

Herbalists were probably our species' first medicine people. The innovative work of today's herbal practitioners is the creative forefront of a flow that reaches back to the beginnings of our ancient species. Herbalists intimately interact with plants and are voluntary stewards of the plant kingdom. Experienced herbalists understand, administer to and teach others about the healing actions of plants, how to harvest these plants carefully and how to make herbal medicine. Herbalists can be found in every healing profession, and most importantly, they are found in many families (more and more families each day). There is no orthodox, stereotypical herbalist or herbalist lifestyle; this is one of the things I love most about my work.

The eyes of language; the language of herbalism

"Language is culture . . . an indispensable vehicle of human knowledge." So Mario Pei points out in his book, *The Story of Language*, as he explores the implacable power that our languages exert on the events of our lives. Mr. Pei portrays how many of our present-day activities are carried on, as they have been carried on for centuries, by the indispensable help of our spoken, written, gestural and symbolic language. "Language is an all-pervasive conveyor, interpreter, and shaper of humankind's social and scientific endeavors. Language enters into, influences, and in turn is influenced by every form of human activity. The most fascinating and mysterious area of language is its connection with the mental processes both of the individual and the social group. It is obvious that everything we do, think and create influences and changes our language, but what is not so obvious, perhaps, is that language in return has a major affect on all our actions and thoughts."

I suspect that language even births and breast-feeds our intuition.

The language that each individual uses reflects his personal science, his chosen methods of investigating his environment and accumulating knowledge. It reflects the nature of his gods, characterizing them as patriarchal or matriarchal, vengeful or compassionate and most importantly, whether they live here on Earth, with us, or are non-residents living somewhere off beyond our sky. A person's language defines his concepts of health and his beliefs about the cause and cure of disease.

Each of humanity's established sciences is a philosophical sub-culture unique unto itself. Each of these sciences is founded on a belief system defining its unique speculation about humanity's relationship to the universe and how the cosmos works through each individual being. There are many established sciences that exist today actively pursuing the reality of Nature and the nature of Reality. Western mainstream science is only one of these sciences. The language of each science uses its unique words to define, illustrate and convey its belief system, its discoveries, its technology and its methods of ongoing inquiry.

The particular scientific language adopted by an individual reflects the relationship the individual has accepted with his universe; consequently the scientific language that an individual chooses to use exerts considerable control on the individual's self-image, his daily life processes and his evolving insights. This language can strongly influence his methods for accumulating further knowledge as well as the ultimate quality of the knowledge accumulated. It is important that one selects with great attention the particular health-care or disease-care science whose language he decides to pursue, for it will deeply affect his comprehension and insight into health-care and the nature of the medicine he or she chooses.

"Tree frog" . . . "wiggle" . . . "Stonehenge" . . . Words are "idea triggers." Once the word is communicated, the trigger squeezed, our senses carry this abstract word symbol to our brain where it ignites an idea in our mind. This idea has been embellished with meaning partially by our direct experience and partially by our acculturation and conditioning. Some words are double triggers igniting not only an idea but also a reflex emotional and even a reflex physical response . . . "IRS" . . . "Nixon" . . . "chocolate" . . . "Rock 'n Roll" . . . see what I mean? Here's another one . . . "congressional-ethics-reform-pay-raise" . . . makes the little hairs on the back of your neck wiggle, doesn't it?

Of course, communicating ideas using the words of the languages of health-care systems works in the same manner . . . "Chi" . . . "star gazing" . . . "vata" . . . "tsentsak" . . . "constitutional remedy" are words used by globally established sciences and systems of health-care. Some of these words may have meaning for the western reader, some may not, but these are words that convey fundamental concepts with significant meaning in the languages of various health sciences. "Disease" . . . "germ" . . . "antibiotic" . . . "doctor" . . . "drug" . . . These are some of our western language's disease-care and health-care words which trigger immediate recognition and response. They have been given meaning due to mainstream medicine's recent dominance in our culture. It is often difficult for us to conceive of the process of health, disease and therapeutics outside the local universe of these western health-care terms.

The word "wholistic," sometimes spelled "holistic" (relating to the whole person), represents a concept just coming into its own in our modern day society as the languages of alternative health-care systems make inroads to our culture's consciousness. Wholistic is a relatively new word, still being culturally defined by each individual's contribution to the concept.

In order for an individual to communicate and use most advantageously an alternative health-care science, it is necessary to openly investigate its unique ideas, giving meaning to the new words and concepts of a different language, often temporarily letting go of some previously accepted concepts and beliefs. Emptying one's cup, so to speak, to receive some fresh tea.

The language of herbalism, like the languages of many other systems of health-care conveys a science of life, transition and dynamic support of the body's innate, self-healing vital energy. The individual who is serious about learning the most efficient use of medicinal herbs for wholistic health-care must attune to a different belief system than that on which mainstream allopathic medical-pharmaceutical science is founded. Conveying an alternative view of the relationship existing between one's self and one's environment, herbalism suggests another way to deal with the internal imbalances and ecological dismays that arise in an individual's life experience. Viewing this imbalance and dismay as merely a pathology, something to get rid of, is only one way of looking at the situation. Wholistic herbal science views it through a wide-angle lens. It looks at the immense panorama of an individual's life, seeing that usually there is more right about a person than is wrong, giving him credit and responsibility for his present state of being. If the current experience of this state is an uncomfortable one or is self-destructive, the individual needs to first recognize and support what is right and then make lifestyle changes to alter what is not. Complementing these changes, herbalism uses the actions of empirically researched whole-plants to support and assist the vital energy operating in the systems of the human body, helping rebalance internal ecology and re-establishing homeostasis. Learning the therapeutic language and skills of herbalism will make it clear how to do this for one's self or for one's family members, keeping in mind, however, that wholistic herbalism uses plants not only as organic chemical remedies but also as uplifting allies that assist the individual to transform his condition, reconnecting in a more comfortable, harmonious way to his internal and external environment. In this book we will be looking at the cause of disease and the phenomenon of healing through the eyes of a different language than that of allopathic medical science and through a vastly different understanding, experience and relationship with medicinal plants.

Built on centuries of people's experience, demonstrating the safety and effectiveness of medicinal herbs, the language of herbalism is primarily a language of doing, not so much a language for explaining the organic technology of how remedies "work." Herbalism speaks of the actions of whole plants on the various systems of the human body; actions such as anti-inflammatory, diuretic, astringent, bitter, carminative, expectorant, adaptogenic and tonic. The language of herbalism is a language of personal independence defining simple tools and techniques of doing things to enhance one's own life and health, not so much a technology of being "done to" by the medical mystique of some other. The language of herbalism readily speaks to doing nothing when simple rest is the necessary factor allowing the body to attend to itself. Ninety percent of the time the normal body spontaneously heals itself given merely adequate rest, pure water and the lack of outside intervention. In other circumstances, herbalism directs one to immediate action harvesting and preparing one's personal medicines or one's family medicines; making herbal preparations such as infusions, tinctures, medicinal wines, liniments and poultices; initiating and experiencing a direct connection with one's own health process.

It is a relatively rare situation when the body needs heroic outside intervention. When intense intervention is necessary, we look to the science and technology of allopathic crisis-medicine. Frequently, wholistic herbalism refers an individual to another appropriate health-care modality to receive insights and support from their unique knowledge, language and skills. To assist our vast population of diverse individuals wholistically, there exists a widely divergent healing community offering a variety of approaches, skills and insights for health-care including herbal, homeopathic, shamanic, allopathic, naturopathic, massage, counselling, chiropractic, meditation and laying-on-of-hands. It all works to support social transformation and personal evolution when fitted precisely to the unique and changing needs of the individual.

When a plant is no longer a plant . . .

Pharmacology is the branch of science that studies drugs, including their constituents, uses, effects and therapeutics. The language of the science of herbalism and the mainstream language of today's predominantly reductionist pharmacology reflect and articulate two different methods of investigation. These sciences reflect different belief systems about human bodies and plants and the relationship between the two. One science is inclined to perceive the nature and actions of a whole plant and how to appropriately use the unique synergy of the plant's diverse properties; the other science more readily perceives the isolated units of the whole plant, analyzing each part separately to determine its pharmacological energy and potential uses. Freely integrating the spirit, insight and technologies of these two sciences in an attitude of cooperation for contemporary plant research could help put our culture's health-care system into the forefront of global research. Using plant preparations (traditionally used plants and newly discovered medicinal plants) by drawing directly from the practical heritage and clinical expertise of herbal science (that exists now in our country and globally) and attuning this with the analytical skills of reductionist pharmacological science will evolve our insight into each plant's health-care potential and give present day humanity full use of nature's curative magic. The long overdue union and coordinated effort of these two sciences for enhancing modern health-care has the potential for equally synergistic magic.

Giving an example of the difference between the languages of these two sciences, illustrating the fundamental difference in the way herbalists and pharmacologists presently comprehend and employ the actions of plants in the healing process, I'm selecting the herbalist's reliable and trusted remedy, Horsechestnut (*Aesculus hippocastanum*), for a model. The therapeutic use of this plant was recently outlawed as unsafe by the government of Canada.

The fruit of *Aesculus* is a safe and gentle herb which has been used for ages by herbalists as an agent to reduce inflammation and to improve the tone and strength of the vessels of the circulatory system, the veins in particular. Consequently it is used as a primary agent in formulas for individuals who are experiencing varicosity, hemorrhoids, etc. It is well known in herbal folklore not to eat the green outer casing of the fruit, for this can cause gastric distress and drowsiness. But founded on literally centuries of observation and successful use, herbalists know that the inner fruit (the nut) of Horsechestnut safely strengthens veins and other circulatory apparatus. This is so because Horsechestnut is a plant containing a highly specific and unique combination of biochemically "Horsechestnut organized" plant constituents that, being thus organized, have a strong affinity for the circulatory system of the human body. Its primary actions on the circulatory system are astringent, tonic and nutrient. The fruit of the Horsechestnut tree is traditionally prepared as an infusion (tea) or a tincture for internal use, or it is administered externally, often combined with Comfrey and distilled Witch Hazel as a compress or a lotion. The bark of the tree is also safely used for its tonic and fever reducing actions.

In contrast, looking at Horsechestnut through the eyes and language of reductionist science, pharmacologists perceive this plant differently. They tend to believe (if they credit the whole herb with any healing action at all) that the pharmacological activity of Horsechestnut is simply due to its tannin, flavone and saponin content. These constituents of Horsechestnut are perceived by western pharmacology as the "active ingredients." Pharmacologists sincerely believe that these "active" constituents can be isolated from the "superfluous," "inert" constituents of the whole plant and that this improves their pharmacological nature; that these "active" plant constituents can be used as molecular blueprints, synthesized by using complex coal-tar molecules in the laboratory, and that these resultant isolated and synthetic molecular forms are more reliable, are more precise to administer and allow side effects to be eliminated. (Thumb through the *Physicians' Desk Reference* [PDR] for endless lists of side effects from virtually every pharmaceutical remedy, to give insight into the actuality of that contention.) Relating solely to these separated "active" parts and based primarily on laboratory animal studies of the actions of these isolated constituents, which are no longer an organized part of the whole plant as herbalists use them, pharmacologists warn against the use of Horsechestnut, pointing out that laboratory research on saponins (one of the identified constituents of Horsechestnut) indicates that they can cause hemolysis (Saponin, when put directly into the bloodstream, acts like soap, lowering the surface tension; consequently the red blood cells burst within the blood plasma releasing their hemoglobin). Certain snake venoms contain saponins, and blowing-up blood cells is how some venoms do their fatal deed.

The saponinic pieces (aescin & aesculin) which are an organized part of Horsechestnut are very weak saponins at that, and have been repeatedly shown by empirical (founded upon extensive experience) herbal science to be perfectly safe when taken orally. In real life saponins cause hemolysis only when they are injected directly into the blood stream by hypodermic devises, such as needles or fangs. The human digestive process quite efficiently transforms saponins into raw materials that the body can use as building blocks to repair and balance itself. According to pharmacologists, medicinal herbs that are also used for common natural flavorings such as Licorice and Sarsaparilla contain saponins, as do Ginseng and Wild Yam. The chemical structure of the hormone precursor saponins (raw materials the body can use to build hormones) of Wild Yam are the plant blueprints that the pharmaceutical industries originally used to create the birth control pill (Presently, due to commercial overharvesting of Wild Yam, Soya bean, Agave and other plants are being used). The vitamin A found in carrots is highly toxic to the liver when it is isolated from the wholeness of the carrot and eaten. Certain constituents of potatoes and tomatoes are also very toxic when these constituents are isolated from these tubers and fruits, but as most of us have experienced, they usually don't harm us when we eat them in their original organized form as whole foods.

Herbalists feel that all plant constituents organized in a whole plant synergistic matrix are more safe and effective, giving fewer unpredictable side effects due to their innate biochemical compatibility with the body's metabolic chemistry. The inert constituents of herbs and vegetables are essential ballasts, balances and buffering agents for the whole organized vessel. Herbalists believe that a whole new arena of basically unpredictable side effects appear when active chemicals are administered in a concentrated isolated form.

Using the separated and isolated constituents of plants, disturbing the natural organization of the plant often gets us into trouble. Herbalists around the world know what whole-plant medicines can do and how best to use them; their science has long standing clinical experience. They can't always tell how plants work, though certainly many herbalists are keenly fascinated with reductionist theories. Isolating, naming and categorizing individual plant constituents supplies supplementary information to the herbalist's knowledge and experience of safe, efficient whole-plant therapeutics. Reductionist science works tirelessly to explain and synthetically replicate the therapeutic actions of plants, and certainly increased knowledge of how and why plants work will enhance the clinician's skill, intuition and effectiveness. But mystery also has intrinsic value in the healing arts. Mystery is appropriate and continues to make up the bulk of human experience. Just as the flight of the bumble bee and the four-winged dragonfly perplexes the aeronautic experts, the synergistic therapeutic actions of whole unadulterated plants often confound the rational precepts of pharmacology and allopathic pharmacy.

Hey bro, what's saponin? . . .

All sciences are creative avenues to knowledge, and all are basically kin to one another, each having a unique window through which it perceives reality. One of the most profound events of any science is the transformational moment when its members realize that a portion of their beliefs are not necessarily clear reflections of reality. It is a true science that can make the shift of collective consciousness allowing it to look at other sciences' beliefs as equally valid windows on what is really out there. When differing sciences seek a common denominator of understanding, are allowed free expression and come together to communicate for mutual benefit, bridges of understanding and cooperation can be built, the evolution of human consciousness well served.

I enthusiastically share the intellectual fascination for studying the parts of plants in an endeavor to understand how nature performs her magic, and my imagination easily sees the importance of this work, but I have to question what's happening when my culture's investigation of isolated bits and pieces becomes a myopic obsession, creating unrealistic state-sanctified fears, distracting society from the original purpose of the exercise; which is to help us prevent and cure disease and feel better.

The priceless ancestral heritage of herbal empirical science knows which plants are safe to use and which ones are not. We have at hand a folk system that has proven common medicinal plants to be safe by the undeniable fact that these plants have been in common use for eons and remain in common use by over 80% of the world's population today. Human beings have been consuming these plants for centuries without obvious ill effects. Continued use cannot have any major new unexpected impact on human consumers. Safety can logically be assumed, and prerequisite animal studies are not needed to prove the safety of common plant remedies. We don't need to outlaw our species' traditional therapeutic lore and processes, as our government has done, by legislating irrational paranoia concerning the safety and effectiveness of common plant remedies, like Horsechestnut. Traditional use of plant medicines is not an "old way" of doing things. It is an excitingly current science that has the unique character of being deeply grounded in the entire history of our species. It is the empirical science that is currently used by over 80% of the rest of the human population outside the U.S. and Canada and by a rapidly increasing number of us living within these borders.

The official North American muteness existing between traditional herbal science and orthodox reductionist science could quickly dissolve, replaced by intelligent, inspirational communication serving our society. Open communication would befriend these two honorable sciences for the common good if it were not for the socially crippling legal restrictions, protocol pressures and polarization placed on health-care research by the Food and Drug Administration (FDA) of the U.S. and the Health Protection Branch (HPB) of Canada which obsessively disallow investigation of folk medicine's plant *materia medica* for finding "new" plants which have major health-care potential. I'm not sure what motivates the rigid narrowness of imagination of our western countries' regulatory agencies, but evidence is revealing that we are not more healthy than developing countries, and our current orthodox pharmaceutical, medical and state-of-the-art clinical research systems are not as effective as our media habitually implies. No single health-care or disease-care science can supply all the requirements of its society's medical needs.

Civilization's experience of extended life span is due to improved hygiene, not to the invention of drugs. We no longer use our public water supplies as latrines, we provide adequate air circulation in our places of work and residence, and we wash our hands and bodies regularly. All this acts to control infectious micro-organisms. Wrapped in the illusion of protecting us from something that we don't need to be protected from, our health protection agencies are not rendering our cultures any true service. They are locking shut the window of a natural science that most other nations on our planet are eagerly looking through, seeking and finding answers to today's difficult health-care challenges. The commercially prohibiting aspects of plant research have been created by the regulatory agencies also. The moment a health claim is made about a natural substance, the FDA and the HPB regard it as a "drug," no longer a food, and it is illegal to make a health claim about anything without FDA and HPB approval. According to a study at Tufts University the cost of obtaining FDA approval of a new "drug," even if it is only flaxseed, is at least 54 million dollars, and since plants are public domain and cannot be patented, no industry is going to spend that amount to "scientifically test" them. Chemical medicines reign commercially superior. Herbs have not been tested simply because it is not profitable to do so in North America. This illustrates one reason for a new "folkloric" category to be initiated which would recognize the viability of traditional uses of U.S., Canadian and foreign plants.

Our nations' health-care systems and each individual's right to freedom of choice in his and her health-care need some original, courageous legislation (or better yet, some courageous elimination of legislation) which will:

- Create a new model of primary health-care which communicates directly with practitioners of traditional medicine;
- Create a new *folk medicine* category further completing the currently insufficient food & drug categories; and
- Preserve and cultivate medicinal plants.

This exercise in common sense would go a long way toward

helping preserve the world's rainforests, home of three quarters of the world's botanical species which are the embodiments of almost all of mankind's yet undiscovered medicines. It would also help preserve the noble aboriginal human beings who are native inhabitants of these rainforests, human inhabitants who are the embodiment of many traditional empirical sciences. They could teach us the actions of these plants once we learn to approach these folks and their environment with caring regard. Researchers throughout other countries of the world are looking for and finding plants with major health-care potential. These researchers are anxious to improve their medical practices by integrating herbal and reductionist allopathic western sciences. They are seeking to modernize and validate herbalism instead of replacing it, while our systems continue to compulsively outlaw folk medicine and shut down all creative support of plant medicine research. At a time in human history when unabated population explosion and immune deficiency are such important issues, almost all discoveries of safe, new male and female contraceptive and immune-modulating plants are Chinese, East Indian and Mexican herbs. This is not to say that plants in the U.S. and Canada don't have equally effective immune-modulating properties, it is just that China, India and Mexico are doing this research, and we are not.

On the other hand, in spite of the existing governments' remarkable lack of vision, herbalism is rapidly regaining substance in the cultures of the U.S. and Canada as we people begin to recall the wisdom of our ancestors and sense the vital interconnection we all share with our planet and her inhabitants. We are reviving the rhythm and melody of our culture's rich and timeless lore, attuning them to a modern tempo. Young healers are rediscovering their roots, traditions & heritage and are preparing medicines in new and different ways. The time has arrived to evolve peaceful creative communication throughout the arts of healing, time to disassemble the archaic inappropriate walls that once were built between people. There is a precedent now. The gov'll catch up.

Herbalism and mainstream medicine

It may not be obvious, but I have deep respect and sincere gratitude for allopathic pharmaceutical medicine when it is prescribed appropriately and conservatively. It is very strong medicine. Modern medical chemistry has accomplished wonderful results, most brilliantly and awesomely displayed in crises, catastrophic medicine and corrective surgery. There is no doubt that the heroic action of pharmaceutical drugs saves lives in the face of serious infection, catastrophic injury and life threatening conditions such as heart failure, kidney failure, or pneumonia. Allopathic medicine can even alleviate certain chronic problems, but these pharmaceuticals are often inappropriately used. They are too strong for most minor conditions such as colds, flu or common childhood ailments and for chronic ailments such as digestive disorders, lung congestion, deficient circulation, arthritis, common nervous disorders or genito-urinary problems, and being of a completely non-nutritive nature, they are not well suited for most preventive care. The aggressive actions of allopathic medicine circumvent the body's normally adequate defenses, and the drugs' powerful side effects hinder the innate ability of the human body to heal itself properly. Consequently, the full cycle of the body's spontaneous natural defense strategy is interrupted, leaving the body's normal defense mechanisms stymied and often lethargic. The original acute disease can reoccur later and become a chronic condition. A more efficient or complementary medicine would give nutritional support to the systems of the body, supplying compatible organic materials for the vital life force of the body to accomplish its normal process of self-healing.

Plants and the human body

Having long since learned to deal with the natural organization of whole-plant constituents, the human body is biologically familiar and metabolically compatible with whole-plant foods and medicines. The body will either use these plant constituents as foods and building materials, or it will actively excrete them. It is this predictable act of excretion by the various organs of the body that give mankind the medicinal uses of the actions of individual plants. Diuretic plants contain constituents that are well known to be excreted by the kidneys, stimulating urine production; diaphoretics are excreted through the skin stimulating sweat and sebaceous flow, while some hepatic herbs are excreted through the liver stimulating liver function and increased bile formation, and so forth (see herbal actions in following chapters). Plants are not ammunition bunkers or vegetable arsenals of medical or nutritional magic bullets.

The tunnel-vision of the isolated "active ingredient" of a plant just does not do what the subtle complexity of the whole-plant does. This includes isolated vitamins, minerals and amino-acids. Albert Szent-Gyorgi, a medical professor and Nobel Prize winner in physiology and medicine, shared his similar experience and appreciation of the organization of nature's whole plants by remarking, "'Organization' means that if nature puts two things together in a meaningful way, something new is generated which cannot be described, any more, in terms of the qualities of its constituents. This is true through the whole gamut of complexity, from atomic nuclei and electrons up to macromolecules of a complex individual. *Nature is not additive.* If this is true, then the opposite is also true, and when I take two things apart I have thrown away something, something which has been the very essence of that system, of that level of organization." Reductionist science and chemotherapy, being relatively new sciences, have so far studied and experimented only with remote pieces of plants. There is much yet to learn about how these pieces, while in their natural organization as whole plants, act on the human body and, in contrast, how these plant constituents after being separated and disorganized by human intervention relate to the body.

Non-poisonous unadulterated herbs traditionally used by herbalists are composed of a complex and subtle biochemistry of organized substances with which the human body has a pristine long-standing biochemical familiarity. Human bodies contain minerals, but for all practical purposes these minerals cannot be taken directly from the soil as food and medicine. They must be obtained from a living or at least a once living cell of either a plant or an animal that previously ate the plant. Plants have the unique ability to take mineral substances from the soil and transform them in such a way that they can, upon digestion, be utilized by the cells and systems of the human body. Plants, having shared a common evolution with human beings, contain these nutritive substances partly in the same composition as they are present in the human system. This compatibility allows direct assimilation of these herbal substances upon digestion. No other chemistry that I am aware of can supplant this remarkably sophisticated organic chemistry that takes place in living plant and animal cells. The action of this whole-plant chemistry in the body's systems is generally quite predictable, having been used and observed by humankind for millenniums. The indications and counter-indications of using whole plant foods and herbal remedies has been well documented and repeatedly demonstrated by our ancestral medicine people. Provided the herbs that one uses are of good quality, harvested correctly, prepared, compounded and prescribed properly based on sensitive, accurate assessment of a person's condition, the actions of each herb are 90% predictable. Experienced herbalists know what whole herbs used singly or in formula can do and what they cannot do. This is our heritage, and this is the art and science that we teach. The 10% variability stems primarily from the individual's lifestyle and how this lifestyle stacks up against the actions of an herb. One cannot expect a lung tonic herb to have much appreciable toning effect on a pair of lungs that are regularly fumigated and upholstered with tobacco tars.

The skilled employment of plant actions in a well diagnosed condition offers modern humankind a powerful materia medica that can be used solely or in conjunction with allopathic diagnosis, medical technology and chemical therapy, supplying the best of both sciences for the health seeker.

Wholism and the use of herbs

Herbs can be used merely for their palliative actions, such as herbal laxatives for constipation, nervine sedatives for tension, carminative deflators for expelling gas, etc., and why not, if this gives quick relief from discomfort? Using herbs for palliation of symptoms does not interfere with the body's normal healing process and does not leave the body with residual toxins as do drugs. But simultaneously, in the same herbal formula, one can also work on resolving the underlying cause(s) of recurring symptoms, working to provide lasting relief. The easy assembly of this type of formulation is a major factor in how herbal medicine performs so well, efficiently rendering its gifts to the human body. Keep in mind, however, that nothing works for every body, for there are many factors that make up each complex human individual. Lifestyle, local environment, diet, sex, habits, age and so on make up the rest of the whole picture of which herbal intake is merely a part of the whole therapeutic formula. Hawthorn berries, an herbalist's most effective cardio-vascular tonic, for example, can never proxy for regular adequate exercises; nor can an herbal adrenal tonic do for the endocrine system what the creative spark of quitting a boring job can do.

Wholistically oriented herbalists perceive humans as complex physical, mental, emotional and spirited beings ecologically interwoven with all life, possessing the innate power to prevent disease and heal afflictions. This style of herbalism bases its therapeutics on working with an individual in the context of this wholeness, helping the person gain relief by somehow resolving the causes of distressing symptoms. Wholism approaches the individual systemically and ecologically rather than merely targeting the palliative removal of symptoms. The use of plant remedies is a significant part of this wholistic therapy, but by no means the totality of it.

To accomplish the ideal, each individual's whole therapeutic formula will necessarily be unique. Certainly, in the context of this book, it is not possible to assess the specific needs of each individual, but the concepts behind wholistic herbal therapeutics will be illustrated giving the reader fundamental guidelines and suggested herbal formulas to use for general relief and renewed health. Using the information which will explain the actions of individual common herbs, the reader can knowledgeably add more personally specific herbs to the general formulas, modifying the blend to more adequately suit the individual, or he can design an entirely original formula.

Please be aware as you explore herbalism that wholistic herbal preventive/therapeutic science is vastly different than, and bares little relationship to, the language of the modern day mass marketing of herbal products. Before buying commercial herbal products, learn to use herbs wholistically and learn to recognize truly high quality herbs (see the section on Herb Quality in this book's chapter "Picking the Right Herbs"). This way you will not be disappointed. Don't swallow corporate hype and flashy packaging that hint of quick cures and mystical panaceas. Herbs used knowledgeably assist, support, inspire, tone, nourish and soothe. You do the healing; appropriate time is a primary wholistic factor assisting you.

Our companion animals and current herbal research

The great psychic closet of our human species contains the bones of many skeletons, most of which today are no longer merely the bones of our own species. Consequently, our companion animal species are rapidly leaving us human beings through the process of extinction. Any conscious, self-respecting being will naturally do this if treated with the overwhelming, exploitive lack of regard that humankind is expressing to its four legged, winged, swimming, hopping and crawling planetary companions. Even the rooted, sporing and leafed companions are leaving us; or maybe it is more accurate to say they are being commercially evicted by us.

Discussion within the herbal community about or relationship to plants and animals and the use of animal testing for herbal research often attains the level of intensity that this issue is currently promoting in the general population. The bottom line for some very dedicated herbalists is that, in an attempt to improve credibility (to mainstream disease-care medical science) of herbs as legitimate medicines, animal experiments have some of the highest current value as evidence. And this is probably true if one is attempting to convince mainstream medical science about the validity of herbal medicine by agreeing to use solely the language of mainstream science. This medical/pharmaceutical language and science is currently committed (philosophically and economically) to using animal test data as primary sources of credibility and legitimacy. However, the empirically validated language and universal practice of traditional herbal empirical science (which is where my particular herbal science's roots draw their juice) have not been and are not necessarily being derived from data acquired from the use of animal testing and vivisection. Many of us herbalists, in my opinion, do not feel the need to validate our science to orthodox medicine, particularly if it requires the harming of animals. We wish sincerely to work in a symbiotic relationship, alongside mainstream medicine within a responsible and compassionate health-care community, but not at the expense of losing our autonomy, wholism and traditional ethics to prove some sort of legitimacy by someone else's rules.

Vivisection is a very recent and radical technique of experimentation, introduced and popularized as "scientific" by the work of Louis Pasteur. Animal testing, in my opinion, is an arrogant and misleading technique that I hope is rapidly coming to its end due to the enlightened review and censure of informed, sensitive human beings. Testing plant constituents or any substance on non-human animal tissue can, at best, only hint to the researcher the direction and extent of the pharmacological activity on human tissue. There are immediately available more reliable and cost-effective alternatives to animal testing that can supply this information such as Agarose diffusion (an *in-vitro* method). This technique is more accurate and 90% less expensive than the Draize test (an eye irritancy test which was developed in 1944 to screen substances proposed for use in chemical warfare). In 1990 the Draize test remains basically unchanged. By direct application of potentially harmful substances into the eyes of rabbits, this test is used to measure the potential irritative effects in the pre-market evaluation of cosmetic and household products. Computer-generated mathematic and mechanical models can be used to simulate many physiological systems. Using data from published studies, they can estimate the LD-50 of a new substance from its chemical structures and properties. These can replace the LD-50 Test (introduced in 1927, it consists of force-feeding a particular compound to a group of animals to determine how much of it will kill 50% of them) as well as simulate countless other archaic and misleading animal tests eliminating the need to poison numerous test animals. *In vitro* research utilizes human epidermal and lymphocyte cell tissue and organ cultures on which agents can be tested for their effect on human organisms. Chemical and physical systems such as enzymes, artificial membranes and robots serve as other reliable alternatives to animal testing. These and many other alternatives are being developed and validated by research scientists working with grants from the International Foundation for Ethical Research. Contact the National Anti-Vivisection Society located in Chicago, Illinois (see resource section), and they'll supply information about these viable alternatives.

Of equal concern to me (I don't want human beings to be involuntarily harmed either) are the highly questionable conclusions that research scientists derive based on the unsubstantial data gleaned from animal testing. The only reliable information we have accumulated from animal research is that animals have proven to be inadequate surrogates for research on humans. Test values vary dramatically from species to species, even from different strains, sex, age and temperament within the same species. Reliance on data accumulated from animal testing poses an unacceptable level of risk to human health. It is too often misleading, giving false promise which results in considerable harm to human beings. *Eraldin*, a cardiotonic drug, was sanctioned for sale to the public and marketed after 7 years of extensive animal testing, but it caused serious eye and intestinal damage to hundreds, killing 18 humans before being recalled. *Thalidomide*, a tranquilizer drug used in Europe to relieve morning sickness and help prevent miscarriage, caused extensive birth defects in human babies, but produced no birth defects in most species of test animals; *Strychnine* can be eaten by guinea pigs and shows no evidence of poisoning, but is deadly poisonous to humans; a Tuberculin "vaccine" developed by Pasteur's peer, Robert Koch, cured TB in guinea pigs, but later it was found to cause TB in humans.

Viable and superior alternatives to animal research exist; no longer can anyone excuse the gruesome tests conducted on our companion animals and the human health risks that are often created. Only after being tested in living human organisms (*in vivo*) by many years of clinical observation can anyone truly determine the actual value (and side effects) of any substance in human health-care. The technology for valid alternatives is at hand; funding organizations and legal precedents, nudged firmly and supportively by public pressure, merely need to refocus and inspire researchers to change their habits.

No information in this herbal has been drawn intentionally from data that focuses on either the isolated components of plants or the effects of plants on the tissue of laboratory animals. I am aware that this is difficult in light of the fact that our English language is infused with the residue of pharmacological information, fashionable medical hypotheses and some current herbal research that has flowed out of the reductionist scientific communities, not all, but so much of which is based on animal tests. However, disconnecting my computer modem apparatus, thus closing my computer's eye to the information pumped out of commercial medical data-banks which thrive on selling worldwide research data gleaned directly from animal testing, I'm withdrawing my support through the market place until I can locate and support an animal-free medical and herbal research data base.

Grizzly bears were my first love, and the threatened loss of their presence on this planet troubles me deeply, but the fear and suffering that screams through the pleading eyes of animal research victims pains my heart even deeper. Beside this personal emotional reaction to companion animal abuse, these are my reasons for boycotting all animal research:

- I believe that our civilization's current disconnection and apparent disregard for its traditions, its myths, its intuition and the planet Earth with all her diverse species are the fundamental underlying causes of humankind's physical and social diseases.
- I am convinced that animal testing is a symptom of this disconnection. At astronomical cost to our society animal testing merely serves the disease-care system of drug, radiation and surgical intervention, rather than a far more practical, economical and compassionate health-care system that researches and teaches improved lifestyle, nutrition, preventive medicine and fundamental environmental caretaking for community-health.
- Modern medical technology has experienced some success treating the myriad disease symptoms of this disconnection, helping palliate symptoms and patch-up humankind, but this is neither cure nor prevention of disease.
- I believe that cruel and degrading treatment of the members of other species as a means to somehow render our species more healthy or more beautiful is folly, and this self-righteous indulgence will neither teach us how to create and maintain health in

our species nor show us the way to prevent disease.

• Today's spontaneous renaissance of the wholistic use of organically cultivated plant foods and medicinal herbs is drawing humankind back to carefully tending Earth as the sole, pristine source of our food-medicines and all other vital resources. This, along with the apparent re-awakening of conscious awareness that every companion species on Earth shares equal status and value, reflects the beginnings of humankind's profound endeavor to re-establish its sense of global community, balance and health.

• I am convinced that by rediscovering and reviving our primal connections with our planet, our ecology, our companions, our wholistic roots and our planetary psyche our species is far more likely to experience healing.

• A more perfect kindness to ourselves and to all species along with intelligent care and use of our environment will prove to be the best medicine for human beings.

I'm not the only sinewy man to feel this way. Mr. M. Gandhi expressed similar feelings, "The greatness of a nation and its moral progress can be judged by the way its animals are treated." Take care of the animals; it's good medicine.

3

The Male Community

While talking with Mr. Rico Baker, co-author of the book, *Conscious Conception,* a man who is deeply involved in the issues around male health-care, the intriguing speculation came up that maleness tends to possess a profound self-sacrifice attitude and stance in life, an attitude that the (adult) male is the most expendable individual in the ongoing day-to-day preservation of the species. Men are expected to die for their family and country. Traditionally, men volunteer and are supposed to be stalwart, self-sacrificing providers and protectors. When escaping imminent disaster it's "women and children first, men only if there is room." Maybe these noble (species-preserving) forms of self-sacrifice are the unique manner by which the male of our species expresses his deepest love. The testosteronic male probably conceived and promoted all these customs.

One can further speculate that this attitude exists at the cellular level, wherein the sperm that makes the male sex baby are more rapid moving and aggressive. As a result they die quicker than the female-producing sperm. It's speculated that they pave the way to the single waiting egg, often to their demise. When ejected, human seminal fluid contains 60 to 100 million sperm per milliliter in a total volume of 3 to 4 ml. Only one of this multitude is needed for fertilization. Although a high concentration of spermatozoa does seem to be associated with better fertility, no one really knows for sure what all the other spermatozoa do. In line with this statistic, spontaneous abortions of male fetuses outnumber those of female, more males than females die during infancy, youth and adulthood, and men die at a more rapid rate than women, albeit from diseases caused by self-imposed stress. Among those humans 65 and older, just 68 men survive for every 100 women.

Another subtle but most significant trait found in men is a certain "dread of being known." An almost sinister, deep-seated dread which manifests a chronic tension over being found out. What we men are probably most afraid of is disclosing to ourselves who we really are (or maybe, who we really are not) and what we most want.

> Only the little boy can tell how it feels,
> how it has felt for so many years.
> Only the little boy and the little girl,
> unveil the wounds of childhood's heart,
> hear,
> understand,
> and let each other be free.
> T.E.S.

A wise and healthy male support system that helps a developing young boy explore his Self and discover what he is all about can facilitate the emergence of a mature and functional male being. And this support system does not exist in our culture .

As infants and young boys we are mostly dependent on Mom for most all of our needs and intimate training. She feeds us, rocks us, teaches us right and wrong, controls us with praises and punishments, yet the issues that are most crucial to developing a sense of male self such as anger, aggression and (male) sexuality are threatening to most women, especially moms. Which man feels that his mother understands or accepts his (testosteronic) aggressive feelings, his anger or his sexuality? It's a rare individual who does. So, a boy develops a fear (or at least a definite lack of spontaneity) of exposing certain parts of his unfolding personality, and in this confusion, he hides a lot of himself from himself at the same time.

Next, a young boy will look to Dad, if there is a dad available. Here we often find a wounded adult male who is dealing with the same or very similar childhood experiences, who is not usually comfortable (even if he makes the time to be) sharing intimacy with his son. The father/son relationship has such rich potential. Currently, however, if this primary relationship manifests at all, it is often a dreary experience with the father not sharing much of what is important to him or how he feels about things, certainly not what one would look back on and call a relationship that was intimate and nourishing. It's a relationship that, apparently, in the present state of our culture, lacks the conscious practice of a common rite of passage, a male to male process of passing on some form of wisdom and male self/community identity that is facilitated by a boy's father giving something of intimate deep meaning and power to his son. Today, instead, many men avoid the simple responsibility of giving even supplementary financial support to their growing sons (and daughters). These men, I assume, received just as little from their fathers.

So, moving on from Mom and Dad, out into childhood's social environment, what significant other is there for a young boy to bounce off of in an attempt to get a true reflection of and male role model for himself? Probably a peer involved in the same search, a group of peers, a hero, maybe a teacher or a coach. Approval seeking becomes the vital game at hand for establishing some sort of a sense of adequate self, perceiving and following other persons' rules, giving up varying portions of one's uniqueness and personal power, selecting and being selected by peer companions, participating and performing, usually through the body's physical skills (or lack of skills), learning all the "right" ways to be recognized and accepted. The young boy's emotional expressions, the ways he reveals his joy, anger, fear, aggression, sensuality, sensitivity and sexuality are shaped by these peer judgments at the same time. But, still the question lingers on into adulthood; *Who Am I*, really? The answer might prove to be inadequate, maybe dreadful (a suspicion the young boy possibly internalized when he lived with Mom and Dad years before), possibly too much to bear. So, maybe it is better to avoid being known, maybe it's safer not to reveal oneself.

Is this the basis of the almost universal difficulty we men have in revealing ourselves to another person, in asking for or receiving help? I don't claim to have the full answer, but I have the question, which I extend in this discussion about male health as a concept that warrants close attention. I feel that herein lies the key to our difficulty with seeking advice in health-care.

Standing behind an often rigid defense against revealing ourselves, we men often place ourselves in a most difficult position, which most likely prevents us from easily entering and becoming involved in a preventive or a therapeutic healing process. When faced with a health problem we frequently sit ourselves on a fence top of lonely procrastination. On one side of the fence we have our heroic, allopathic, scientific medicine which, as previously discussed, serves us well for treating our acute emergency symptoms. It's tolerable to wake up between clean white sheets after being carried off the playing field, from a wrecked car, after a heart attack or after being mauled in a field of war. All that is required is to surrender the wound for treatment and adapt to the damage sustained. We can usually handle those heroics. However, when we are required to deal with the progressive symptoms of chronic ill-health, there arises the premeditated necessity of relating to another person, most likely another male, at an intense level of closeness. Allopathic methods of diagnosis and use of heroic medicine for serious male disorders are most often painfully uncomfortable. Often disfigurement and/or dysfunction follows the allopathic techniques of treating chronic pathogenic symptoms (i.e., the frequent side effects of impotence and infertility resulting from surgery for prostatic cancer due to the severing of the bundle of microscopic nerves that control erections). So, when faced with the awareness of a chronic condition, the thought of going to an allopathic physician is usually overwhelming, often intolerable, readily disregarded and put off day after day.

On the other side of the fence, if we will even turn our heads and look at the so-called "non-scientific" alternatives, we find the natural, wholistic healing processes (the alternate medicines discussed previously). In their search for a cure, a common modus operandi found in most of these alternate schools of healing asks an individual to reveal much of himself (to himself) or herself (to herself) to determine the cause of the dis-ease condition. This is a difficult and often an emotionally painful process for any individual to sustain, especially a male individual, so this too is disregarded and put off. In general, the male finds himself trapped on his fence top by his own history of choices and cultural conditioning.

The fact that disclosing one's self in one way or another is a necessary part of the healing process, makes it essential for the health practitioner who wants to have an effect on male clients to understand how, under what circumstances and with whom males let themselves be known. This is an issue that urgently summons the focused attention of all schools of the healing community. There are ways to make it safer for a male to initiate his health-care. Exploring the information and considering ideas presented on these pages, we can adopt techniques that help us develop more insightful and effective male health-care. A women health practitioner told me that she often suggest herbs and other modalities that will support the man's "drivenness." She nourishes or treats the nervous system and adrenal glands before any other specific therapy is suggested. There are insightful ways to acknowledging and nourishing more specifically our male energy and the male spirit.

Concurrently, in a preventive mode, I strongly suggest that we reach out to male childhood and adolescence and develop a deeper understanding of these intimate, integral processes, initiating cultural support systems for our male children. While attending a potlatch (a northwestern coastal Indian spiritual gathering, feast and ceremonial distribution of gifts) in Alert Bay, British Columbia, Canada, I witnessed a native Indian man give his spirit name, his spirit dance and his spirit song to his adolescent son. During this festive gathering, in the presence of their clan members, the father passed to his son an ancient cultural heritage, a direct connection with his clan's traditions and science, personal recognition and wise spiritual ground on which the male youth could place his young feet. Watching this as a guest and reflecting on what I received from the male society of my boyhood, I felt personally deprived and culturally impoverished.

Re-establishing in our culture some form of male rite-of-passage experienced between father and son would create the vast heart of a strong male support system for our growing boys and for ourselves. I'm suggesting here, that we do some family homework. That we reach back and salvage family and cultural tradition; that we honor this tradition with ritual, song or story and pass this on to our young children; that we re-empower our personal connection with our family's ancestry and heritage; and carry forth this awareness as a bonding agent between our present living relatives and the new arrivals, allowing each child a stronger sense of belonging and a feeling of personal identity and self-worth. If there is no family tradition or rite-of-passage in memory left to salvage then initiate one and commit to the profound value of its energy. If your children don't pass it on to their children, pass it on to your grandchildren. I am the father of three daughters. I gave each of my daughters, Bre, Ajana and Shannan a coming of age ring when they started their menstruation cycle. Their mother and I expressed and ritualized our love and respect for them as whole, self-empowered, dynamic female human beings, and I know they felt honored, even though at the time they received the acknowledgment shyly. The significance of the occasion, the giving of the ring and the ritual will grow in meaning as our daughters grow on into their womanhood. We initiated this as a family tradition that I hope my daughters will nourish and carry on through their daughters and granddaughters and so on. If they don't, I will. To young grandsons I will (try to) give meaningful gifts and the intimacy and wisdom of another male spirit. I feel strongly that all of our adolescent sons need a similar ritualistic experience; a ceremony of honor, recognition and helpful cognizance of the meaning of their dawning arrival to manhood.

The current male spirit, young and old, is a most worthy candidate for cultural compassion. We fathers, grandfathers, sons, brothers, the male community, need to take a close look at ourselves, our role in the evolution of the human species and the evolution of our planet, our personal and collective power, and prepare ourselves to give something of direction and heart to each of our sons. Maybe, simply a story, a vision, a dance, a journey together or a song, a male song or sharing one's male fears; letting a male youth hear from a male adult that it is okay to feel fear, anger and confusion; that it is okay to own these feelings and to ask help from others, especially when feelings of fear and anger are confusing. Share some intimate, meaningful ritual passed from father to son. I suggest that it be, at least in part, a ritual of forgiveness, peace, prosperity, male power/responsibility; a simple ritual of heartfelt mutual awareness, of caring (re)connection with each other, with the planet Earth and her diverse companion species.

Show boys respect and caring between males. When men learn to like men, we will stop the wars.

〜4〜

Female – Male Herbal Heritage

Along with the obvious and enjoyable differences, there are far more similarities between the male and female body than appear on the surface. The
most salient difference, aside from the distinct angles, curves and organic
plumbing, is that men produce up to 10 times more testosterone hormone
than do women (30-200 mcg circulating as compared to 5-20 mcg in
women). This gives males greater capacity for developing body size and
muscular bulk. It also creates the male's commonly more aggressive, more
yang energy. Possibly this hormone, manufactured predominantly in the
male testicle, is the root cause of the more reckless, seemingly disinterested
and preoccupied attitude the male displays toward his body and health-care.

     Secondly, men ejaculate as compared to women who menstruate
and lactate. Sperm is a bio-chemically precious and costly fluid energy that
most males relinquish probably too freely. This expenditure of energy and
the nutrients involved must be monitored and replaced or the male creates
self-depletion and debility. Practice of non-ejaculatory sex is recommended
by many of the eastern schools of medicine for maintaining a balanced
nutritional economy as a means of retaining a man's health and vitality
(more about this later).

     In face of the relative drought of commonly available information
about the use of herbs for promoting male health and for treating male
health problems, men who wish to employ herbs and other natural health-
care modalities can derive some practical information by studying the
folkloric use of traditional "female" herbs and natural therapies. Males who
intend to practice natural health-care can be assisted by identifying the
similarities that exist in male and female organ tissue and thereby co-reap
the mutual female-male heritage of traditional herbal medicine. In line with

this possibility, I will list some of these feasible similarities. In the following chapters I will focus on the obvious differences in the male body pursuing ideas about the cause and cure of specific male problems; introduce three hypotheses that I offer as fundamental concepts for developing male health-care programs; and discuss wholistic herbal methods to deal with prevention and treatment of problems that manifest in the male system.

Male and female sexual organ anatomy look dramatically different, one being nearly the reverse of the other. However, in terms of how these genital organs developed, they are very similar, having evolved from the same tissues in the developing fetus. Workshop discussions generated from the information I have gathered and opinions I have formulated about the similarities that conceivably exist in male and female bodies have occasionally unnerved, for whatever reasons, some men who were involved. Please hold in mind that these concepts are ideas to consider; they are not dogmatic truths. Being aware of these similarities, we can tap into the extensive herb-lore that exists for female care and develop comparable understanding for male care. The similarities are:

- The prostate (the anatomy and physiology of which will be discussed later) can be interpreted as a male uterus which does not overtly display a monthly cycle appearing not to refurbish itself cyclically. As an endocrine-dependent organ it, in one sense, is also thought by some physiologists to be the counterpart of the breasts in the female. Either way it is an organ of nourishment.
- The activities of both the testicles and the ovaries are governed by the hormones of the pituitary gland. Sterility in either sex is often due to deficiency of a pituitary hormone, the need of the entire endocrine system to be nourished.
- The testes produce the male hormone testosterone as well as the female hormone estrogen. Some of the estrogen secreted in the male may come from the adrenal gland, but at least 80% comes from the testes. And likewise the female ovaries secrete testosterone. Both the mature ovary and the testes are about the same size, approximately 1-1/2 inch long.
- Testicles are ovarian tissue that has dropped down. Certainly when a male suffers a blow in the testicles much of the pain is felt up in the vicinity where the ovaries are located in a female's body, which is where the testes are located in the unborn male

child before they drop down into the scrotum. They hang out in the scrotum, so they can keep cool. Body temperature is a little too warm for generating active sperm. Body temperature is just right for nesting an egg.

- Erectile tissue is found around the opening of the vagina, in the clitoris of the female and the penis of the male as well as in the nipples of the breasts of both sexes.
- The clitoris and the penis are homologous tissue and neurologically similar. Just different in design.
- The penis has a glans (head) and the clitoris has a glans. The penis has a foreskin and the clitoris has a clitoral hood. The glans of the penis is, in fact, an internal organ which the foreskin is intelligently designed to cover and protect throughout a man's life. The clitoral hood protects the clitoris and should not be surgically removed either.
- The male scrotum and the female major labia are of homologous tissue.
- Anecdotal information outlining numerous instances of men suckling infants is published in a text titled *Anomalies and Curiosities of Medicine* by G. Gould, M.D. and W. Pyle, M.D., Julian Press, N.Y., 1956. Male nipples obviously exist for some remote reason.
- And, in answer to the often asked question, "Why is there pubic hair on men and women?" Well, it (they) receives, traps and holds the male and female scent, dispersing it in wafts of subtle pheremonic seduction as hormonal interest is aroused. This probably holds true for underarm hair as well. I have no published source for that information, but it's the only explanation I've heard so far that makes good sense.

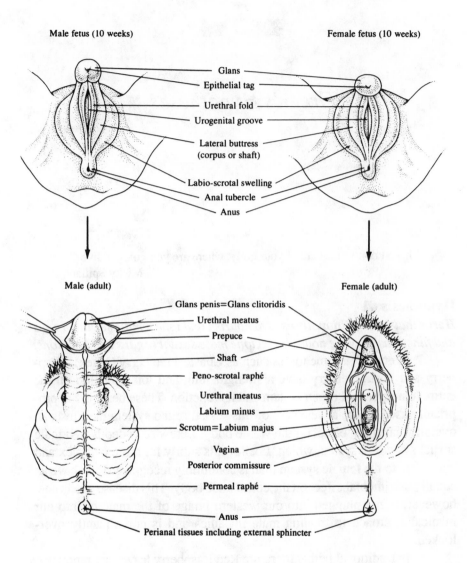

Male fetus (10 weeks) Female fetus (10 weeks)

Glans
Epithelial tag
Urethral fold
Urogenital groove
Lateral buttress
(corpus or shaft)
Labio-scrotal swelling
Anal tubercle
Anus

Male (adult) Female (adult)

Glans penis=Glans clitoridis
Urethral meatus
Prepuce
Shaft
Peno-scrotal raphé
Urethral meatus
Labium minus
Scrotum=Labium majus
Vagina
Posterior commissure
Permeal raphé
Anus
Perianal tissues including external sphincter

Comparative anatomy of male and female external genitalia illustrating
similarities (homologeous tissue) that exist between these organs.

5

Green's Hypotheses

"If you don't take care of your body, where are you going to live?"
Micky Spillane

Hypothesis #1

Herbs that are traditionally used to nourish and tone female sexual organs and functions likewise nourish and tone male sexual organs and functions.

"Female" uterine tonics such as Chaste Tree berry (Vitex), Raspberry and Partridgeberry have a strengthening and toning action on the entire female sexual organ system and its function. These herbs are appropriately used where a weakness of this sexual organ system manifests an overall weakening effect on the whole body. Likewise, a debilitated male sexual system (a system which, I believe, is subtly far more complex and congruent to the female system than is commonly recognized) can have an equally detrimental effect on the entire male body. This disease syndrome, however, is not plugged into our western image of the male or into our medical approach to treating male maladies and is consequently overlooked.

In traditional herbal literature Red Raspberry leaves are renowned as a uterine tonic and enthusiastically recommended for pregnant women to drink daily as tea before, during and after parturition. I have seen no mention in herbal literature of using this herb for male organ toning, except in an animal herbal written by Juliette de Bairacli-Levy. In her classic animal herbal, *Herbal Handbook for Farm & Stable*, she mentions that this herb is an acclaimed tonic for all male animals and a treatment for sterility. I have been told that the Arabs regularly feed Red Raspberry leaves to their prize stallions as a tonic, and I would wager that these desert equestrians

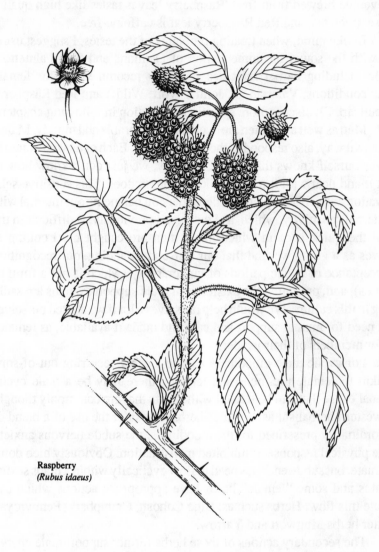

Raspberry
(Rubus idaeus)

seldom refuse a cup of this tea for their own personal tone and pleasure. A hot beverage brewed from fresh Raspberry leaves tastes like high quality Chinese green tea, and Red Raspberry leaf is caffeine-free.

In like mind, when treating problems of the testes, I suggest using along with the sound recommendation of Damiana and Saw Palmetto a formula including herbal remedies regularly recommended for female ovarian conditions: Valerian, St. John's Wort, Wild Yam, Red Raspberry and Scullcap. I'll discuss more specific formulation in following chapters.

Men as well as women are cyclically vulnerable and moody. Males, in their own way, also respond to the moon phases. Each of us who honestly observes ourself knows this is so. Generally, we just don't know how to accept it and deal with it (take it) like a woman does. This sensitive self-observation and self-acceptance is dependent on balancing our internal with our external sensitivity, which, as I discussed previously, is difficult in the face of the quick pace in which many men are caught up. Looking at ourselves as a group we find that our self-understanding, our recognition and acceptance of cyclic periods of vulnerability (which is not a form of weakness), and, presently, the existence of male support systems are sadly lacking in this culture. We would help ourselves a lot if we alerted ourselves to this need for mutual support and care and made it available, as females have for members of their gender.

For cyclic male moodiness and noticeably recurring out-of-sort-ness akin to female pre-menstrual tension, there may be a male cyclic hormonal cause that can be treated with plants that are commonly thought of in western herbalism as "female" herbs. Consider the use of a blend of herbs ordinarily prescribed for the moodiness, the subtle nervous anxiety and the physical response of inhibited menstruation. Obviously men don't menstruate, but subtle energies need to flow cyclically within a mans sexual apparatus and some "female" herbs have appropriate actions which can facilitate this flow. Herbs such as: Blue Cohosh, Crampbark, Pennyroyal, the bitter herbs Mugwort and Yarrow.

The secondary actions of these herbs further support male energy during subtly stressful periods. Yarrow, for example, while it strengthens and tones the genito-urinary system also has a strong affinity for the cardio-vascular system dealing with hypertension. So, this herb is appropriately used to simultaneously nourish the reproductive organs and the heart. If an individual tends toward a sluggish digestive system, choose Mugwort in addition to or in place of Yarrow. Mugwort also has a normalizing affect on the reproductive system, but it is more stimulating to the digestive system and helps ease tension which often plays a role in nervous indigestion.

During female menopause herbalists recommend the use of combinations of Chaste Tree berry and Wild Yam as hormonal aids; with Red Raspberry, and Partridgeberry as uterine tissue tonics, Black Cohosh as a relaxant and normalizer and St. John's Wort as a nerve tonic with the possible inclusion of Damiana, Saw Palmetto or Ginseng if the individual's sexual organs and energy are run down and weak. Do men experience a change of life? Ask their immediate family members.

A man's change of life is not a loss of his manlihood, his sex appeal or his maleness. On the contrary, it is a refining and maturing of his maleness. Through this normal transition a male's strength becomes more supportive of life in general. He becomes more gentle, freed of many rules, and can allow himself more behavioral options. His matured emotional strength allows him to perceive more clearly, rely on more patience, be more understanding and therefore more accepting. He moves himself from a primary arena of physical strength and competition and steps into the courtyard of functional wisdom, compassion and compromise. If all goes well, that is. Many of us men fight the transition all the way. This natural process is not introduced and explained to us during our youth. Instead, it crowds into our life like the shadow of a stranger. We are not helped by any shared folklore or support system, so often we feel quite isolated and profoundly frightened. Comprehending the multi-faced transitions of the male psyche is man-kind's final frontier, not space.

While a male's menopause is not as hormone altering as the female's, it can call for similar herbs to facilitate rebalance during these changes in life. A combination of herbs for a man experiencing male menopause will do well to include:

- Wild Yam for hormone building assistance
- Black Cohosh for a relaxant and normalizer;
- Saw Palmetto for a reproductive system nutrient;
- Damiana as a prostate tonic, anti-depressant and nutrient for sluggish sexual organs;
- St. John's Wort and Oat for nerve tonics to help deal with any depression and other stress due to the changes.
- And sometimes Chaste Tree berry. Normally I would not recommend this progesterone/estrogen promoting herb for men (especially not for young men and boys who are in the process of

developing their male physical and emotional bodies), but in some cases it can be helpful for older men who are going through a testosterone/estrogen redistribution.

A story was shared with me by Amanda McQuade-Crawford, M.N.I.M.H, herbal practitioner, about a patient of one of her British teachers. The patient was too strongly resisting this change. He had become so distracted and distraught by the thought of aging and "getting old" that he complained too much and became irritable and fussy. It was suggested that he take Chaste Tree berries for awhile. He did so and was enabled to work through this (for him) difficult transition. The actions of Chaste Tree berries can help a man settle into this transition (wherein he gets more in touch and comfortable with his female side) by helping him to establish an appropriate arrangement of his hormones for functioning in this ensuing phase of malehood. Use the herb for a few weeks, its actions are slow and gentle.

It is most helpful to design herbal formulas to fit as much as possible the full spectrum of a man's unique needs. As you treat a primary symptom or condition also take into account other body systems as well, especially the cardio-vascular and the nervous system. A man might require Yarrow and Hawthorn to support his heart and circulatory system, Wild Oat or Scullcap as nerve system tonics and Mugwort as a bitter flavored digestive aid that has a reproductive organ affinity.

Therefore, a general combination of herbs that is well suited to nourish, tone and help balance the male reproductive, digestive, circulatory and nervous systems is equal parts of:

Red Raspberry leaves
Wild Oat
Black Cohosh
Yarrow
Damiana
Wild Yam
St. John's Wort
Saw Palmetto
Mugwort

The addition of Licorice and/or Sassafras can enhance the flavor of this combination if desired. Make a tea or a tincture of these herbs and take 1 to 2 times a day, 3 to 4 days a week for a few months or until equilibrium has been established (Please refer to the chapter, "A Technology of Independence" for preparing teas and tinctures).

Hypothesis #2

The predominant avoidance and lack of the daily bitter flavor experience in western diet is a subtle, primary cause of male and female sexual organ and immune system deficiencies.

It is my opinion that the nearly complete lack of bitter flavored foods in the overall U.S. and Canadian diet is a major contributor to common cultural health imbalances such as PMS, other female and male sexual organ dysfunctions, hormonal imbalances, migraine headache, indigestion, liver and gallbladder dysfunction, abnormal metabolism, hypoglycemia, diabetes, etc. The only bitter flavored items commonly eaten in this culture are coffee and chocolate (both of which are usually highly sweetened before taken) and the hops in beer (bitter stouts or dark bitter beers, etc. are not often advertised and rarely imbibed in this culture). "Salad," which was originally a small daily serving of bitter greens taken before meals to stimulate appetite and digestion is now, in America and Canada, merely watery, no longer bitter (see Wild Lettuce in the "Male Herbal" section of this book), nearly tasteless hybrid lettuces covered with sweet, salty and/or tangy dressings. Currently however, there is a gustatory craze circulating through the big cities which is re-instating the prestige of bitter greens into the salads of gourmet restaurants.

The taste sensation of a bitter flavor is quickly ushered by the tongue receptors and sensory nerves to the central nervous system where it reflexively stimulates the exocrine and endocrine glands. There is a general stimulation of the flow of digestive juices from the stomach, liver, pancreas and duodenum which in turn stimulate appetite, digestion and assimilation. Accompanying this, the bitter action appears to help the intestinal walls repair any damage by stimulating their self-repair mechanisms (bitter action which stimulates flow of stomach acid is contra-indicated when secretions of stomach acids are not wanted, e.g. hyperacidity, hypersecretiveness or gastric ulcers. However, after the healing of an ulcer begins, bitter action helps to speed up the healing). Bitter action also aids the (frequently overworked) liver to perform its detoxification functions and increase the flow of bile, which directly assists proper bowel function. An active liver in turn helps regulate the hormones. The action of bitter flavor effects the pancreatic secretions that regulate blood sugar. There is evidence that the bitter action, as it stimulates action and sensations within the entire physiology of the being, has a marked anti-depressant psychological effect along with a subtle grounding effect on one's consciousness. It is impossible to remain in a depressed state with all the internal secreting and squirting going on in the gut and glands due to the stimulating effect of bitter flavor.

The mistake of eliminating the bitter flavor from our daily experience is like eliminating one of the colors from the rainbow light spectrum. It is nutritionally important and intriguingly enjoyable to recultivate the appreciation of bitter flavors which can concurrently diminish the inordinate health threatening thirst for sweet and salty flavors. It's my opinion that the habit developed throughout our lifetime of avoiding bitter flavored foods and herbs has created a chronic dysfunction in our livers and our organs of digestion, assimilation and excretion creating secondary hormone imbalances. Consequently, menstrual pains are the norm, as are prostate problems in the later years in most males along with other diverse symptoms resulting from poor digestion, inadequate nutrient assimilation and sluggish peristalsis. In my experience prostate problems can be an indication of the need for liver cleansing and toning.

Hand-in-hand with the avid avoidance of bitter flavors in the diet, the North American psyche refuses, in general, to deal with the (bitter) "shadows" of its life, routinely projecting the darker side of its own nature onto others (individually in relationships and nationally in foreign policy). We Westerners seem quite unwilling to deal with the difficulties and more bitter struggles of life. We look predominantly toward sweetness and the "American Dream" of living happily ever after. We refuse to look at and accept the darker aspects of our own personal (and national) being. The "Punk-Thrash-Metal" music popular with today's youth is experimenting with looking at and acknowledging the shadows that exist in a human soul. Presently this dawning psychic awareness of a generation is being commercially exploited, but like all other youth sponsored insights its nature will mature and be assimilated into the collective psyche of the general population as were the "peace," "love" and "anti-war" concepts of the '60s youth movements and their music. Our culture is at the threshold of identifying, accepting and relating to its shadows in order to become more whole and more accepting of itself (and others). Concurrently, I foresee bitter foods and the appreciation of the bitter flavor coming back into popular use along with the diminishing of our culturally salient sweet lust and experience of obesity.

To date, we have created a throw-away society (including disposable relationships and disposable companion species) which has left us

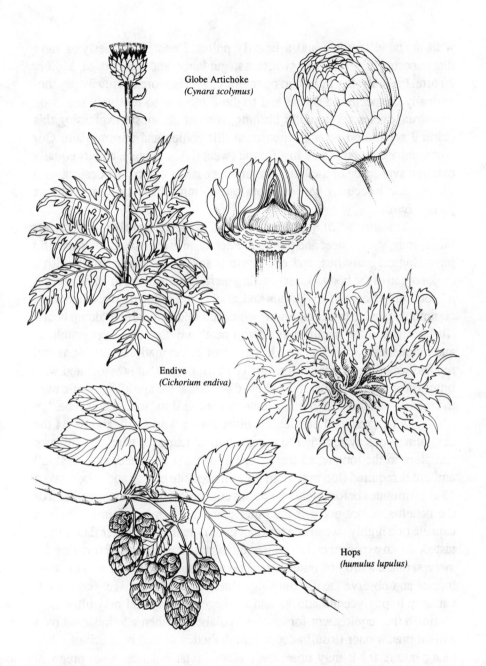

Globe Artichoke
(Cynara scolymus)

Endive
(Cichorium endiva)

Hops
(humulus lupulus)

with unstable families and a heavily polluted nest. Our lifestyles have disconnected us from the sweetness, guidance and support of Mother Nature. Possibly, the female in our culture, who is more obviously psychologically connected to caring and to the Earth due to routinely recurring menstrual cycles and to child birthing, is most obviously expressing this cultural separation through menstrual difficulties and uterine pain. Our community's predominant lust for the sweet flavor (sugar), and its equally extreme avoidance of the bitter flavor are possibly symptoms dealing with the psychic insecurity we feel from our cultural disconnection with our planet, Earth.

Traditional Chinese Medicine (TCM) identifies five main tastes: bitter, sour, salty, sweet and pungent. Each taste is accredited with specific physiological activities, and each taste is said to have an affinity with a major organ of the body. Bitter taste is generally considered in TCM to elicit a "cooling" effect which "drains and dries," and bitter flavored herbs are commonly used to treat conditions which are said to manifest "damp heat." Illnesses that often manifest as "damp heat" are digestive/liver problems and biliousness, as well as a wide variety of inflammations, infections and red and weeping skin conditions. In TCM the organ that is associated with bitter is the heart. The heart is believed to "house the spirit" and "rule over the mental faculties," and bitter remedies are said to "tone the psyche."

As I explained previously, bitter flavor works reflexively via the central nervous system due to a neurological response triggered by taste receptors in the tongue, so the bitter flavor must be tasted. Only a small amount is required (too much can give an opposite effect) and is best taken 15 to 20 minutes before meals for its appetite promoting influences. Most of the benefits do not occur if the bitter plant is taken in a form, such as a capsule or a highly sweetened tea, that does not allow the bitter flavor to be tasted. As an experiment, next time you experience a (routine?) craving for sweets, place a drop of bitter herbal concentrate (tincture or tea) on your tongue and observe the diminishing effect it has on this sweet scenario. It can stop hypoglycemia attacks and the urge to binge and may ultimately diminish the requirement for insulin in diabetics when administered by a skilled practitioner (insulin dependent diabetics should be cautious when using bitters for it may upset their blood sugar balance; also, pregnant women should take care not to use too much bitter for this action can stimulate contractions in the uterus; bitters are also contra-indicated for excess menstrual flow and during painful menstrual cramps).

As most bonafide bartenders know, the best remedy for the hang-over is a squirt or two of Angostura Bitters taken in a small glass of water. Angostura Bitters is an aromatic herbal compound containing, amongst other harmless vegetables extracts, the bitter herb, Gentian. And likewise, as many experienced hangover heroes and heroines know, this little bitter cocktail gives blessed, quick relief. The bitter flavor stimulates the flow of internal juices helping the body to more quickly detoxify itself and feel better. The spirit within is soon ready for still another night of sweet partying and the self-abuse of alcoholic over-merriment.

Some common bitter herbs are Gentian, Dandelion leaf, Mugwort, Blessed Thistle, Globe Artichoke leaf, Chickory, Chamomile, Centuary, Hops, Goldenseal, Yarrow, Wormwood and Agrimony. Delightful bitter salad herbs are Cress, Endive, young Dandelion greens, Wild Lettuce and Beet greens. My dad, who used to toss together some delicious salads when I was a young boy, always told me that a truly great salad must include some bitter and some sour flavored greens. That was my first herbal lesson.

Hypothesis #3

The lack of simple exercise in both sexes is a second cause of male and female sexual organ and immune system deficiencies.

Our ancestors lived by strength and endurance in an admittedly less comfortable environment. To survive each day brought tasks that required vigorous physical action. Survival meant running and climbing after one's dinner or running, screaming and climbing to avoid becoming dinner. Physical fitness was a necessity. Each of us has inherited the physical requirements that resulted from our species' genetic programming. Merely 2 to 3 generations ago our grandparents walked to evening dances, hung up clothes to dry, walked up stairs, walked to work, shovelled snow, cut and split firewood, raked leaves, pushed lawn mowers and ironed clothes with an 8 pound iron. Today most folks do none of these activities and much less. The average adult today hardly has to move a muscle group. We merely flick switches, turn keys, watch screens, click remote controls, push gas peddles, sit, talk, listen, write and type. Of course, life continues to give us adrenaline rushes which excite an immediate and urgent fight or flight reaction, and this creates a sizeable problem for our body and emotions because our life styles often do not provide us the opportunity to physically express or act out this adrenaline-induced condition. Picture the individual sitting in his or her automobile, locked in traffic, frustrated and stressed by the highway congestion. When an incident suddenly occurs that makes the adrenaline flow what is there for the physical body systems to do to act it all out? Usually nothing but merely pushing on the gas peddle, honking the horn and maybe rolling down the car window to voice a few succinct and graphic phrases. The body is frequently left with the frustration and the stress of energy that goes unexpressed. All too seldom any more do we lift, run, climb, push, stretch, pull, strain or grunt (except maybe during an attempted bowel movement). Regular, vigorous exercise uses up this energy in a healthy way for our times.

The highly visible multitudes of roly-poly, soft-drink generation children hanging out at fast-food kitchens and gaping at TV screens demonstrates that sedentarianism (and nutritional nonsense) is not reserved merely for adults. The American Alliance for Health, Physical Education, Recreation and Dance surveyed physical education in all 50 states and compiled the following picture of our culture's young folks: Half of our growing children are not getting enough exercise to develop a healthy heart and lungs. Forty percent of our young children (ages five to eight) are already obese or have elevated high blood pressure, high cholesterol levels and live an inactive lifestyle. One third of all school-age boys and one half of all school-age girls cannot run a mile in less than 10 minutes (some probably can't run a mile). Only one state, Illinois, has a physical education requirement. I see this cultural peculiarity as the precursor for a lot of low self-esteem. Quoting Bill Wood, author of *Marty the Marathon Bear*, "With 40 percent of America's children facing the risk of heart disease, the question should be: Why isn't youth fitness a bigger priority?" Bill Wood's book is written for children ages 8 to 12, showing them the importance of how health, fitness and nutrition can improve self-esteem, self-discipline and self-image.

Franz Steinberg, in his work *The Immobilized Patient*, (Plenum Medical Co., New York, 1980) viewed the role of inactivity in the production of disease from a unique perspective. He studied the effects on the body's circulation, respiration, bone tissue, skeletal muscle, joints and emotions created by the physician's tendency to prescribe extensive bed rest and immobilization (casts, traction, etc.) to patients. His study vividly illustrates the effects on the body and psyche that occur due to a medically imposed extreme lack of motion. Some of these effects are: The stroke volume of the heart is reduced while the heart rate accelerates, consequently the ability to adapt to physical effort diminishes rapidly; the ability of the bronchial tree to rid itself of foreign material and of excess mucus is very much affected; calcium is released excessively and eliminated as calcium salts in the urine, leading to true osteoporosis; skeletal muscles weaken, lose tone and atrophy due to decreased fiber size; stagnation of the intercellular fluid of the cartilage decreases nutrition to the joints causing limitation of motion; drives, expectancies and motivation to learn are greatly diminished by immobility, while emotions are expressed in various ways including apathy, withdrawal, frustration, anger, aggression and regression; and there is a dulling of sensory processes and progressive dulling of the intellect. This medical study is most interesting in showing the body's natural organic, inorganic, mental and emotional responses to an imposed environmental sedentary condition. From this perspective we can observe and more clearly understand why relatively similar symptoms develop in individuals and cultures that accept and indulge in a prolonged sedentary (immobilized) lifestyle. It seems reasonable, based on Dr. Steinberg's findings, that our modern society's dramatic increases in metabolic malfunctions, degenerative diseases, prostate and menstrual problems, adult and juvenile delinquency, hypertension, neurosis and drug abuse, violent and non-directed energy, learning problems, obesity, etc. may be pernicious symptoms of the chronic immobility inherent in our culture's extremely sedentary life-style.

Doctors Kraus, M.D. and Raab, M.D. in their work *Hypokinetic Disease* (Charles C. Thomas, Springfield, Ill., 1961) have coined the term "hypokinetic (caused by insufficient motion) disease" to describe the vast array of disease and disorders that may be caused or influenced by our sedentary lifestyle. Kraus and Raab feel that a tremendous transition has taken place in the biologically short period of time (only a 100 years ago hard labor was a necessary part of the lives of the majority) that has transpired from primitive man to today's domesticated citizens; a transition from an active and physically strenuous life, subject to privations and hardships of climate to an extremely well protected but caged (akin to Steinberg's immobilized patients) existence. They feel it is highly unlikely that such a change of environment and mode of living can take place without major reactions of the organism. The great adaptability of the human body and mind to new circumstances is one of our outstanding qualities, but we can function only within certain limits. Lack of exercise constitutes a cause for a deficiency state comparable to avitaminosis. Kraus & Raab believe that this lifestyle interferes with the biological function of action and that this interference is physically damaging to human beings.

This idea is based on the view of the body as essentially active and dynamic in nature. The system that has been mostly suppressed is the skeletal muscle system which makes up 40% of our body's weight and has important roles which go beyond mere locomotion. The action of these striated muscles profoundly influence circulation, metabolism and endocrine balance. It directly affects the structuring of our skeletal system and posture and serves as an outlet for emotions and nervous responses. Exercise plays a great role in how we handle stress and moods. The lack of physical response causes tension (non-directed energy) due to insufficient expression. This tension manifests as disease with symptoms such as degenerative cardiovascular derangement, obesity, metabolic malfunction, endocrine malfunction, gastro-intestinal upset, skeletal muscle dysfunction (their research discovered that 80% of all lower back pain was due to muscular deficiency resulting from lack of physical activity), degenerative disease, neurosis, depression, anxiety, etc.

Sometimes we experience inner emotional weather fronts. We may feel sorry for ourselves, confused, ungrounded. This is a valid state of mind, and we can take time to sort out the gloom and focus on what is truly bothering us. But we don't want to flounder in such states for too long. One of the best antidotes is to go and work out. Get physical. Move in Tai Chi. Exercise stimulates the production of endorphins, which give us a sense of well-being. During this experience our body helps our mind and moods to uplift. Visualizing yourself well and whole, the mind helps the body. When you are having fun and laughing, the body and mind are getting it on together, enjoying life. Today, with all the focus and social value our western culture places on youth, regular exercise is a daily deposit into one's youth savings account, and it's being discovered that exercise keeps you youthful in more ways than one. A study by researchers at Bentley College, Waltham, Mass., summarized in *Men's Health* magazine, found that master swimmers reported frequencies of sex typical of people 20 to 40 years younger. For swimmers in their forties, the monthly average was 7.1 times. For those aged 60 and over, the average was 6.7 times a month. If nothing else, you must admit that .1 sex or .7 sex could contribute some interesting new dimensions to your sex life.

Physical frailty in people of even very advanced ages is treatable with exercise. In a pilot program conducted by a group of physicians from Tufts University in Boston, frail, institutionalized men and women under-took regular (supervised) weight training to improve their strength and mobility, thereby reducing their susceptibility to injury in falls and other accidents. Some of the men and women improved their strength threefold to fourfold in an eight-week period, all of them became stronger than they had been many years previously. This can greatly enhance the ability of older people to live independently, replacing nursing homes with home exercise rooms, Tai Chi in the parks and nature walks in the country.

A sidelight on this issue is an observation that Ryan Drum, Ph.D., an herbalist, wildcrafter and herbal brewmaster shared with me about individuals he calls "sitters." He observed that men who complain of prostrate problems (and possibly women with chronic uterine cramping) are frequently those who sit in chairs for long hours. Sitting in a chair is not a normal position for the human body. Remove the chair and the person of course will fall. This imbalanced position causes tension. The fear of falling onto the back and tail bone causes a tension of the buttocks and perineum that no longer registers consciously. When continued over a span of years, this holding reflex compacts the prostate and creates chronic prostate congestion and subsequent infection. Squatting or sitting cross legged in the yoga full or half "lotus" position will expand the area and help relieve this condition.

Exercise and stretching are essential for male internal organ and overall body wellness. As a self-administered preventive medicine, regular proper exercise coupled with sensible nutrition helps prevent the following all too common complaints:

- Arthritis by keeping joints mobile and active
- Osteoporosis by keeping bone tissue dense and strong
- Heart disease by improving and maintaining cardiovascular efficiency
- Poor circulation by increasing blood flow
- Muscle atrophy by stimulating muscle strength and tone
- Mental and emotional illness by relieving stress
- Poor self-image by doing something about it
- Impotence by reducing the probability of diabetes
- Immune system weakness and lethargy by increasing resistance
- Cancer by reducing body fat levels.

This is an impressive list of potential benefits by anybody's standards.

❧6❧

A Technology of Independence

Before the Great Cultural Amnesia Attack (GCAA) of the industrial revolution, most family members knew how to use herbs. The *materia medica* of herbalism is free, once an individual (re)learns to recognize local medicinal plants (aka "weeds") and (re)learns how to harvest and prepare them correctly.

A *simple* is a single health-enhancing plant. A *simpler* is one who knows how to use these plants. The techniques of making herbal medicine remain simple.

The materials necessary are minimal
- measuring cups
- glass, stainless steel or porcelain tea pot and sauce pans (avoid aluminum cooking vessels as you do red ants)
- electric coffee bean grinder (a post-Edison mortar and pestle) for powdering dried herbs
- electric blender for mixing fresh plant preparations
- glass jars and other glass containers having good, tight-fitting lids (especially save all amber glass containers for storing herbs and herbal preparations)
- fine mesh kitchen sieve and natural, undyed, cotton muslin cloth for straining and filtering
- assorted funnels, rubber spatulas and stirring sticks
- kitchen scale that indicates metric weight
- food and herb dehydrator — not essential, but extremely useful (After you have owned one and used it for a while, it becomes essential.)

How to Prepare
Infusions (tea)
Put one heaping teaspoonful (a teabagful) of cut, powdered or crushed herb leaves and/or flowers (the tender more delicate plant parts) into a preheated cup, pan or teapot (approximately two teaspoonsful if using a fresh undried herb); add boiling water, stir, cover, and let steep for 10 minutes; strain and drink. You have made a natural medicine called an herbal infusion, or call it herb tea. You need to use this infusion within 24 hours. It deteriorates rapidly. Standard dosage is 1 cupful 2 to 3 times a day.

Some mucilaginous herbs such as Marshmallow and Slippery Elm are best prepared as cold infusions. This process extracts the most mucilage from these herbs, and these constituents don't coagulate in the cold water solvent (menstruum). To make a cold infusion, simply place the cut or powdered herb into a container of cold, distilled water, stir it well, let it steep 5 to 12 hours until the water is slimy, and strain. Adding a little maple syrup gives it flavor.

Decoction (strong tea)
Put one heaping teaspoonful of cut, powdered or crushed dried or fresh undried herb seeds, root, rhizomes and/or bark (the tougher, woodier plant parts) into a saucepan and add 1-1/2 cup of cold water; place on low fire; bring to boil, cover and simmer 15 minutes; strain and drink. This is an herbal decoction. You can keep this decoction approximately 72 hours if you refrigerate it. Standard dosage is also 1 cupful 2 to 3 times a day.

Concentrate (very strong tea)
You can continue to simmer a completed decoction, evaporating the tea down to 1/2 or 1/4 the original volume, and you make an herbal concentrate. Concentrates are considered more potent due to their condensed form, so they are often used to prepare compresses and syrups.

Syrup
To make an herbal syrup, begin with an herbal concentrate. To approximately 1 pint of this concentrate add about 2 to 4 tablespoons of raw honey and 2 to 4 tablespoons of vegetable glycerine (alter these amounts depending on the consistency you desire). Tinctures can be added to syrups by adding 2 tablespoons of the tincture to 1 cup of the syrup. Store in the refrigerator. The honey and glycerine will preserve them for approximately

a year. Syrups are generally used to treat coughs and sore throats, because they coat the throat lining, keeping the herbs in contact with the throat tissue (think of a syrup as a sweet, flowing poultice). Standard dose is approximately 1 teaspoonful as needed.

Tincture

Combine approximately one ounce of powdered dried herb (powder the dry herb by grinding it in the electric coffee grinder) with 1 pint of 80 or 100 proof alcohol (vodka, gin, brandy, whichever you prefer) in a glass jar, stir well and cap the jar tightly. If you choose to use a fresh undried herb, cut it into small pieces, put it in a blender, cover it with a 100 proof alcohol and blend it all to a pulpy mash. Pour this mixture into a glass jar; shake vigorously once or twice a day, for 14 days (this is very important to keep the extraction process most active). After two weeks, strain out the liquid through muslin cloth and squeeze as much liquid out of the remaining pulp (the marc) as possible. Discard the marc into a compost pile and store the deeply tinted liquor in a dark cool place in a tightly covered jar (preferably a light-retarding amber brown jar) which has been appropriately labeled. You have made an herbal tincture. This tincture will keep for years. Standard dosage is 15 to 40 drops 3 times a day. Some practitioners suggest 1 to 4 ml 3 times a day (a ml is about 25 drops).

Note: If you wish to eliminate most of the alcohol from each dose, drop the dose to be taken into 1/4 to 1/2 cup of boiling water and simmer 2 minutes, cool and drink. This will not impair the quality of the tincture.

Liniment

The method you use to make a tincture is the same method you use to make an herbal liniment, only with a liniment you can use rubbing alcohol* in place of the beverage (ethyl) alcohol. If you do use rubbing alcohol, be sure to label your liniment: "For external use only."

---

* Note: I have been informed by one experienced herbal practitioner that rubbing alcohol is a nerve poison and is not a good medium to use as a medicine. It penetrates the dermis (the fibrous inner layer of the skin which is well supplied with nerves and blood vessels) and, he feels, the net result of contact use is toxic and harmful. The best alcohol to use is 190 proof ethyl alcohol which can be purchased in some states. A brand named *Everclear* is a good 190 proof grain alcohol.

Glycerite

To make a concentrated extract which is similar to a tincture but has no ethyl alcohol content, you can make a glycerite. This can be made using fresh or dried herbs as follows:

When using a fresh undried herb, first cut the herb into small pieces, place into a blender and add pure vegetable glycerine, enough to cover the herb. Blend the mixture until the herb is well-blended with the glycerin. Initially it will be difficult to get the herb into the blades of the blender, use a blunt ended wooden stick to assist you; persevere and be careful of the blender blades. You may need to add a little distilled water to dilute the syrupy glycerine, but this is not usually necessary when using fresh plants, for they bring their own water to the blend. Use as little added water as possible. After the herb and glycerine are well blended, proceed the same as if making a tincture (see Tincture, p. 54).

When using a dried herb, first crush the herb well or powder it in an electric coffee bean grinder. Place this in a jar. Prepare a mixture of 6 parts glycerine to 4 parts water. Stir this mixture well to blend the glycerine and water. Pour this liquid onto the powdered herb, enough to saturate the herb, stir thoroughly, proceed the same as if making a tincture.

Your final preparation, after it has been strained, must contain *at least 50% glycerine by volume* in order for the glycerine to be an adequate preservative. Most commercial glycerine contains approximately 5% water; allow for this in your calculations. This preparation will store for one to two years if prepared correctly. Standard dosage is 15 to 40 drops taken internally 3 times a day. Note: Mucilaginous herbs such as Comfrey and Marshmallow do not lend themselves to this form of extraction.

Oil Infusion

Put dried powdered plant parts into quality cold-pressed olive oil and stir well, creating a mixture having the consistency of mud pies that will drip off a spoon but are not too runny. Keep in a warm place approximately 100° F. Stir or shake this blend frequently throughout the day for 10 days. While the mixture is still warm, strain out the oil through cotton muslin cloth. Press remaining oil from the marc (this step can be a messy process, so be sure you are in a patient mood before commencing, and have wipe-up materials at hand). Store in a covered jar in a cool place. You have made a soothing medicinal herbal oil infusion.

Salve

Put 1/2 ounce (14 grams or about 2 tablespoons) of pure beeswax shavings (do not use large whole chunks, as this requires over-heating of the herbal oil) with 1/2 cup herbal oil infusion into a small saucepan; place over low heat and warm until the beeswax is melted. Test for desired consistency by dipping a spoon into the mixture, removing the spoon and letting the mixture harden on the spoon. If, upon cooling, the mixture becomes too hard, add a little more oil to the warm mixture which is still in the pan; if too soft, add a little more beeswax. Re-test until the consistency is perfectly to your liking. Remove the oil/wax mixture from heat; pour into container with lid; allow mixture to harden. You have made an herbal salve. Tightly covered, these keep indefinitely, but it's best to keep salves relatively cool. Apply directly to skin as needed.

Suppository

Suppositories are designed to be inserted into the orifices of the body. They act as carriers for any herb that is appropriate to use for treatment. Suppositories can be shaped to use in the ear, nose, rectum or the vagina. Most commonly they are used for insertion into the rectum (the most direct route for treating the prostate) or the vagina. Their form is usually cone-shaped, with a rounded apex (torpedo-like), about the size of the first two joints of your little finger (approx. 30 grams). Their consistency should be such that they will retain their shape at ordinary room temperature, but will readily melt at body temperature liberating the herbs contained therein. Cocoa butter is an excellent base to use for it fulfills both the above requirements, and it is easily attained. If you dwell in a very warm climate, it may be necessary to add a small amount of beeswax to raise the melting point of the cocoa butter (about 6 parts cocoa butter to 1 part shaved beeswax).

To prepare a suppository using powdered herbs: Handmake a mould by shaping aluminum foil into the length and shape you need for the suppositories. (An easy way to shape foil is to form it around a medium width writing pen and crimp the two ends of the foil. This will mould a long suppository which can be cut to appropriate lengths once it has cooled.) Grind the herb(s) to be used to a fine powder. Use an electric coffee bean grinder to powder the herbs if necessary. Melt cocoa butter over low heat. Mix the finely powdered herb(s) with melted cocoa butter. Herbs vary in texture and "fluff," so it is difficult to give exact proportions. Begin by mixing equal parts by volume (example: a level tablespoon of herb powder to a tablespoon of melted cocoa butter). Hold aside some extra herb and cocoa butter in case they are needed to adjust the final consistency of this mixture. Pour the final mixture into the aluminum foil moulds and let it cool. You can now use the suppositories or store them for a while in the refrigerator for future use.

Employing a liquid extract in a suppository form requires the use of a base other than cocoa butter.

To prepare a suppository using liquid herbal extracts (i.e., infusions, decoctions or tinctures): Handmake your aluminum mould as above. Measure the following proportions of liquid herbal extract, vegetable glycerine and gelatin. (Gelatin is an animal product):

Liquid extract	40 parts
glycerine	15 parts
gelatin	10 parts

Soak the gelatin in the liquid extract for a half hour, then dissolve the gelatin by using a very low heat. Add the vegetable glycerine to the mixture and stir well. Using a water bath or a double boiler, heat the mixture to evaporate the water. The final consistency of the suppositories will depend on how much water is removed. If all the water is removed, you end up with a very firm consistency. Pour the final mixture into the aluminum foil mould and let it cool. These suppositories can also be stored for a while in the refrigerator for future use.

Compress (fomentation)

Dip a clean, freshly laundered, white cotton cloth into a warm herbal infusion, decoction or tincture (even an oil infusion, if you can live with the mess). Wring out excess liquid and place on an injured or stressed body part. You have made a healing herbal compress. Cover this compress with a recycled plastic vegetable bag and then a blanket, hot pad or hot water bottle if added heat is appropriate.

Poultice

Crush, bruise, pummel, chop, juice, or — in an emergency — merely chew up fresh plant parts and lay them directly on injured, stung, bitten or otherwise stressed body parts. Wrap with a clean cloth to hold herbs in place. Or moisten powdered dried herb with hot tea and place directly on body. You have made an herbal poultice. Apply poultices thick and wet (but not runny wet); this is when they draw and soothe most efficiently.

A "part" of an herbal formula

When putting together a formula, herbalists design the formula and communicate its composition by referring to numbers of "parts." *Example:* For treating an irritated prostate gland, mix 2 parts Saw Palmetto, 1 part Echinacea, 1 part Damiana, 1 part Yarrow, 1/8 part Ginger. The question often arises: What is a part? Is it a gram, an ounce, a cupful, a shovelful, a truckload or a drop? It can be any of these measures. You retain the proper proportions as long as each measure used to make up "a part" is the same measure as each of the other measured "parts" in the mixture. It all comes down to how much mixture you wish to ultimately make. If you chose shovel-fulls as a measure for each "part" in the sample formula, you'd end up with enough mixture for all the prostates in the NFL. So, a more reasonable measure to use is the (Avoirdupois - 16 oz. to the lb.) ounce when compounding bulk herbs or the (32 ounce to the quart) fluid ounce for blending liquid extracts (metric measures are much better to use, but we won't pursue that issue here). Referring back again to the sample formula, you would blend together 2 ounces Saw Palmetto, 1 ounce Echinacea, 1 ounce Damiana, 1 ounce Yarrow and 1/8 ounce Ginger, ending up with 5-1/8 ounces of the formula. If you only want half that amount, make each part = 1/2 ounce. It doesn't matter what measure you use, a household coffee scoop works fine as a (volume) "part" measure, just use the same measure throughout.

As you can see, making herbal medicines is a relatively simple process. Selecting the appropriate herbs to successfully treat a condition is the rest of the art and science of Herbalism, and that is what the scope of this herbal is prepared to help you learn. If you become interested in learning further techniques and insights into making herbal medicines, including harvesting, drying and storing herbs, you may be interested in sending for *The Herbal Medicine-Maker's Handbook*, a booklet I prepared for students attending the California School of Herbal Studies. To order, send $6.95 U.S. plus $1.50 postage to: Shake Your Tinctures, P.O. Box 39, Forestville, CA 95436.

7

Picking the Right Herbs

Perspectives

In following chapters, I will discuss issues pertaining to specific male
health problems, outline appropriate herbal formulas and give suggestions
for relevant lifestyle alterations. But rather than merely build herbal fires for
you, so to speak, by giving you a formula for this and a formula for that, I
am going to introduce a concept that lays a wholistic foundation for using
herbs in a western model. With a grasp of this simple concept, you can build
your own fires as needed, insuring yourself greater health-care self-sufficiency. Understanding this concept allows you to employ ingenuity in using
herbs; to exercise your autonomy. The formulas I give you, or any other
formula you find, can be customized to treat more specifically your unique
condition. Most importantly, with this fundamental understanding you can
design and prepare original formulas using the common herbs that grow
locally or are available at the local herb store. If there is no herb store in your
community, you can purchase high quality herbs through mail-order. There
are small cottage industry herb companies that are preparing excellent high
quality herbs, herbal extracts, herbal formulas and aromatherapy products
for mail-order purchase. (See Resources, p. 253.)

It has been remarked to me that, what most people want is to be able
to look up their symptoms in the index of this book and be directed to a page
on which they will find a quick 'n easy herbal cure. A habit, hope and
illusion we have picked up from living in a society that basically offers
mostly an extensive disease-care medical/drug system. I have been told that
many men won't use this book if it does not lay out herbal devices and
techniques that will "fix" them, requiring minimal effort on their part to care
for themselves. If this is truly what you are seeking, then please, don't

59

bother with this book or any other book to serve that purpose. If you do, you will be disappointed, for a system of dial-a-cure won't work, and I do not wish to contribute to any illusion that it can.

Please try not to be annoyed by having to read through this book for the information you seek. I've made it more than just a rap about disease and herbs. I think the ideas I hold out to you are vital to our male health and are worthy of your time, contemplation and discussion.

Easy (just take a pill) cures for human ills have been marketed to the naive consumer for years now, not only by the drug industry and its salesmen, but also by alternative schools of therapy that teach an allopathic-like "drug" approach. I've yet to witness or hear of a successful quick-cure for any chronic or constitutional health problem. Aside from a miracle, healing these conditions requires some time and commitment to self-care. Miracles do happen mind you, but even they require some efficient work.

I will discuss herbal remedies and other health-care techniques that can give blessed relief, but they need to be used with some understanding of, and cooperation with, the regenerative process that is being set into action. Sustained effort is required to allow this process to take hold and "work." There is no magic-bullet cure in quality health-care. There is magic, however. The experiential magic is woven as you commit yourself to participate directly in your own healing. We men are remarkably capable of this, but we need to quit wasting time and energy looking for effortless cures or for someone else to do it for us. Making necessary changes in lifestyle, using the herbs and the assistance of a competent practitioner, when necessary, and getting on with actualizing personal transformation are priority endeavors in health-care. I am not promising that the formulas and herbal information I give you are anything more than integral parts of this process. I will promise, that if you take the time to read and understand these chapters and employ the techniques for yourself, you will become healthier. You will make yourself stronger. You will resume conscious control of your health and vital energy, enriching all facets of your male body and your male psyche.

Herbal Dynamics

When I began studying herbal therapeutics, it was not made clear to me to, first, learn the *actions* of each herb. Like learning a new language, one must first build a little vocabulary. Then he can start exploring and playing with the language. The energetic actions of herbs comprise the vocabulary of herbal therapeutics. The actions are an herb's known thera-peutic abilities. It is a mistake to ask, "what herb do I take for... ?" or "what herb will cure my ... ? " Herbs are far more clever and practical than that. Each herb has energies that can be used for treating a wide variety of conditions.

As I briefly discussed in the chapter Recycling Our Heritage, the effects of an herb on the human body are quite predictable. This predictability has been made possible for us by humanity's timeless history of observing the actions of each herb as the herb has been used internally and/or externally by myriads of human beings. These well documented actions of an herb are readily outlined in most herbal texts, but they are rarely understood by the modern day reader and are casually regarded as peripheral information. The average reader tends to look for a "hit-medicine" that can be taken to eliminate a particular condition. We western individuals are strongly conditioned to approach health-care in this manner, but this is the manner in which allopathic science deals with disease, using a potent drug to override and counteract a body symptom. Individuals seeking alternatives to allopathic heroic chemical drugs turn to herbalism for its plant *materia medica*, but then usually continue to approach the use of these herbs in an allopathic fashion. This is not the most efficient method for using herbs. Instead, one needs to reconsider the relationship inherent between the energy of herbs and the requirements of the human body which is a spontaneous self-healing organism. Normally the actively healing body does not need something to be done to it, but rather it readily uses allied supportive energy (herbal actions) and biochemically appropriate nutrients to supplement its inherently competent, self-healing, vital energy.

Understanding and employing the supportive actions of individual herbs (e.g., tonic, bitter, astringent, demulcent, carminitive, etc.) composes a major portion of the practice of herbal therapeutic science. Learning and understanding the particular system(s) affinity of each herb makes up most of the rest of this therapeutic art.

Each herb embodies an "action" or "bio-medical energy" (usually many actions), and, concurrently, each herb also has a natural affinity for, or kinship with, one or more of the systems of the human body (e.g., the circulatory system, the urinary system, the immune system complex, the nervous system, the musculo-skeletal system, etc.). It is these actions and affinities that supply the systems of the body with the supportive energy and nutritional reinforcements that are most helpful during the healing process.

Recall from the previous chapter, for example, the natural affinity identified by folkloric empirical science that Horsechestnut has for the circulatory system and its bio-chemically tonic, astringent and nutrient actions on that system. Learning and understanding the actions and the affinities of an herb is fundamental knowledge which empowers the herbalist to use plants as reliable tools for assisting the healing and prevention of human maladies. This intimate knowledge of the actions and affinities of our planet's herbs is the heart and soul of the rich folkloric heritage that has been handed to us by our ancestors. Our ancestors were extremely bright, observant, resourceful, clever people, equal to us current folks. We stem from intelligent, intuitive and clever elders. In my experience, the wisdom, accuracy and durability of their empirical health-care science is exceptionally trustworthy, safe and effective.

Using an Herbal

One finds information about the "actions" and "body system affinities" of an herb by reading an herbal. There are many books being published about herbs and herbalism today, but few that are written by experienced, knowledgeable herbalists. It is strongly advised that the reader seek out truly accurate herbals from the current glut of books about herbs that have become fashionable to publish. In the Resource section of this book I have listed for you some of the herbals that I use and value most highly.

While referencing an herbal, the reader is confronted with a blend of information that the author has selected to illustrate his or her particular herbal emphasis. As you peruse various herbals, you can note the primary bent of the authors. Some herbalists emphasize the botany and cultivation of herbs, for this is the aspect of herbalism that intrigues them most; some the more therapeutic/medicinal aspects of herbs and others the natural habitat, harvesting and medicine-making details. But whatever is the author's particular experience and pleasure, the information shared is commonly organized in the following general order:

Common Name: Horsechestnut
Botanical (binomial) name: *Aesculus hippocastanum*
Plant Family: *Hippocastanaceae*
Parts used: (Gives the part of the plant that is used therapeutically)
Fruit and bark

Description: (This section gives a fairly detailed macroscopical and often microscopical description of the plant to help the herbalist accurately identify it) The trunk is very erect and columnar . . . bark is smooth and greyish . . . large leaves are divided into 5 or 7 leaflets, spreading like fingers from the palm of the hand . . . flowers are mostly white with reddish tinge growing in dense, erect spikes . . . fruit is a shining chest-nut brown nut having a bitter taste . . . the fruit has a large green husk, protected with short spines which split into 3 valves when it falls to the ground and frees the nut . . . . (M. Grieves)

History: Horsechestnut is indigenous to Persia and north India . . . was introduced into Central Europe in the 16th century . . . now common to many parts of the U.S . . . extensively cultivated for shade and ornamentation . . . (Felter-Lloyd, Shauenberg)

Flowering season: May – June

Collection season: Ripe nuts are collected in September and October as they fall to the ground; the bark is harvested in early Spring season.

Cultivation & Habitat: Generally raised from the nuts sown in early spring . . . thrive in most soils and situations but do best in a good sandy loam . . . .

Actions and medical uses: (Also termed "properties," "affinities" or "virtues") The fruit is a circulatory tonic and astringent. The bark is tonic, astringent, febrifuge, narcotic and antiseptic.

Specific indications: (The specific uses of the herb's actions and affinities are discussed) The unique actions of Aesculus are on the vessels of the circulatory system . . . increasing the strength and tone of the veins in particular . . . used internally to aid the body in the treatment of problems such as phlebitis, varicosity and hemorrhoids (D. Hoffmann). A remedy for congestion and engorgement. Nerve pain in the viscera due to congestion. Soreness of the whole body, with vascular fullness, throbbing and general malaise . . . rectal uneasiness with burning or aching pain (Felter-Lloyd).

Combinations used: (An herb often combines particularly well with certain other herbs in the treatment of specific conditions, so usually both the combination and the condition are discussed) Combines well with Hawthorn, Yarrow and Prickly Ash for internal use to treat varicosity. Combines with Witch Hazel for preparing a lotion to use externally on varicose veins or hemorrhoids.

Constituents: (A list of isolated chemical constituents theorized to be most relevant to the action of the plant) Saponins, tannin, flavones, starch, fatty oil, the glycosides aesculin, aescin and fraxin.

Precautions: Do not inject extracts hypodermically.

Preparation and dosage: (Discusses common preparations of this herb and general dosage)

Infusion: 1-2 full teaspoons of the dried fruit steeped in a cup of boiling water for 10-20 minutes. Drink 1 cupful three times a day.

Tincture: take 1-4 ml of tincture three times a day. A ml of tincture is about 25-30 drops.

Externally: This plant is used as a lotion for the above conditions and is also appropriate for treating skin ulcers.

Folkloric uses: Traditional uses of the plant which have been preserved unreflectively amongst the people.

Toxicity: Eating the leaves or green outer casing of the fruit can lead to symptoms of gastro-enteritis, reddening of the skin and drowsiness.

Other uses: Shade and aesthetic ornamentation. The seeds or "conkers" are used by English children like marbles.

And sometimes a picture:

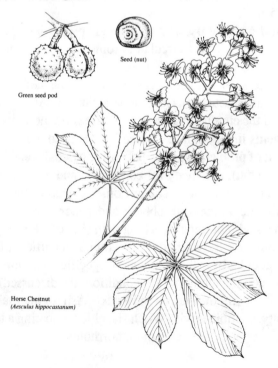

Seed (nut)

Green seed pod

Horse Chestnut
(*Aesculus hippocastanum*)

Few herbals will speak to all the attributes listed above, the format of each being custom designed by the emphasis of the author, but all of these attributes are commonly used in some combination throughout the herbals of our culture. The one category of attributes, however, that you will always find is the "Actions." This is the most important empirical information given and is often the most misunderstood and confusing to the student. Some herbals will present a long list of actions, which leaves one more frustrated than informed. It frequently appears that a particular herb is good for just about everything, which can leave one in a state of dismay due to over-saturation. Unfortunately, what has not been defined, and is often not understood, is the particular body system (eg., digestive system, respiratory system, lymphatic system) or systems that each herb has a natural affinity with. In some cases, different parts of a particular plant (leaf, root, flower, seed, etc.) provide different actions and have affinities for different systems of the body. But in many herbals this information is all lumped into one amalgamated list and becomes nearly useless as a practical guide.

What will help a learner most is to study and recognize the actions of an herb in relationship to its natural "body systems affinity." This affinity between an herb and a body system can also be thought of, or visualized as, a biochemical kinship, a natural spontaneous relationship or a mutually attractive force. From centuries of human observation, the herb has demonstrated a consistent, predictable affinity with a particular body system, and the herb's actions cause a specific effect or action on that system. Ginkgo, for example, will move to the peripheral-vascular systems and other outlying regions, dilate the blood vessels, and voila! increased blood and oxygen ultimately get to the brain; a Horsechestnut fruit extract, having a natural affinity with the circulatory system, will move to the vessels of this system and act to give them strength and tone, while an extract of its bark will readily cruise to the rectal arena and supply astringent action for congested hemorrhoids (varicose rectal veins), a true friend indeed.

So it is imperative that individuals who choose to use herbs for their personal and family health-care become familiar with the 'action' words of the language of herbalism that introduce them to the unique attributes of each individual herb. An herb can then be used most appropriately with the greatest efficiency. Combinations of herbs can be formulated to work synergistically in a more wholistic approach, treating not only the obvious symptoms, but at the same time, supporting all the other systems and related problems that make up the more subtly contributing pieces of the whole picture. Each herb has an array of actions and affinities, so a knowledgeable person can take care to cleverly combine herbs such that they enhance each other's actions and also cover a range of problems. With the understanding of the actions and affinities of a few herbs one can devise a specific strategy for toning, balancing and cleansing individual human systems, treating simultaneously the causes as well as the symptoms.

An example formula for treating a prostate infection will illustrate this approach.

- The actions of Saw Palmetto are tonic, nutrient and antiseptic, and this herb has a strong affinity for the reproductive system and the nervous system. It acts to nourish the nerves and tone and strengthen the male reproductive system particularly the prostate gland.
- Echinacea is an overall systemic (works throughout the whole body) anti-microbial, lymphatic, alterative and immune enhancer.
- Damiana is a nerve tonic, prostate tonic, urinary antiseptic, anti-depressant, and it is mildly laxative. It too has an affinity for the reproductive system and the nervous system.
- Yarrow is astringent, bitter, urinary antiseptic, diuretic, dia-phoretic aiding the body to deal with fever, also having an affinity for the circulatory system, directly assisting in normalizing blood pressure.

Using the combined actions of these four herbs, we can create at once a strong glandular tonic which is astringent and strengthening for a debilitated and, most likely, swollen prostate gland. In all cases of infection the body's natural resistance is not functioning correctly. This may be caused by stress, constipation or inadequate diet, so we have included bitters in this formula to help stimulate appetite and the secretion of all the digestive juices. We have included immune enhancing herbs with genito-urinary system antiseptics to support the overall immune system, especially targeting the prostate. We also have circulatory system and nervous system tonics with an alterative herb. These herbs support circulation, nerve impulses and blood conditioning respectively, with a mild laxative action present if needed.

So, by taking advantage of the specific actions and system affinities of these herbs, we are attending to the major symptom, the infected prostate gland, while also enhancing the health of the nervous, circulatory and digestive systems and firmly assisting the body's overall systemic immune action. If there is discomfort and pain Crampbark and/or Black Haw can be added to the formula. These two herbs are both nervine, analgesic and antispasmodic having an affinity with the reproductive system. If flavor is an issue we can add Fennel seed to the formula. It is a delicious tasting herb having carminative, aromatic and antispasmodic actions. Fennel has an affinity with the entire digestive tract, stimulating appetite and digestion, while relieving flatulence.

So a herbal remedy specific for treating infection in the male genito-urinary system which simultaneously nourishes and strengthens supportive systems combines the above herbs as follows:

Saw Palmetto	2 parts
Echinacea	2 parts
Damiana	1 part
Yarrow	1 part
Crampbark	1 part

I suggest including Saw Palmetto and Echinacea in 2 parts, because they possess the primary properties that are required to treat the prostate infection.

Prepare a pot of tea (using 1 rounded teaspoon of this formula per cup of water) and drink 1 cupful 3 times a day. In place of taking a tea, you can take the herbs as a tincture blend, combining the individual plant tinctures in the same proportions, using 30 to 50 drops of the blended liquid formula 3 times a day.

With proper diet, adequate exercise and rest, a blend of herbs similar to the above formula can profoundly assist a man to rid himself of prostate infection and sexual organ debility. Preventive care will then become the key to his continued better health.

Herbal Actions

Now that there no longer exists even a wisp of doubt about the importance of knowing the actions and affinities of the herbs one uses, I will list and discuss some of the main actions of herbs. Reductionist science has undertaken difficult research to determine the plant constituents that are responsible for these actions and has classified these constituents according to their chemical groups and physiological properties or effects. Thus, for example, plant *gum* and *mucilage* constituents are said to give rise to the soothing demulcent and emollient actions; the *tannins* give rise to astringent and hemostatic actions; while some *saponins* are believed to give rise to anti-inflammatory and expectorant actions. Using this reductionist insight and technology to determine the chemical constituents of herbal medicines which are newly introduced to us by the regional folklore of the plant's native environment, we can gain valuable hints as to the actions of these new plants. At the same time, when experimenting with these plants therapeutically, it is important to keep in mind the herbalist's perspective that the integrity and therapeutic value of a medicinal herb remains biomedically unique only when the herb's individual constituents remain in the context of the natural organization of the hundreds of synergistic biochemical constituents contained by the whole herb.

There are approximately 120 different actions that have been identified through the ages. However only about 40 of these actions are commonly considered. In the specific context of male health-care we need to be most functionally cognizant of the following:

Tonic

I am presenting this action first for it is perhaps the most important contribution herbal medicine can make in the process of natural healing. Tonic herbs stimulate nutrition by improving the assimilation of essential nutrients by the organs, improve systemic tone giving increased vigor, energy, and strength to the tissues of either specific organs or to the whole body. This is the central essential action to consider when devising any healing therapeutic formula. The other herbal actions work symbiotically with toning to evolve relief and full healing. Each of the tonic herbs has a specific system affinity which is discussed in the "Male Herbal" chapter. The list of tonic herbs is long. To name a few: Alfalfa, Coltsfoot, Oats, Damiana, Hawthorn, Saw Palmetto, Nettles, Garlic, Goldenseal, Calendula, Dandelion, Cleavers, Horsechestnut, Ho Shou Wu, Burdock, Bearberry, Angelica, Dong Quai, Ashwagandha, Ginseng, Hyssop, Oregon Grape, Motherwort, Scullcap, Vervain, Wild Yam, Raspberry, Sarsaparilla, Yarrow, Yellow Dock.

Adaptogen

This is a timely new action concept that is unique to herbal therapeutics. Adaptogenic or hormonal modulating actions increase the body's resistance and endurance to a wide variety of adverse influences from physical, chemical and biological stress, assisting the body's ability to cope and adapt. Adaptogens are non-toxic and possess normalizing actions. For example adaptogens tend to normalize high or low blood pressure, under active and over active adrenal glands and possibly other endocrine glands, and high or low blood sugar. This adaptogen action appears to work through hormonal regulation of the stress response which in turn has a modulating effect on human immunity. Siberian Ginseng, Chinese & American Ginseng, Schizandra, Ashwagandha, Licorice and possibly Devil's Club, Stinging Nettle, Suma and Astragulus.

Alterative
Herbs that have this property gradually restore health and vitality to the body. They have been referred to as blood cleansers. They help the body assimilate nutrients, eliminate metabolic wastes and restore proper function. Alterative herbs are used to help treat infection, blood toxicity, skin eruptions, impotence and chronic degenerative conditions: Burdock, Red Clover, Nettle, Cleavers, Oregon Grape are merely a few of the commonly used alterative herbs. Nature is generous with these health builders.

Analgesic, Anodyne
These herbs relieve pain when administered orally or externally, but they are not narcotic: Scullcap, Valerian, Passion flower.

Antacid
These herbs neutralize excess acid in the stomach and intestinal tract: Fennel, Catnip, Dandelion, Slippery Elm, Mullein, Meadowsweet (clears symptoms of hyperacidity).

Anthelmintic
These herbs destroy or expel worms from the digestive tract: Garlic, Onion, Wormwood, Rue, Thyme.

Antibilious
These herbs help remove excess bile from the system and help relieve biliary conditions or jaundice in the body: Centuary, Balmony, Barberry, Dandelion, Goldenseal, Yarrow, Turmeric.

Anticatarrhal
These herbs eliminate or counteract the build-up of excess mucus and catarrhal buildup from sinus or other upper respiratory parts: Eyebright,

Echinacea, Garlic, Black Pepper, Cayenne, Sage, Hyssop, Goldenrod, Yarrow, Yerba Santa.

Anti-emetic
These herbs lessen nausea and help relieve or prevent vomiting: Balm, Peppermint, Ginger, Fennel, Dill, Gentian, Meadowsweet.

Anti-inflammatory
Moderate inflammation is the body's appropriate reaction to infection, injury or irritation, resulting in enhanced tissue repair and containment of invaders. One does not always want to lessen this inflammation, but often finds it more efficacious to stimulate it by using rubifacients or systemic vasodilators. (See rubifacient and vasodilator actions below). One uses anti-inflammatory action to combat extensive or too painful occurrence of inflammation. Anti-inflammatory herbs include those having demulcent, emollient and vulnerary actions when applied externally: St. Johnswort, Calendula, Arnica, Licorice, Chamomile, Wild Yam.

Antilithic
These herbs help prevent or dissolve and discharge urinary and biliary stones and gravel. For urinary system kidney and bladder stones: Gravel Root, Hydrangea, Dandelion, Cleavers, Buchu, Goldenrod, Corn Silk, Uva Ursi. For gallbladder: Oregon Grape, Chaparral.

Anti-microbial
These herbs help the body's immune system destroy or resist pathogenic micro-organisms: the green, unripe Black Walnut hulls, Echinacea, Chaparral, Garlic, Goldenseal, Wormwood, and herbs high in volatile oils such as Anise, Caraway, Clove, Eucalyptus, Myrrh, Peppermint, Rosemary, Thyme.

Aphrodisiac
These herbs help correct conditions of impotence mostly by strengthening sexual excitement and desire. They tend more to stimulate sexual arousal than to improve performance. The combined use of alteratives helps restore proper function: Damiana, Saw Palmetto, Ginseng, Sarsaparilla, Yohimbe.

Aromatic
These herbs have a salient, usually pleasant odor, which stimulates the gastro-intestinal system (see carminative action) and are frequently used to improve the aroma and taste of medicines and foods: Lavender, Peppermint, Angelica, Cardamon, Cinnamon, Dill, Citrus Peel.

Astringent
This action promotes greater density and firmness of tissue by precipitating protein and condensing the cellular structure of the tissue, contracting and firming relaxed weakened tissue such as piles and prolapsed organs. Astringency can reduce excessive discharge of fluids like diarrhea in the intestines; blood hemorrhaging from the lungs and kidneys or excessive perspiration from the skin. These herbs include: White Oak, Pipsissewa, Horsechestnut, Partridgeberry, Witch Hazel.

Bitter
These herbs stimulate the secretion of digestive juices benefiting the digestive process. They stimulate the activity of the liver and pancreas, aiding the elimination of toxins: Gentian, Hops, Artichoke, Mugwort, Dandelion.

Carminative
This action excites intestinal peristalsis, promotes the expulsion of gas, soothes the stomach promoting digestion and relieves gripping (severe cramping pain) in the gastro-intestinal tract. These herbs are rich in aromatic volatile oils: Anise, Fennel, Chamomile, Peppermint, Caraway, Ginger.

Cholagogue
This action promotes the discharge and flow of bile from the gall-bladder into the small intestine. This is beneficial in treating gall-bladder problems. Bile helps disinfect the bowels and can have a laxative effect, as bile naturally stimulates peristalsis elimination. Cholagogues include: Barberry, Goldenseal, Dandelion, Oregon Grape, Wild Yam.

Demulcent
This action relaxes and soothes the tissue of the digestive tract upon direct contact, and triggers reflex mechanisms that travel through the spinal nerves effectively reducing inflammation and irritation in the respiratory

and urinary systems. These herbs are mucilaginous, gelatinous, soothing and protective: Comfrey, Marshmallow, Slippery Elm, Mullein, Corn Silk.

Diaphoretic

Fever is a very appropriate defense response of the body for dealing with infection. Contrary to accepted medical technique, stimulating a fever is often highly beneficial. This acts to increase sweat bringing the heat and inflammation outward to the surface of the skin, cooling the skin by evaporation of the sweat and concurrently facilitating the excretion of waste matter. These herbs induce increased perspiration, dilate capillaries and increase elimination through the skin: Elder, Yarrow, Osha, Ginger, Peppermint.

Diuretic

These herbs increase the elimination and regulates the flow of urine. For best results, drink lots of pure water while using diuretics: Dandelion, Couchgrass, Uva Ursi, Plantain, Horsetail.

Emetic

Emetics cause vomiting, helping the stomach to empty. To produce this effect, these herbs usually need to be taken in large doses: Lobelia, Ipecac, Boneset.

Emollient

Applied to the skin, these emollients soothe, soften and protect externally much like demulcents do internally: Comfrey, Chickweed, Plantain, Slippery Elm, Marshmallow.

Expectorant

These herbs support the respiratory system in removing excess mucus.
Stimulating expectorant – These herbs stimulate the nerves and muscles of the respiratory system to manifest a coughing syndrome, causing expectoration by encouraging the loosening and expulsion of mucus: Elecampane, White Horehound.
Relaxing expectorant – These herbs reduce tension in lung tissue, often easing tightness, allowing natural coughing and flow of mucus to occur: Coltsfoot (excellent for children), Gumweed, Licorice, Hyssop.
Amphoteric expectorant – These herbs can stimulate or relax the respiratory

system, using the body's wisdom to determine which is necessary: Lobelia, Mullein, Horehound, Coltsfoot, Elder, Garlic.

Febrifuge
These herbs assist the body to reduce fevers: Angelica, Catnip, Elder Blossom, Peppermint.

Hemostatic
These herbs are internal astringents that arrest hemorrhaging: Bayberry, Blackberry, Cayenne, Shepherd's Purse, Goldenseal.

Hepatic
These herbs strengthen and tone the liver, stimulating its secretive function, and causing an increase in the flow of bile: Oregon Grape Root, Agrimony, Dandelion, Goldenseal, Wild Yam.

Hypnotic
These herbs have a powerful relaxant and sedative action and help to induce sleep: Hops, Valerian, Wild Lettuce.

Hypotensive
These herbs reduce elevated blood pressure: Crampbark, Onion, Garlic, Yarrow, Hawthorn berries and flowers.

Laxative & Aperient
Laxative herbs stimulate bowel action, promoting evacuation: Cascara Sagrada, Yellow Dock, Rhubarb root.
Aperient herbs have a very mild laxative action: Dandelion root, Boneset, Beet root.

Lymphatic
These herbs support the health and activity of the lymphatic system: Cleavers, Calendula, Echinacea.

Nervine
These herbs effect the nervous system, having either a tonic (Oats, Damiana), relaxing (Chamomile, Hops) or stimulating (Coffee, Yerba Mate) effect.

Pectoral
These herbs have a general strengthening and healing effect on the entire respiratory system: Elecampane, Coltsfoot, Comfrey, Mullein, Yerba Santa, Anemopsis.

Rubefacient
When applied locally to the skin, rubefacients cause gentle irritation, promoting capillary dilation and increased circulation in the skin, drawing blood from deeper areas of the body. Drawing blood from deeper areas of the body relieves inflammation and congestion in these parts, often reducing pain. These herbs are useful for treating acute sprains, chronic arthritis, rheumatism and other joint afflictions: Stinging Nettle, Mustard seed, Cayenne, Horseradish, Black Pepper.

Sedative
These herbs calm the nervous system by lowering the functional activity of an organ, or by reducing stress and nervous irritation throughout the body: Valerian, Scullcap, Passion Flower, Black Cohosh.

Sialagogue
These herbs promote the secretion and flow of saliva from the salivary glands: Echinacea, Gentian, Prickly Ash, Black Pepper.

Stimulant
These herbs warm the body, quicken the circulation, break up obstructions and congestion, increase energy and possess a notably intense energy: Cayenne, Ginger, Horseradish, Mustard, Wormwood.

Styptic
These herbs arrest or reduce external bleeding due to astringent action on blood vessels: Yarrow, Horsetail, Cayenne, Bayberry, Plantain.

Vasodilator
These herbs expand blood vessels allowing increased circulation: Ginkgo, Feverfew, Siberian Ginseng, Ginger, Cayenne, Bayberry.

Vulnerary
These herbs help the body to heal wounds and cuts, and are applied

externally: Comfrey, Calendula, Chickweed, St. Johnswort, Marshmallow.

The Systems Affinity of Herbs

Each system of the body has plants that are particularly suited to it, plants that have a natural affinity with it. So, we find that within each of the action categories listed above there are plants embodying that action which carry the action to a particular body system. To illustrate this the following lists of body systems will name some herbs that carry anti-inflammatory, demulcent, bitter or astringent actions to these systems.

Herbs that carry *anti-inflammatory* action (reduces pain and discomfort) to
> The **circulatory system**: Hawthorn berries, Horsechestnut, Yarrow and Lime Blossoms.
> The **digestive system**: Chamomile, Peppermint, Fennel and Ginger.
> The **musculo-skeletal system**: Willow and Meadowsweat
> The **nervous system**: St. John's Wort.
> The **reproductive system**: Lady's Mantle and Blue Cohosh.
> The **respiratory system**: Licorice and Coltsfoot .
> The **skin**: St. John's Wort, Calendula, Chickweed, Arnica and Plantain.
> The **urinary system**: Corn Silk, Goldenrod and Marshmallow.

Herbs that carry *demulcent* action (soothes and protects) to
> The **circulatory system** (generally does not require demulcent action; however, Horsechestnut and Linden blossoms applied externally have a soothing emollient action on the blood vessels.
> The **digestive system**, (the anti-inflammatories will have a more direct therapeutic value on this system than demulcents): Slippery Elm.
> The **nervous system** (demulcents have direct value only when applied to the skin for nervous conditions like shingles): Slippery Elm, Marshmallow.
> The **reproductive system**: Marshmallow root, Mullein, Licorice and Coltsfoot.
> The **respiratory system**: Mullein, Marshmallow root, Plantain and Licorice.
> The **skin**: Marshmallow root, Comfrey, Plantain and Chickweed.
> The **urinary system**: Corn Silk, Couch Grass, Bearberry and Marshmallow leaf.

Bitter herbs that affect
   The **circulatory system**: Yarrow, Gentian and Goldenseal.
   The **digestive system**: Gentian, Artichoke, Goldenseal and Yarrow.
   The **musculo-skeletal system**: Bogbean.
   The **nervous system**: Chamomile, Hops and Mugwort.
   The **reproductive system**: Goldenseal.
   The **respiratory system**: White Horehound, Goldenseal.
   The **skin**: Goldenseal.
   The **urinary system**: Agrimony, Burdock and Bearberry.

Herbs that carry *astringent* action (tone and strengthen) to
   The **circulatory system**: internally Bayberry; externally Yarrow,
      Horsechestnut and Arnica.
   The **digestive system**: Agrimony and Oak Bark.
   The **musculo-skeletal system**: Agrimony.
   The **nervous system**: Rosemary.
   The **reproductive system**: Raspberry.
   The **respiratory system**: Sage, Goldenrod and Yarrow.
   The **skin** (externally): Witch Hazel and Oak Bark.
   The **urinary system**: Bearberry, Horsetail, Yarrow.

With these four actions, a skilled herbalist can basically perform most of the therapeutic work he or she might need to accomplish (especially when dealing with the digestive system). The *anti-inflammatory* action helps reduce inflammation, pain and discomfort. *Demulcents* soothe and protect. The *bitter* element stimulates normal internal secretions, counter-acting physical (and to a certain extent emotional) depression, while the *astringent* action can reduce excess discharge, toning and giving strength to body tissues. Of course the many other actions and affinities of our herbal materia medica are equally as important to understand and learn to use. The scope and intent of this male herbal is not to undertake an in-depth discussion of all these actions and system affinities. I recommend that one acquire a small collection of practical herbals which will provide a diversity of information and experience contributing to a well-rounded foundation of herbal knowledge. An excellent herbal text that teaches most thoroughly this western "actions and systems affinity" approach to herbal health-care is *The Holistic Herbal*, written by David Hoffmann, M.N.I.H.M., Medical Herbalist. A supplementary booklet titled, *Herbs, Actions and Systems*, prepared by Amanda McQuade Crawford, M.N.I.H.M. and David Hoffmann, which is based on course material for the California School of Herbal Studies is a short guide to herbal remedies, relating their actions and affinity for body systems. (Please see list of suggested herbals and other informative publications in the Resource section of this herbal.)

Herbal Specifics

True to the nature of Nature, there are those plants that can act entirely outside their recognized actions and systems affinity. Wild Yam, for example, has been experienced as a specific remedy for the pain and discomfort of diverticulitis (an inflammation in abnormal pouches which have been formed along the border of the colon wall). This would not be known by studying its normal actions, but based upon folkloric knowledge herbalists find that it has exceptionally helpful energy for this specific condition. Agrimony is a specific for treating appendicitis, when it is used in time. Red Sage taken as a tea internally and used as a mouthwash is a specific for treating mouth ulcers. Gumweed is a respiratory anti-spasmodic, while Mugwort is a digestive and reproductive system bitter, but the combination of these two herbs prepared for external application creates a traditional Poison Oak allergy remedy. This knowledge of the use of certain herbs as "specifics" is a specific gift of folkloric wisdom.

Herbal Light Show

Using one's inherent ability for direct knowing is a gift of one's own wisdom that must be trusted when selecting herbs for health-care. The more one acquires therapeutic knowledge and experience by studying and working with herbs and people, the more frequently one's intuition brings the two together in a successful experience. The practical use of intuition in times of crisis and healing is a quality that we tend to let go of in face of the onslaught of authoritarian information that continuously bombards us. But let your intuition not be denied. All scientific knowledge and hypotheses are inspired by the proverbial "flash" of insight. Like healing, intuition is a basic human function. Trust it, please.

About "male herbs"

Panax ginseng is probably the western world's most reknowned eastern "male herb." However, Ginseng renders actions that are equally effective for treating a female's condition when appropriate. Historically, the exotic and expensive Ginseng root was restricted exclusively for use by the male in ancient Chinese cultures and consequently through the ages, acquired its global "male herb" reputation. In a somewhat similar fashion *Dong Quai* acquired its "female herb" reputation. Based on the ageless insights of Chinese herbalism, Ginseng root is classified primarily as a Chi (Qi) tonic (please see glossary for discussion of Chi). *Dong Quai* is classified primarily as a blood tonic. The use of Ginseng is indicated in cases of deficient Chi and *Dong Quai* is indicated in cases of blood deficiency, both for either men or women. However, more often than not, men suffer from deficient Chi due to their "drivenness" and tendency to overwork, and women suffer from deficient blood due to their cyclic menstrual flow. Over the ages the bitter-sweet Ginseng root became known as the male's revitalizing medicine and the sweet warming root of the *Dong Quai* plant was endowed with the reputation of having wonderful gynecologic effectiveness. Keep in mind, however, that occasionally a man will manifest deficient blood and a modern woman deficient Chi.

Note: If you plan to use *Panax ginseng*, please be aware that cultivated Ginseng is the most heavily sprayed herb on the commercial herb market due to its susceptibility to hosting fungus growth and the high labor cost through the seven years required to mature it for harvest. It is recommended to use the wild-cultivated Ginseng grown commercially in unsprayed woods.

There is likewise a western herb (although Ginseng is also indigenous to the West) that is often referred to as a "male herb." Its name is Saw Palmetto (*Serenoa serrulata*– synonyms: *Sabal serrulata, Serenoa repens*), and like Ginseng its actions can be equally appropriate for promoting female health. This herb was highly valued by American Indian herbal science and later used extensively by the Eclectic physicians of the U.S. (The Eclectics were a prominent school of medical doctors who used primarily herbs and other natural remedies from 1880 to 1930.) This is a uniquely important nutritional herb for modern day males to be aware of and to use. I would like to discuss in some detail its remarkable nutritive and preventive properties.

The part of the plant that is used is the ripe berry of this Southeastern USA and Southern California palm tree. These palm berries are easily acquired and are best used when only partially dried or as a tincture of the partially dried berries. Saw Palmetto berries, when used regularly, directly influence the entire male reproductive apparatus, but especially the prostate gland. Saw Palmetto berry extracts have been shown to prevent the conversion of testosterone to dihydrotestosterone (DHT) in the prostate gland and also increase the breakdown and excretion of DHT (see section subtitled "The Prostate" in the chapter titled *Specific Male Problems* for discussion about the possible role DHT plays in prostate enlargement). Male organ symptoms that indicate this herb's use are: enlarged prostate with throbbing, aching, dull pain (a pain which often feels like it might be originating in the rectal area); discharge of prostatic fluid; discharge of mucus or a yellowish, watery fluid, accompanied with weakened sexual power; also for symptoms of testicle infection (orchitis) when associated with an enlarged prostate. Continued use of Saw Palmetto greatly benefits women who manifest ovarian enlargement, with tenderness and dull aching pains, weakened sexual activity, and small undeveloped mammary glands. Quoting from the work of Finley Ellingwood, M.D., *American Materia Medica Therapeutics and Pharmacognosy,* this herb "may be given with confidence in wasting of the testes in the early stages. It relieves irritation of the bladder, correcting the irritable character of the urine, increases the muscular power of the patient to expel the urine and produces a sense of relief, that is in every way gratifying and satisfactory. In the treatment of impotence in young men who have been excessive in their habits it can be relied upon with positiveness. It will increase sexual power in those newly married who, having been anxious concerning their sexual strength or ability, have become suddenly almost entirely impotent after marriage." Take the Saw Palmetto extract in doses of from 20 to 30 drops 3 to 4 times a day, combined with nervines such as Scullcap and Valerian to help relieve any anxiety impotence. (I've been told by some men that sometimes drinking a glass of good dark malt liquor before making love will effect the same cure for temporary anxiety impotence. The bitter Hops & malt used in the dark brew relaxes the anxious spirit as does the Scullcap and Valerian.)

In addition to Saw Palmetto's genito-urinary corrective qualities, it acts to relieve irritability of the entire nervous system by stimulating the nutrition of the nerve centers. It soothes local irritation of the urinary system, stimulates digestion, and encourages assimilation. If you decide to use this herb and set out to purchase it, don't be distracted by herbal high-technology marketing. Cherish your self-sufficiency. Saw Palmetto is very effective taken as a simple alcohol/water extract. It does not require high tech methods of preparation or extraction like freeze drying and liposterolic processing to unlock and release its actions. Simple plant extracts of this

Palm berry have nourished and healed humans for centuries.

Please refer to "The Male Herbal" section of this book for specific information about each of the herbs mentioned above.

Herb Quality

Herb quality is an important issue when it comes to picking the right herbs for herbal therapeutics and health maintenance. Discrimination is most necessary when selecting an herbal product, for the fact that it is herbal is not enough. For effective health-care it must be "high quality" herbal. Many people assume that if it is an herb it is organically grown and properly harvested. This is not necessarily so. Many herbs are grown for the commercial market using standard agricultural techniques and chemical fertilizers, sprayed with pesticides and fumigants, harvested and dried without regard for the proper plant part to be used. (For example, often flowering tops provide the medicinal actions in plants, but the parts harvested and sold will include a large percentage of extraneous leaf and stem, all of which may have been harvested incorrectly by machinery, over-heated when oven-dried in large batches and stored for long periods of time.) Plants must be harvested and processed carefully to ensure the quality of their constituents, and plants gradually lose their potency when stored too long or in unsuitable conditions.

Once you have picked and processed your own fresh herbs you will know what high quality herbs are like. It is always best to prepare medicine from herbs you have harvested and dried yourself, but this is not always possible. When selecting an herb from a source other than yourself use your senses to determine its quality. It must show excellent color, it should release a strong aroma, and it must have flavor. Not necessarily good tasting flavor, but intense flavor. These are all signs of herbal vitality. If the plant looks like lackluster hay with hardly any aroma or flavor, question its worth as a healing agent. Liquid extracts should also be scrutinized and expected to pass the same sensual tests.

If you hear from someone that herbs don't work, you can be assured that the individual either used the wrong herbs for the condition or used poor quality herbs. (See Resource section for a list of herbal outlets that have excellent reputations for preparing high quality herbal products.)

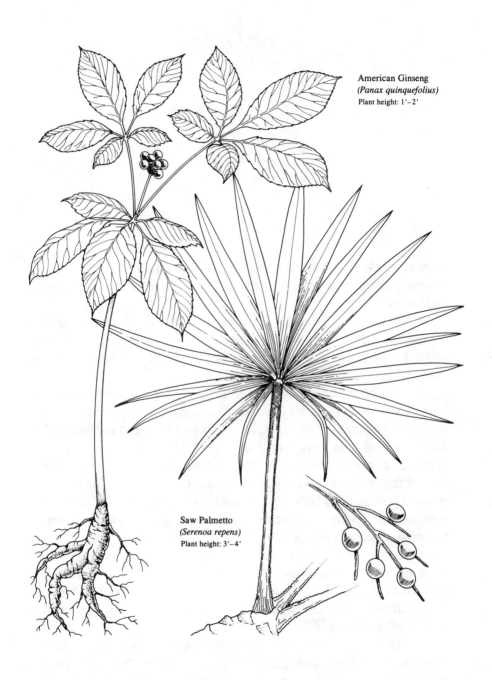

American Ginseng
(Panax quinquefolius)
Plant height: 1′–2′

Saw Palmetto
(Serenoa repens)
Plant height: 3′–4′

✄8✄

Specific Male Problems

Broken Hearts — the number one killer of males.

In order to stop breaking our male hearts we will have to start breaking our male rules.

The heart is an organ of receptivity and stress management. It is recommended by all systems of medicine to tune in regularly to the feelings and functions of the heart and take care of this strong but highly sensitive muscle.

The heart is the chamber of feelings; feelings for one's self and for other beings. There is some melancholy statistical evidence backing up a rumor that beginning at a certain age little boys are hugged and held 60% to 80% less than little girls. The exact age that this cultural phenomenon begins is of minor importance. The fact is, this cultural inheritance is unfortunate for the heart at any age. I think that little girls should be held as much as possible, and little boys should be held just as often. The fact that men act emotionally reserved and don't hug as spontaneously as women probably begins at some point in little-boy-hood when they no longer get hugged enough. Giving and receiving affection through the sensual medium of hugs communicates the feelings of the heart and ultimately nourishes this sensitive muscle.

Honor your tears, which are nectar of the heart; they can quench your emotional thirst.

These ambrosial secretions are harvested during moments of happiness and experiences of frustration, grief and pain. They are a healthy response to life's stimulations, helping us rid ourselves of the emotional and physical residues of stress. The human capacity to cry is universal, and this cathartic release is sanity enhancing. It has been theorized that suppressing tears may even increase one's susceptibility to illness. Certainly the necessary task of walling off one's emotions in order to suppress tears can be a contributing factor in hypertension and other complications of the heart. Except when chopping onions, men have been big boys and "not cried" for centuries now, and male cardiac-disease statistics show that this role-playing has taken its toll. Our current cultural prescription for "being a man about things" does not include in the formula permission to cry, even privately. So we'll have to muster the testosteronic organs to give ourselves this permission. Supportive male comrades can allow this of each other. When I see another man cry, my heart is often moved by his self-esteem and by this expression of his heart's power. We all know what it is like to be emotionally isolated, for manly appearance's sake. I feel that crying in times of critical stress, empathy, deep joy or grief is a sincere manly response.

Six Principles that Help Keep Your Heart Safe

1. Put your emotional life in balance.

Express your feelings, both the positive and the negative feelings, but especially express the caring ones. Feelings and expression of truthfulness, compassion, outrage, understanding, righteous anger, gentleness, forgiveness, love and joy are the songs of your life.

2. Laugh and play frequently (again).

Try to balance productive, creative ambition with relaxing, playful frivolity. Playing helps normalize the blood pressure and is equally as productive in life as is work. But, somehow (rumor has it, it was 16th century Rev. John Calvin's idea) a negative value got placed on play for adults, particularly male adults. In place of celebrating life with frequent vignettes of frivolity, we often use work as a socially sanctioned drug to avoid feeling and to avoid other pleasures of life.

It's time to change our culture's stuffy, self-denying definition of play from "the activities of childhood" to "the frequent spontaneous frivolity of the lifelong child in each of us." Dancing at noon is the surrender of one's pessimism. Let's shed some of our medieval adult armor and put some giggles back into our folklore. A moment of timely frivolity is looking into the somber face of chronic adult seriousness and saying, Gotcha! "Don't be silly," you say. "Why not?" I ask you. Because if you're having fun and smiling, you must not be working hard enough, right? The emphasis on work in our society is so great that most men define their "self" and unquestionably base their masculine self-concept on their work role, to the extent of often having a routine hand in polluting and despoiling their planet and local environment with the surly excuse that, "It's my job." I suggest that when one is truly having fun, be it at work or play, he is most closely in touch with his true self.

Playfulness and frivolity are attitudes that must courageously cut through social conventions to find their expression. Men, at the time of "falling in love" are allowed to play because they are allowed to be intoxicated with the new relationship. They can also play with their children, at least while their children are young. And of course sports allow men a modified form of play, but not usually a form that imaginatively reaches beyond the male-role confines and really gives a spritely, heart-touching unique experience in life. The following components of playfulness (as defined by a number of spirited psychology majors who, I assume, went out and had themselves a heck of a good time playing, then rushed back to the psych lab and light-heartedly wrote down everything they could remember about what they had just done) are ingredients that make the most powerful medicine for the heart:

Non-violence,
Non-competitiveness (admittedly a tough one),
Emotional and physical spontaneity,
Non-goal or task orientation,
Creativity,
De-emphasis on external control and evaluation,
Self-acceptance (that is not contingent on ones behavior or performance),
Joy,
Fun, Humor and Pleasure.
You remember: *Play.*

Beneath which stack of paperwork
lies concealed
our enchantment?
T. Elder Sachs

Laughter : Laughter is music of the heart. Like the fragrance of flowers, laughter dissolves anger, soothes anxiety, lightens depression and enriches all relationships. It is consistently the human being's best medicine.

Norman Cousins, author of the book *Anatomy of an Illness As Perceived by the Patient* which documents his return to health from a usually progressive, painfully crippling spinal disease called ankylosing spondylitis, described how daily doses of self-prescribed laughter facilitated his healing. Cousins reported in his best-selling book that just 20 minutes of hearty belly laughter (from doses of old Candid Camera and Marx Brothers clips) brought him two hours of pain-free sleep, with no unwanted side effects. Medical tests confirmed that after each laugh session his crippling inflammation subsided a little more. He described the physiological and psychological effects of laughing as "internal jogging," a form of sedentary aerobic exercise.

Studies on laughter designed by William F. Fry, a psychiatrist associated with Stanford University, have shown that laughing 100 times a day is equivalent to about 10 minutes of rowing or each hearty laugh is good for about 6 seconds of rowing. Laughter increases respiratory activity, oxygen exchange, muscular activity, and like aerobic exercise, it appears to stimulate the production of alertness hormones called catecholamines which in turn trigger the release of endorphins in the brain, and that these endorphins foster a sense of relaxation and well-being and dull the perception of pain. Catecholamines also enhance blood flow which can speed up the healing process and reduce inflammation. There is also some evidence that laughter enhances the immune response by reducing hormones that suppress immunity. This life is temporary, and it's even more temporary if you don't take good care of your heart, so don't be too serious, you miss all the fun.

3. Reject violence with your whole heart.

This is the only way we men can empty the jails and war-machines and erase the tiresome invented borders between our homes and countries. It nourishes one's heart to break the malodorous rules of how men are supposed to be, ultimately freeing our sons from the yoke of war and teaching them to be truly free men. We may even teach our countries how to live prosperously without requiring an enemy.

4. Exercise!

Exercise alone may be the most effective non-drug method for normalizing blood pressure. Exercise helps keep the excess fat pounds off, develops the muscle pounds and assists the heart by providing the rhythmic contraction and relaxation of the skeletal muscles which help circulate the blood and lymph. Keep in mind that each extra pound requires extra yardage of blood vessels which the heart has to service. Ten minutes of rowing is equal to 100 laughs. All men, particularly men 40 years and older, also need to stretch daily. It requires no equipment other than your flesh, bones and connective tissues and merely 15 to 20 minutes for a session. Systematic stretching feels good and keeps us supple. There are many books that discuss and illustrate stretching routines. One that I have often used to instruct me is *Yoga* by Richard L. Hittleman, Warner Books, N.Y., 1974. When my back hurts or begins to get stiff, I go to this book and renew my stretching practice. In a remarkably short time (5 or 6 days) my body is functioning much better, and I feel more integrated and grounded. Please see chapter titled, "Green's Hypotheses." Check hypothesis #3 for further propaganda promoting exercise as humankind's health panacea.

5. Eat simple, delicious, unadulterated foods and liquid.

Enjoy a health supporting diet that is based upon a variety of starches embellished by fruits and vegetables. An excellent resource that teaches a practical diet for promoting a healthy heart is the work of John A. McDougall, M.D. (see resource section in this book). Eat foods that supply high quality balanced fiber, foods like whole unadulterated grains (not merely the separated "bran"), nuts, seeds, vegetables and fruits. Select foods that are low in cholesterol and fat (both vegetable and animal fats). Avoid excess proteins, salt, simple sugars, additives and processed-refined foods. Develop a habit of drinking plenty of good pure water (avoid fluorine like you do no-see-ems). At parties, especially when you're dancing a lot, drink crystal clear cool water; it's a great beverage, particularly when sipped from a fashionable wine glass; try it next time. At work, set a glass pitcher full of water on your desk each morning and drink the contents throughout the work day. You can create a delightfully refreshing drink by adding a sprig of freshly picked Mint, Lemon Balm or Lemon Verbena to your pitcher of water.

6. Include the cardio-vascular nurturing herbs in your daily diet.

Our species has been eating and rubbing its skin against herbs since our primitive ancestors left the primal slough. The human heart recognizes and trusts these plant allies. Herbs that are specific foods for nourishing, strengthening and toning the heart muscle and its related blood vessels are: Hawthorn berries, blossoms and leaves (cardiac tonic and vascular tonic),

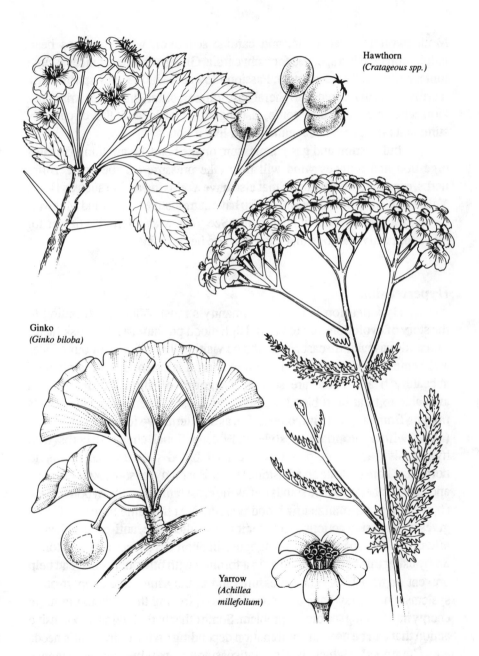

Hawthorn
(Cratageous spp.)

Ginko
(Ginko biloba)

Yarrow
(Achillea millefolium)

Motherwort (cardiac tonic, and cardiac sedative), which reduces heart palpitations and is a specific for tachycardia, Ginkgo (cardiac tonic, vascular tonic, peripheral vaso-dilator), Passion Flower (sedative, anti-spasmodic), Yarrow (vascular tonic, peripheral vaso-dilator, bitter, diuretic, astringent), Horsechestnut (vascular tonic, astringent), Garlic and the circulatory stimulants Ginger and Cayenne if you like it hot.

Indigestion and gas put pressure on the heart, so anything that aids digestion and reduces wind will help take pressure off the heart. Bitter herbs, especially those bitters that also have a relaxing action such as Hops, Valerian, Camomile (all of which also have carminative action) and Mugwort can play a specific role in heart care. (See "The Male Herbal" chapter for other supportive actions that each of these herbs offer.)

Hypertension

Hypertension is modern humanity's most salient contribution to the story of evolution (or creation). High blood pressure, a major risk factor for cardiovascular disease, seems to be visiting the majority of our offices and homes. Obviously, blood pressure control is essential for maintaining a healthy heart. There are several categories of allopathic medication available to treat high blood pressure, but most of them have side effects ranging from fatigue to impotence. So, as an alternative for male health care (along with appropriate lifestyle and occupational changes) herbs with hypotensive action help reduce elevated blood pressure, appearing to normalize both systolic and diastolic levels. For many reasons, both aesthetic and non-aesthetic, Garlic stands out as the most famous of the hypotensives. (It even helps normalize low blood pressure.) At the same time that Garlic gives hypotensive actions to its user it is also alterative, anti-catarrhal, anti-microbial, anti-spasmodic, cholagogue, diaphoretic, expectorant and tonic. So by using this herb as a food or in a formula with other herbs one can help prevent or treat high blood pressure, and at the same time support other systems which may have a minor weakness, freeing the body to put more energy into healing the bigger problem. Some other herbs having hypotensive action that can be used in combination depending on the individual's needs are: Crampbark (which is also antispasmodic, nervine and astringent); Yarrow (anti-microbial, astringent, bitter, diaphoretic and diuretic); Onion (anti-catarrhal, anti-microbial, diaphoretic, expectorant, hepatic, tonic and vulnerary); Hawthorn berries (cardiac tonic, digestive); Siberian ginseng (adaptogen) and Vervain (anti-spasmodic, cholagogue, diaphoretic, hepatic, laxative and nervine).

Other non-drug techniques to help keep the cardiovascular system strong and the blood pressure mellow are:

- Limiting sodium intake. Modern human beings eat up to 10 times more sodium than our primitive ancestors did. These relatives apparently didn't suffer from chronic hypertension. They also ate about 15 times more potassium than sodium. Today we eat far more sodium than potassium. A low sodium, high potassium diet seems to be the better way to eat. Fresh fruits and vegetables, Plantain, Dandelion and the sea vegetable, Kelp, are all high potassium foods.

- Keep all oils at a minimum in your diet, but especially eat less saturated fat. This does not mean that one should eliminate all saturated fats. Our ancestors ate meat, but it was wild meat and contained only about 5% fat which was predominantly unsaturated fat. Today's domesticated animals' meat contains about 25+% fat, most of it being saturated fat (along with the residue of growth hormones and antibiotics commonly fed to commercial livestock). The important thing to remember is to balance the intake of saturated fats with the intake of unsaturated fats. The body requires a balanced intake of both these fats to increase the efficiency of their metabolism. This can be facilitated by adding "unrefined" safflower, canola, sesame, sunflower, wheat germ, almond or peanut oil to your diet. These oils are all excellent sources of unsaturated fats. Ban margarine from the kitchen and dining room as a food impostor. Instead mix safflower, canola or sesame oil with butter and use this blend as a more balanced food, but eat even this only occasionally in small amounts. Be aware that lard, palm and palm kernel oils are extremely high in saturated fat content. Try putting sesame oil, chives and a little apple cider vinegar on your baked potato in place of butter. I've grown to like the taste of this combination, which I use 3 out of 4 times that I eat a baked potato. And it makes the 1 out of 4 times I use straight butter on my potato even better.

- Lose weight when necessary. Obesity (definition: presently weighing in at 20% over desirable weight) causes high blood pressure, elevated serum cholesterol and excessive secretion of insulin, which can lead to diabetes, which in turn can lead to impotence, depression and so on. Exercise and enjoy aerobic activity regularly, which in itself reduces blood pressure independent of dietary changes and weight loss.

- Limit alcohol. Alcohol consumption seems to be the most common cause of curable high blood pressure (and highway slaughter).
- Smoking and coffee. Throw away the cigarettes and once in a while have a nice hot cup of coffee. Neither coffee nor cigarettes seem to cause high blood pressure, but nicotine causes other pathogenic changes that lead to heart disease. We have to have something if we can't enjoy butter any longer, so a ritualistic cup of coffee (a touch of bitter) seems to be the lesser of all dietary evils, and it's the last legal high we have left. Coffee is a stimulating nervine, a good medicine for those who require this particular herbal action. However, if your nervous system is greedy for this relatively mild drug you will do well to also feed yourself some nervous system tonics, such as Wild Oat, Scullcap and St. John's Wort. This way you give your nervous system nutritional support while you push it with caffeine. Cut down on using sugar and cream in your coffee; develop an appreciation for its inherent bitter flavor. Bitter is one of coffee's most positive actions, but bitter flavor must be tasted (not hidden) to be effective.

Arteriosclerosis

Arteriosclerosis, alias hardening of the arteries, is not really a condition of the arterial tissue getting hard*, it is the "gunk" that has been laid down by one's lifestyle along the inner surfaces of the arteries that is hardening. Gunk is the vulgar word for the more scientifically sophisticated word, atheroma. Atheroma is a plaque, a combination of cholesterol and a lot of other greasy stuff that can be deposited anywhere in the body. Adrenal hormones that are secreted due to stress, but which are not appropriately

---

*Note: Arteries are formed as various layers of tissue. The initial hardening effect of these tissues is inspired by an individual's elevated blood pressure which sends the blood coursing through the arteries. This heightened rate of blood current eventually inflames and wounds the arterial tissue. Over these wounded areas atheroma plaque is laid down and ultimately hardens. To further deal with this inflammation the body eventually lays down a protective deposit of calcium, at which point one could say that the arteries, in fact, do harden.

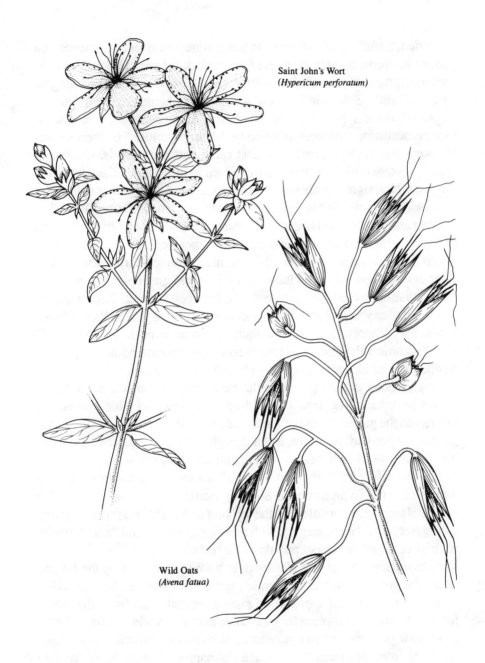

Saint John's Wort
(Hypericum perforatum)

Wild Oats
(Avena fatua)

expended, contribute significantly to this plaque formation. Sometimes you can see atheroma lying in the sclera (the white of the eye). It looks like little cream colored bumps on the inner corners of the eyes. In time atheroma gets hard and brittle. Sclerosis is a word which means hardening, thus "atherosclerosis" depicts hardening of atheroma. Atherosclerosis is a disease process occurring anywhere in the body. "Arteriosclerosis" is atherosclerosis occurring in the arteries, blocking these vascular tunnels. Obviously blood pressure is directly affected by reduction of the inner diameter of the arteries which significantly inhibits blood flow and by the loss of elasticity of these vessels which puts additional work load on the heart. The key to treating arteriosclerosis is, like with most degenerative conditions, diet and lifestyle. To summarize a lot of dietary data, meat, eggs, dairy, salt, excess oils, tobacco and alcohol are no-no's and high complex-carbohydrate, high fiber low fat diets which include lots of fruit and green plants along with adequate routine exercise (to help the body expend adrenal juices) are the yes-yes's. But you probably already know that. What you might not know is that the "phytosterols" that are abundant constituents in all green leafy plants significantly lessen cholesterol build-up in human bodies, supplying a sane form of balanced fiber as well. After exercise, regular eating of a variety of good quality greens is the best preventive medicine. When it comes to reducing cholesterol build-up by eating vegetable greens, the more wild the greens the better the action. Stinging Nettle is the king of the greens, the pot-herb of choice, and although it requires protective gloves to harvest this formidable herb, even the tiniest of tongues and most delicate of lips can safely enjoy the rich flavor of this tender-when-steamed wild-harvested herb. To prepare wild Stinging Nettle :

Harvest as a whole unit the top bud and first two leaves of young spring Nettles; fill a cooking pot with these fresh Nettles and then fill it with water; put the lid on the pot and slosh the herbs around; pour out the water and place the potful of wet Nettles over a low flame; replace the lid and steam the greens until they are tender. Eat the hot steamed Nettles with a wisp of forbidden butter or a good tasting vegetable oil (or both). Some folks add a touch of apple cider vinegar as one would with spinach greens, or sprinkle on some tamari soy sauce, and be sure to drink the Nettle juice left over from steaming. This annual culinary experience is Springtime herbalism at one of its finest moments.

Also include Garlic in your diet. Eating 3 cloves of Garlic a day will cut cholesterol build-up in half. It will also cut your social life to pieces. So you might want to either cook the garlic or marinate it to remove its obstinate odor. Cooking Garlic does not destroy its beneficial action for atheroma control. It does, however, kill Garlic's anti-microbial action. Marinating Garlic greatly reduces its non-social aroma but tends to leave its anti-microbial action intact. One method for making delicious marinated fresh Garlic is to combine:

> 1/2 cup of fresh peeled whole *Garlic* cloves
> 1/4 cup tamari soy sauce
> 1/4 cup raw honey
> 1/4 cup pure water

Put all ingredients together into a glass jar and cap it tightly. Place this in a refrigerator and let it age for at least one month. This will keep indefinitely. Eat the whole marinated cloves, at least three a day.

An equally delicious way to eat Garlic is to prepare it in fresh pesto. This adds to Garlic's actions the immune-enhancing actions of fresh Basil along with the nutrients of olive oil, and it is socially acceptable to eat lots of it with friends. To make fresh pesto combine:

> 1 and 1/2 cup of stripped, fresh Basil firmly packed
> (can substitute 1/2 cup of Nettles and/or Parsley for 1/2 cup
> of the Basil)
> 3 to 5 cloves of peeled Garlic
> 1/3 cup of extra virgin olive oil
> 1/4 teaspoon sea salt
> 1/3 cup shelled pine nuts
> 1/2 cup grated Romano or Parmesan cheese

Put all the above ingredients, except the olive oil, into a blender or food processor and blend until smooth paste is formed. Then with the machine running slowly, add the olive oil and blend. Makes about 1 cup of pesto. This is a flavor intense, high oil content food; eat it in moderation.

To herbally treat and/or help prevent arteriosclerosis there are four basic herbs to keep in mind whose actions have a great affinity for the cardio-vascular system—Hawthorn, Linden, Ginkgo and Yarrow. Formulating these four herbs to deal with hardening in the arteries, along with other appropriate herbs to deal with an individual's overall symptom picture, will prove to be of great value. Remember to treat the person, not merely the disease symptom.

In this situation Hawthorn is the cardiovascular tonic of choice. The action of the blossoms and berries of this plant tone the cardiac muscle and the arterial tissue, giving the circulatory system essential strength to help deal with this condition. Linden, also a cardiac and vascular tonic, is a specific for this condition. The flowers of this plant are vasodilators with nervine actions that relax the arterial walls, dilating the blood vessels, reducing the blood pressure by assisting a greater volume of blood flow. Ginkgo is another specific for treating this cardiovascular condition. It has tonic and peripheral vasodilating actions supporting those of the previously mentioned herbs. Yarrow is the fourth herb that enhances this basic formula. It is a mildly bitter, multi-talented herb, having an affinity for numerous body systems; in this case having a beneficial hypotensive, astringent and diuretic affect. Use these four herbs in combination as a basic formula:

Hawthorn berries and/or flowers	2 parts
Linden flowers	1 part
Ginkgo leaves	1 part
Yarrow flowers	1 part

Add additional plants to this basic formula to work more wholistically with the individual's full symptom picture (See "The Male Herbal"). Continue to alter the formula appropriately as this symptom picture changes.

Stress

Although stress is not specifically a male problem, it does run rampant in our gender. The word stress comes from the Latin *stringere* meaning, to bind tight. This is probably the ancestral word to our current descriptive terms, up tight and strung out. Stress is the response of our mind and body to any demand. Stress can be seen as an external or internal stimulus, or it can be seen as the body's and mind's response to some factor.

Closely observing the dynamic process of stress, a "General Adaptation Syndrome" has been theorized by a researcher named Hans Selye. In his work he has identified three phases to an individual's reaction to stress.

- The Alarm Phase wherein one experiences the initial adrenaline rush reaction.
- The Resistance Phase wherein the body recovers to a level superior to the pre-stress state. This includes adrenal, liver and nervous system responses.
- The Exhaustion Phase where eventually there can be a depletion and breakdown of any recovery that was demonstrated in the

Resistance Phase due to a continuation of exposure to the stressing factor(s). Initially the adrenal gland swells in response to deal with stress, then it exhausts after chronic stressful conflict.

An individual experiences both a physiological response and a psychological response. Physiologically there is nervous system activity and release of adrenaline/noradrenaline into the blood stream by the medulla of the adrenal glands. The body's response to these two hormones includes increase in heart rate and blood pressure; mobilization of liver based energy stores; and peripheral vaso-constriction which releases blood for required muscle use. This is basically the fight or flight response. Psychologically the fight or flight response is accompanied by emotions such as anxiety and/ or fear and the activation of coping mechanisms. In general there are two basic methods used to cope with stress: change or palliation. Either the relationship with the stressful environment is changed by escape, if possible, or by preparations made to soften the effects of an anticipated stressful event. This may include palliative strategies, such as denial and intellectualization that are used to soften the impact of stress once it has occurred. If the coping strategies succeed, the anxiety state tends to subside. If they fail, a wide range of psychological responses can result, such as withdrawal or depression, depending on the emotional bent of the individual. Of course each individual responds to a similar stress differently, for there are many factors affecting a person's response, such as previous experiences, information or lack of information regarding the issue, the individual's psychological and physiological differences, available social support systems and personal control.

Long term unabated stress tends to have a "grinding down" effect on an individual, usually culminating in illness of some form. Stress is often an occupational hazard especially in shift work, long hours, physically adverse conditions, boring and repetitive work or responsibility and deadline pressures (book manuscript deadlines for example).

Short Term Therapeutics for dealing with stress

Herbal therapeutics aimed at short term symptomatic alleviation of the impact of stress reduce symptoms in the body and help break distressing cycles.

Nervine relaxants, such as Black Cohosh, Cramp Bark, Camomile, Scullcap and Lavender help soften the physical reactions to the experience of anxiety. However if the individual is suffering physical anxiety due to the unexpended energy of adrenal secretions, physical exercise is the best medicine, and relaxants would be counter-productive.

Nervine hypnotics help induce deep healing sleep and have nothing to do with hypnotic trances or opiate drugs. Valerian, Passion Flower, Vervain and Hops are appropriately used when sleep is needed. Catnip, Lemon Balm, Camomile and Red Clover are particularly suited for children.

If there are accompanying physical digestive disturbances, such as colic, cramping or gas, these calmative, anti-spasmodic herbs have an affinity for both the digestive and the nervous system: Camomile, Lemon Balm, Peppermint, Wild Yam, Fennel, Marshmallow.

Cardiovascular implications call for tonics such as Hawthorn and Ginkgo along with anti-spasmodic and hypo-tensive nervines that have affinity with the circulatory system: Motherwort and Linden blossoms.

If there is breathlessness, this can spiral down into an asthma attack. To help alleviate respiratory symptoms that accompany stress anxiety, employ the action of pulmonary anti-spasmodic herbs such as Gumweed, Wild Cherry bark, Lobelia or Wild Lettuce.

If the skin responds with flushing or eczema, use a mixture of distilled Witch Hazel and Lavender essential oil for a topical application. Mix 10 drops of Lavender essential oil to 1 oz. of distilled Witch Hazel.

Therapeutics for dealing with long term stress

Therapeutics aimed at dealing with the long term "grinding down" effects of stress usually require at least two weeks or more to elicit relief. Ideally they help an individual cope with the stressful situation by helping to change the situation.

To tend to the psychological issues of long term anxiety, the use of nervine herbs such as Wild Oat, St. Johnswort, Vervain and Damiana are required. The criteria to use in selecting the most appropriate tonic herb will be the secondary actions of the herb that will most appropriately serve the individual. Wild Oat also has anti-depressant and vulnerary actions, St. Johnswort is anti-inflammatory and sedative, Vervain is anti-spasmodic and hepatic, while Damiana is urinary anti-septic and laxative.

If depression occurs as a symptom of long term stress, anti-depressant herbs like St. John's Wort, Damiana, Lavender, Lemon Balm can help break this cycle. The bitter herbs Mugwort and Vervain will stimulate internal vitality that can alleviate depression.

Usually the immune system is depressed by long term stress

reaction. Immune system tonics such as Astragalus, Echinacea, Pau d'Arco and Myrrh give strong support to this complex system. Use of the adaptogen herbs Siberian Ginseng, Ginseng, Licorice or Suma for supporting the adrenal glands as well as the overall immune system is extremely important for the stress adaptation and somatic rehabilitation process.

Non herbal, non medical therapies for alleviating the effects of stress are many, and all of them are most pleasant:

Massage, the therapeutic touch of human hands, is nearly an essential for reducing deep and surface body tension. It is also uniquely therapeutic for the mind and emotions. Once the members of our western cultures learn that sensuality is not the same as sexuality and that sensual therapies such as massage, hydro-therapy and exercise are essential for dealing with high stress lifestyles, legitimate therapeutic massage will thrive in the American and Canadian cultures. Meanwhile, the deeply relaxing touch of legitimate massage therapists can provide the primary preventive therapy for stress related illnesses. If a full body massage does not appeal to you at first, try a foot and hand massage. This experience in itself is a piece of heaven; then you can progress to back, neck and shoulder massage. Soon shyness and misinterpretation will dissolve along with stress and tension.

Meditation, probably the most efficient practice for promoting serene inner quiet and physical relaxation, is a simple discipline to develop. There are many teachers of this technique for stress reduction and many books available to introduce one to the power of meditation to facilitate spiritual and physical self-care.

Sharing troubles, asking for the family's ideas and help to deal with the stress of family management and financial matters works wonders in many ways. Expressing one's fears and apprehensions with immediate family members is not commonly considered the appropriate technique and strategy for male providers in family dynamics. Yet, asking for help and advice from family members during difficult times goes a long way to relieve stress and isolation, and at the same time, it allows the family members to experience a healthy intimate bond as a functioning unit. As a young boy, I would have been thrilled and honored if my dad had occasionally shared his fears and concerns with me and asked me for my opinions and help to pull the family through. This would have touched my heart deeply and would have been my coming of age ceremony as a young maturing male.

Stretching, Tai Chi and Yoga exercises help the body "let go" of residual tension. This gives the body's musculo-skeletal system increased extension and flexibility, allowing life to physically "feel better" and helping prevent injuries.

Aromatherapy full body baths employ the relaxing sensual aromas and herbal actions of pure plant essential oils with the soothing action of warm water. Add 2-3 drops each of Marjoram, Rosewood, Ylang Ylang and Sandalwood directly to your full bath of warm water. Agitate the water well to disperse the oils before entering the water. Then lie in the aromatherapy bath, soak for 20 minutes and feel stress seep out of your body systems. If, on the other hand, you might require a comfortable stimulating affect, use Rosemary, Geranium, Clary Sage and Lemon essential oils.

Gardening heals the gardener and the environment as it weeds the human Spirit of mental and emotional anxieties. I have on my desk a Lila Productions greeting card designed by Amie Hill which says, "We come from the earth, we return to the earth, and in between we garden." This is probably the most wholistic herbal formula offered in this book. Gardening literally puts one back in touch with Mother Earth, and touching her body attentively helps heal our troubles and wounds. Even city gardening in clay pots and planter boxes provides anti-stress herbal medicine. It is important to grasp the full scope of gardening, and to comprehend the re-connection to a balanced life that gardening can offer us. To help reduce stress, one needs to evolve this plot to a stress-reducing garden of peace and tranquility. One needs to avoid turning his garden into a theatre of war. Weeds and wild animals are companions on this planet. They live and eat with us, not against us, so peaceful stress-healing gardening needs to flow compassionately with the whole planetary-family unit. Poisoning "weeds" and kill-trapping or shooting animal "invaders" will neither relax us nor enhance the spirit of the garden. There are ecologically compassionate methods to manage a garden, and this peaceful experience and management of a garden reduces stress, reconnects us to Earth and honors life. Gardening is a means to whatever end one chooses, if one keeps focused on the desired goal. May we bring flowers forever to our friends.

Sensuality is a primary method for reducing stress by employing the abundant free therapies of nature. I have discussed the virtues of massage by human hands. But massage only works for one who will *receive* the touching, and often this intimate human connection is difficult for some folks. Taking your shoes and socks off and shuffling around barefoot in grass (especially dewy grass at night — when you can't fall asleep), running along the seashore in the wet sand or walking on smooth warm pebble stone renders sensual touch to the feet that is equally therapeutic and stress reducing. Removing your clothes and allowing the warm sunlit air to touch your skin, letting the cooling breeze blow through your hair or soaking in warm healing waters or warm beach sand are sensual experiences that relax and nourish the conscious inner being. Smelling the exotic aromas of forests, deserts and wetlands, hearing the musical sounds of wildlife and running streams and seeing the profound beauty of Earth's diverse and abundant natural wonders reminds us of why we are here on this charming and exotic little planet and how we can change some things to enjoy our life more fully. Surrounded by the habitual distractions and sedentary comforts of common electronic and mechanical technology, we simply forget about freedom and the free healing of being sensually in touch with raw nature.

> In order to design a more perfect car,
> I took off my shoes
> and went for a walk.
>
> T. Elder Sachs

Also keep in mind the frequent experience of internal sensuality. One of the most important attributes of experiencing love, humor and laughter is that IT FEELS SO GOOD.

Ulcers

In time, prolonged stress will have a marked impact on the stomach and small intestines, causing a breakdown in the linings of these organs. The protective mucous membranes lose their ability to deal with the emotional and dietary stress placed on them, the acids and digestive enzymes of the organs reach the organ walls and painful gastric or duodenal ulcers can develop. Herbs can readily heal these conditions, but the ulcers can quickly return if the stressful environment that has set up the symptoms is not altered.

Although conditions leading to gastric ulcers are a little different from those that manifest duodenal ulcers, the treatment is similar for both kinds. It is important to observe a low fiber diet during the acute phase of the illness. Reduce the intake of protein foods because these foods are the most difficult for the stomach to process. Temporarily reducing dietary proteins will give the stomach less work, so it can heal and repair itself. Once the symptoms are reduced, fiber foods and a variety of proteins can be slowly reintroduced into the diet. Avoidance of alcohol and nicotine is important. Also avoid the general use of bitters during the acute phase as these stimulate the secretion of stomach juices. After the healing has commenced the use of bitters is appropriate. The bitter action will then act to strengthen the linings, invigorate and promote healing of the stomach and intestines.

Along with appropriate diet and systematic reduction of stress, the actions of herbal remedies can quickly soothe, heal and renew the intestinal linings. Demulcent herbs such as Marshmallow root, Comfrey root and Slippery Elm bark are used to soothe the ulcer and the inflamed tissue surrounding it. The vulnerary action of these same herbs provides a strong healing effect to inflamed surfaces. A Slippery Elm gruel (or Slippery Elm tablets) is a soothing, strengthening food to introduce at this point. It supplies welcome, pain relieving, demulcent action to the ulcerated stomach and duodenal walls, and it is an easily digested, highly nutritious food. To prepare this gruel, simply mix 1-1/2 to 2 rounded teaspoons Slippery Elm powder in 1 cup cold water and let this soak several hours or over night. A little maple syrup can be added to give flavor. Drink 1 to 3 cups a day. Another method for preparing Slippery Elm gruel is given in Dr. John R. Christoper's classic herbal, *School of Natural Healing*. He makes a smooth paste of 1-1/2 teaspoons full of Slippery Elm powder with 1 full teaspoon of raw honey; brings 1 cup of raw milk to a boil and stirs in the Slippery Elm mixture as the milk reaches the boiling point. Remove this from the heat and stir 5 to 10 seconds. Drink 1/2 to 1 cup 3 times a day.

The specific mucous membrane healing properties of Golden Seal are always called on for these conditions. It also provides general tonic action for the entire body. Astringent action of Agrimony, American Cranesbill, Bayberry or Meadowsweet is used to strengthen the tissue and to help stop any bleeding that may be occurring in the stomach. Meadowsweet also settles the stomach and reduces the impact of overacidity. The carminative and nervine action of Hops, Valerian or Chamomile will aid digestion and help calm stress and nervousness. To safeguard against any infection that may be lurking due to a debilitated immune system or low vitality, the alterative and lymphatic actions of Echinacea are most reliable. So good herbal therapy for treating intestinal ulcers can consist of the following two basic formulas:

Formula #1

Marshmallow root	2 parts

Comfrey root	1 part

The cold infusion of these demulcent herbs is much more mucilaginous and soothing than a tea or tincture. (See Technology of Independence chapter for preparing cold infusions.) Drink 1 cup 3 times a day.

Formula #2

Golden Seal	1 part
Plantain	1 part
American Cranesbill	1 part
Echinacea	2 parts
Chamomile	1 part
Meadowsweet	1 part

Prepare these herbs as a tea and drink 1 cup 3 times a day before meals, or take 15 to 40 drops of a mixture of the combined tinctures (in hot water to evaporate the alcohol) 3 times a day before meals.

In conjunction with these herbs drink a 4 oz. serving of pure Aloe vera juice or Cabbage juice 3 times a day. Their actions are soothing and healing to the stomach and intestines.

These herbs will heal the ulcer, but one must take note of the signals the body is giving. An ulcer is an intense sign of self neglect. It is essential at this point to re-examine one's goals and purpose and immediately alter one's lifestyle. There are many valuable techniques to help do this.

For further information on stress control and herbal therapeutics please read the book, *Successful Stress Control* written by David Hoffmann, Inner Traditions, Vermont, 1987. It is an excellent wholistic resource.

The Prostate – chronic trouble maker for males

It is said that "men push their worries into their prostate," our uniquely male chamber of silence where we store our most private concerns. What is a prostate (often called "the male gland")? Where is it, and why is it there? How can it be taken care of? Few people can answer these questions. Few men ever ask them until they become painful questions. And yet, a majority of men have trouble with their prostate gland sometime in their lives.

The prostate gland is a chestnut shaped organ, partly muscular and partly glandular, having basically an outer and an inner mass of prostatic tissue. The normal prostate is a little over 1-1/2 inch (4 cm) wide and about as long, approximately the size of a walnut. It sits just below the bladder, next to the rectum and surrounds the urethra (the urinary exit tube) in the male genito-urinary system. It is undeniably a most mysterious gland. The prostate is an endocrine-dependent organ; however, knowledge of its endocrine relationship remains a blur to science. Castration or the withdrawal of male sex hormones (androgens) produces atrophy of the gland. The administration of androgens following castration delays the development of atrophy, but administration of estrogen, the female sex hormone, also delays atrophy of the prostate. No satisfactory explanations have come forth to explain this phenomenon of opposing hormonal influences exerting a similar effect on the male gland. One interesting theory, reported in a pathology text book written by Stanley L. Robbins, M.D., suggests that the outer mass or zone of prostatic tissue is the "male prostate" and is responsive to androgens, whereas the inner zone is a "female prostate" responsive to estrogens. Based on this view of the prostate it might be more understandable why it is that the development of abnormal enlargement of the prostate in older males usually arises in the inner mass which appears to respond to the decrease in androgen secretion and the relative increase in estrogen levels. However, adding to the general confusion surrounding the whys and wherefores of the prostate, there are other medical theorists who suggest that it is the work of excess testosterone build-up in the prostate that stimulates prostatic enlargement in a man's later years. I'll discuss that theory a little more in the following section.

The most obvious function of the prostate gland is to secrete a milky protein fluid which is discharged into the urethra at the time of the emission of semen. This prostatic fluid mixes with the semen during ejaculation helping to transport sperm out of the body. Prior to puberty the prostate gland does not secrete any fluid. Beginning at puberty prostate secretion is continuous, and even during periods of sexual inactivity a small amount of prostatic fluid is deposited into the urethra daily and passes with the urine. If, for whatever reason, the prostate enlarges or inflames and swells, the urethra running through a hole in the prostate is pinched off, like pinching a drinking straw, which obstructs the flow of urine causing the urine to stagnate, back up and distend the bladder. If the urine further backs up into the kidneys it can cause renal damage. These are a lot of potential problems due to an organ that appears to perform such a relatively minor function. It must have a subtle covert function that our sciences haven't as yet detected . . . And there must be more compassionate therapies than the common reaming out with steel devices.

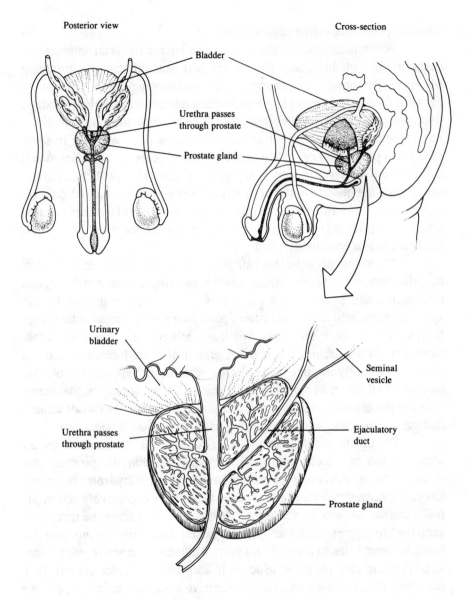

Posterior view

Cross-section

Bladder

Urethra passes
through prostate

Prostate gland

Urinary
bladder

Seminal
vesicle

Urethra passes
through prostate

Ejaculatory
duct

Prostate gland

The Prostate Gland

Benign prostatic enlargement (BHP)

A common problem that affects men later in life is an enlargement (hypertrophy) of this gland that causes pain and difficulty in urinating (dysuria). This condition, occurring in approximately 50% to 60% of men between the ages of 40 and 59 years, is often referred to as benign prostatic hyperplasia (BPH); hyper = excessive, and plasia = formation. The condition has a tendency to be progressive; however, this is not always so. In some men it can progress very slowly over a period of years, and in other men it can progress slowly and stop at any point. Further clinical befuddlement arises from the observation that in some cases a greatly enlarged prostate causes hardly any trouble and in other cases a slight enlargement causes great discomfort and difficulty in urination. Genetics and lifestyle are most likely the major contributing factors.

There appears to be three stages of prostatic enlargement. The first stage is characterized by the stream of urine growing thinner and the urge to urinate increasing. Some men will notice that it takes more time for the sphincter muscle to relax and urine to pass. Many men remain at this stage for the rest of their lives, and this stage is very responsive to herbal treatment. In the second stage, the retention of urine increases, and the bladder never fully empties. The urine that remains in the bladder is referred to as residual urine. In stage three the residual urine increases, stagnates, distends the bladder creating back pressure and eventually causes kidney damage and uremia. At this stage surgical intervention is necessary.

Prominent medical theory suggests that BHP is caused by an accumulation of testosterone in the prostate. Within the prostate this testosterone is converted to a compound called dihydrotestosterone. Dihydrotestosterone in turn causes cells to multiply excessively and eventually causes the prostate to enlarge. Testosterone is a hormone that helps keep healthy aggression intact. When a male retires from his professional work, he often loses an arena for his normal constructive active aggression, so he needs to keep his lifestyle active to keep from being too retired. This may help him avoid accumulating excessive testosterone in the prostate gland.

The following story about the prostatic-herbal adventures of a normal healthy man was given to me by herbal educator and author, Kathi Keville. "Peter had a typical case of enlarged prostate which the doctors classified as 'normal' for his 55 years. An active man, he also noticed a slight decrease in energy and a new tendency for occasional cold or flu. He began taking a combination of Saw Palmetto berry, Sarsaparilla, Siberian Ginseng, Marshmallow root and Echinacea extracts. He used 15 drops twice a day. Six weeks later he went for a check-up. Not only was his prostate almost normal, but his doctor sensed a renewed "vigor". In six months, the prostate was normal. Peter continued taking the herbal combination, 15 drops once a day, but after eight months he began experiencing symptoms again. He increased his dose back to the 30 drops and symptoms again disappeared. During the course of treatment Peter developed a urinary tract infection, so he took a course of Oregon Grape root, 10 drops 3 times a day, along with his regular combination. The infection was rid of in four days." Kathi has found that Oregon Grape often works as an excellent substitute for Golden Seal in treating genito-urinary infections. In other cases where there is abnormal prostate growth, an addition of Chaparral has proved very effective.

Prostititis

Prostitis is inflammation or infection of the prostate gland. This can in turn inflame the prostatic urethra and ultimately the bladder. This completed scenario is referred to in the university-trained doctor's language as prostatocystitis.

The common symptoms of an inflamed, infected and/or an enlarged prostate gland are similar: There is an aching pain in the area of the prostate; pain on sitting; frequent dribbling; urination can be difficult with difficulty starting stream and difficulty emptying the bladder; sometimes blood will appear in the urine and often there are chills and fever. Causes often boil down to stress (usually, but not only, sexual stress), excesses in diet (especially excess consumption of alcohol and caffeine products), lack of regular physical exercise and as a secondary infection caused by another infection such as tooth abscess, venereal disease, etc. If prostate infection is the result of another infection, of course the primary infection must be attended to concurrently and the immune system bolstered.

In addition to using appropriate herbal and nutritional therapy, congestion of an enlarged prostate can be relieved by the use of a firm seat on chairs and by avoiding cold, dampness, long rides in automobiles, trains, etc., hard bicycle seats, alcohol (especially heavy beer drinking because of sheer volume and delay in urinating), caffeine, cooked hot spices which appear to irritate the prostatic urethra, and sexual excesses. The call to urinate must be acted on immediately for the bladder must never be permitted to be overdistended. Intentional urination every couple of hours may avert overdistention of the bladder. Extreme difficulty in urination may be relieved by sitting down in a tub of warm water to urinate. A drink of water several times through the day produces dilute urine that helps flush the bladder outlet. Drinking lots of water throughout the day is good for the heart, the genito-urinary organs, the skin and all the other body tissues as well.

An insight shared with me by Roy Upton, an herbalist skilled in Traditional Chinese Medicine, points out that retention of urine due to not responding to "the number one call of nature" reduces the tone of the genito-urinary organs including the male prostate gland, eventually leading to problems such as urinary incontinence, premature ejaculation and increased susceptibility to urinary tract infection. This is an atonic habit, the action of which is somewhat like blowing up a balloon too large, stretching and weakening the walls. Young children should be trained and supported to respond immediately to the call to pass water (as well as immediate attention to bowel movements). They should not be required to "hold it" until a parent or classroom teacher says "okay, go" at his or her leisure.

Non-medical/non-surgical treatment of these prostate problems requires focus and perseverance. Natural healing takes longer, but it is well worth the time and self-commitment. Keep in mind that as you treat these symptoms systemically using herbs, diet and exercise, you are at the same time nourishing and normalizing your entire physical body. Modern allopathic medicine and surgery tend to the symptom, not to the deficiencies or excesses that caused it. Each man experiencing a prostate problem must make his own decision as to how he wants to treat and care for the condition.

Suggested herbal/nutritional treatment of prostate conditions goes as follows:

1. Relax. Relevant evidence has been acquired by Dr. Ira Sharlip professor of urology at the University of California at San Francisco demonstrating that relaxing the body's muscles is the core of a successful method of treatment for chronic nonbacterial prostatitis. Dr. Sharlip points out that an abnormal increase in the tone of the urethral sphincter muscles due to stress is one cause of male prostate dilemma. The urethral sphincter muscles are those that we use to close off the flow of urine. Learning stress management techniques, enjoyable exercise, pulling worry back out of the prostate and, if necessary, using herbs like Valerian, Crampbark and Scullcap that help relax muscles, assist the successful employment of this technique.

2. Drink lots of pure water. Avoid drinking cold beer.

3. Eat lightly. Eat a diet which is substantial in whole grains, steamed vegetables, fresh fruits, miso based soups and sea vegetables such as kelp, nori, hiziki etc. This diet provides your body with a variety of foods that are relatively easy to digest, so it can tap into a wide range of vitamins, minerals and other essential nutrients to revitalize and heal the prostate.

4. Seeds are a most valuable food for developing prostate health. Throughout the day chew up to 1/2 cup of pumpkin seeds (*Cucurbita pepo*). Pumpkin seeds are a natural mucilaginous source of zinc and linoleic acid (vitamin F). This is important for respiration of internal organs and to help decongest the prostate gland and lessen residual urine. Other important seed foods for males are poppy seeds (best eaten as whole grain poppy seed cake), sunflower seeds and sesame seeds. These are easily added to your diet as a sunflower seed butter (spread) or sesame seed butter. Be sure these seeds and seed butters are fresh when you buy them and keep them refrigerated, so their oils do not turn rancid.

5. Supplement your diet daily with vitamin and mineral supplements: 800 I.U. of vitamin E (mixed tocopherols), a calcium/magnesium supplement 400-600 mg., zinc picolinate or amino chelated zinc 20-50 mg.

6. Apply hot and cold packs to the prostate area. This is the area between the scrotum and the anus. Crushed ice wrapped in a face towel makes a simple ice pack. Apply the hot to cold in a ratio of 4:1 (i.e. Apply the hot pack for 4 to 8 minutes, then follow this immediately with the cold pack for 1 to 2 minutes). Do this routine 2 to 3 times a session, two sessions a day, or as often as you wish. This technique does a remarkable job of reducing inflammation (not just on the prostate, but anywhere on the body where inflammation is experienced), and it gives blessed relief. Take the time and trouble to do it for yourself.

7. Herb teas and tinctures can provide soothing demulcent action to an inflamed and/or swollen prostate. At the same time they can be highly nourishing and toning to the whole male system, bringing circulation to the genital area and providing effective cleansing and anti-microbial action. As exemplified by the following formulas, the strategy to consider when tending to the symptoms of an enlarged prostate should include the following herbal actions:

- Male reproductive system and prostate tonics: Saw Palmetto, Siberian Ginseng, Suma.
- Genito-urinary system tonics and astringents to strengthen and

heal the overall system. Choose tonic/astringent herbs that also give anti-microbial and vulnerary actions: Yarrow, Horsetail, also Buchu, Dandelion.

• Diuretics to prevent excess build-up of urine in the bladder due to an enlarged prostate, to prevent potential back-up of urine into the kidneys and to support preventive measures: Hydrangea, Couch Grass, Cleaver, Cornsilk, Watermellon seed, also Pipsis-sewa.

• Immune system enhancers that help the body's defense system build resistance: Echinacea, Astragalus, Siberian ginseng,

• Urinary system anti-microbials are used even when there is no obvious symptoms of infection. This helps insure that no infection stresses the urinary tract: Oregan Grape, Echinacea, Uva Ursi, Couch Grass, Saw Palmetto, also Pipsissewa.

• Demulcents to soothe and protect the urinary system: Couch Grass, Corn Silk, Marshmallow, also Comfrey.

Each day brew and drink alternately a total of 2 cups each of the following 2 herb tea formulas:

An infusion (steeped tea) of

Cornsilk	1 part (diuretic/demulcent)
Couchgrass	1 part (very soothing demulcent/ astringent/diuretic)
Organic watermelon seeds	1 part (soothing anti-inflammatory diuretic)

A decoction (simmered tea) of

Echinacea	3 parts (immune enhancer/anti-microbial)
Saw Palmetto*	3 parts (prostate tonic/ nutrient)
Marshmallow Root	1 part (promotes tissue healing)
Uva Ursi	1 part (urinary antiseptic/astringent)
Horsetail	1 part (astringent/specific for benign prostate enlargement)

---

* Many people find that Saw Palmetto berries taste disagreeable. I surely do. So if you prefer, take Saw Palmetto as a tincture (25-40 drops) with each of the two cups of the decoction. Placing the tincture in a glass with a little water and a 1/4 teaspoon of vitamin C powder renders the Saw Palmetto flavor much more agreeable due to the sourness of the vitamin C.

Hydrangea Rt.   1 part (gravel solvent-antilithic/astringent)

Often, during the times of prostatic complaints, a man's vital energy is also depressed due to accompanying digestive and/or circulatory deficiencies. If these problems are part of the symptom picture, include Hawthorn berries and Yarrow in the above formulas. These plants have therapeutic actions and affinities for both the circulatory and digestive systems.

If the individual can't seem to get on top of the prostate and urinary tract symptoms, he most likely requires some deep immune system nourishment and some adaptogenic stress handling assistance. In this case use immune system enhancing herbs such as Astragalus, Siberian ginseng, Echinacea and Suma with the nutritional, sexual organ tonic herbs Saw Palmetto and Damiana.

If infection is suspected in the prostate gland or in the genito-urinary system (characterized by a burning pain when passing water as well as pain in the groin area before, during and after urination*) combine Saw Palmetto with Oregon Grape and Echinacea (add Fennel to improve the flavor). Take 2 to 3 cups of this combination as a tea or take 25 to 40 drops of the combined tinctures 3 to 4 times a day.

Currently, German phytotherapists are recommending the use of suppositories inserted rectally for treating irritated or inflamed prostate. They are observing excellent results. The formula used is equal parts of Saw Palmetto berry and Echinacea root. They recommend inserting the suppository before going to bed. (See the chapter, Technology of Independence, for instructions on how to prepare herbal suppositories.)

8. Last, but definitely not least, exercise your pubococcygeal (PC) muscle regularly. This is best done by learning the Kegel Exercises, a private workout routine.

Kegel Exercises

A well developed pubococcygeal muscle is essential for male and female sexual health. This muscle runs between the pubic bone in front and the coccyx (tailbone) in the back. To locate this muscle work up a good flow of urine and while the flow is full close it off. The muscle you automatically

---

* Note: Excessive use of Mustard, Horseradish and other sharp-tasting culinary herbs can cause irritable burning sensation in the penis during urination. Acute episodes may resemble the bladder discomfort of infectious cystitis.

tighten is the pubococcygeal muscle. Muscles grow strong with exercise and become flaccid without it. This muscle needs to be well developed to maintain sexual control and keep the prostate supple. As the muscle is exercised, a greater flow of blood services the genitals and the supporting organs. As the muscle grows stronger, erections come more easily, sexual endurance is increased and the prostate gland is strengthened and toned.

Back in the '40s a gynecologist named Arnold Kegel developed an exercise program to help women who had problems with bladder control. It was soon discovered that these exercises not only created good pelvic health facilitating control of bowels and bladder, but they also helped develop and nourish the entire genital system, in men as well as women. Routine performance of Kegel exercises is one of the finest techniques for increasing reproductive organ health, sexual performance and pleasure.

A man or a woman can do Kegel exercises anytime, anywhere, while standing in a long line waiting to get seats in an overrated movie, while waiting for teenagers to get out of the bathroom, while stuck in traffic or when just hanging out reading comics. Probably the best time to do Kegel routines is while lying in bed, just before or just after sleep. Lying still, you can comfortably concentrate, visualize and experience the entire set of genital apparatus being exercised. You can feel Kegel exercises reach right down and touch the prostate, bringing invigorating massage and circulation to the often stagnant terrain lying in the mature male gland, tilling the prostatic soil so the actions of the therapeutic foods and herbal formulas can more easily take root and nurture the male gland. Think of this as "genital jogging" without the need to buy a lot of expensive equipment (well, maybe a walkman). Pardon me for going on and on about this, but I want to get your attention here. This is probably the single most important, simple, self-healing action you can provide for your prostate, your fertility and your sexual potency.

There are three parts to these exercises:

- *Slow clenching* of the PC muscle. You squeeze and clench the PC like you do when stopping urine. Hold it clenched for a slow count to three, then relax.
- *Rapid clenching.* Repeatedly clench and relax the PC as rapidly as you can.
- *Pushing out.* Bear down with moderate pressure as if forcing urine or a bowel movement. This uses a number of abdominal muscles along with the PC.

Like any muscle, the PC tires quickest when weak. Begin with a small number of repetitions then gradually build up the count. Quit before tiring the PC, but give it some good daily exercise. At first you might find that you cannot keep your PC tightly clenched during the Slow Clenches or you cannot do the Rapid Clenches very smoothly. This is because the PC is weak; you've gotten to it just in time. It might be best for some individuals to scatter the exercises throughout the day rather than doing them all at once. Begin conditioning your PC muscle by doing 10 Slow Clenches, 10 Rapid Clenches and 10 Pushing Outs. Consider this to be 1 set of exercises, and do 5 sets every day for the first week. In the second week increase each set to 15 Slow, 15 Rapid and 15 Pushes, and continue to do 5 sets a day. Continue increasing each set by 5 of each exercise until a set includes 30 of each exercise. Then continue to do at least 5 sets a day each day to maintain muscle tone and prostate massage. You will experience healthy changes quite soon.

I recommend two books that discuss these and other exercises in detail: *ESO, Extended Sexual Orgasm*. Alan Brauer and Donna Brauer, Warner Books, N.Y. *Taoist Secrets of Love; Cultivating Male Sexual Energy*. Mantak Chia, Aurora Press, N.Y.

Malignant prostatic enlargement

Prostate cancer in men is very similar to breast cancer in women. Both of these cancers are best prevented with a low-fat, high carbohydrate, high fiber diet. Adopting this diet is essential for assisting any form of treatment. There exists basically two biological forms of prostatic cancer: a "localized form" which is the most common form and consists of a small incidental lesion, and an "advanced form" which is a much less frequent form that may metastasize and cause terminal harm. It has been assumed by the allopathic medical profession, without significant proof, that the localized form will inevitably become a clinically significant lesion. If prostate cancer is diagnosed, keep in mind that this is a slow-growing cancer. Qualified help is essential and the coordinated assistance of a variety of healers may be required to help you manifest remission as the initial step of a continued self-healing. With the wide variation in the inherent growth potential of tumors, many of the small localized lesions may have persisted for some time and may continue to persist as such for years. Treatment by radical prostate surgery is as ineffective as mastectomy is in breast cancer surgery. Each person is unique and must be treated individually. Consider treating a malignant prostate condition wholistically with diet, herbs, attention to psychological factors, strong emphasis on building and maintaining general health and a strong immune system, use of alternative health-care sciences and lifestyle changes before panicking and immediately resorting to allopathic heroic techniques of surgery and radiation therapy. To my knowledge the medical profession has no studies to refer to in treating this form of cancer systemically and nutritionally. They only have studies which compare radiation treatment with chemotherapy and surgical treatment. Locate a trained herbalist, Oriental Medicine practitioner or other natural therapy practitioners and get a second, third and fourth opinion on treatment. Use your time wisely, positively and calmly. You have time, you have available help and you have your powerful human potential to heal this condition.

Aromatherapy treatment for inflamed prostate

It is helpful to apply herbs and essential oils directly on the inflamed prostate area. One way to get herbs to the prostate is by means of an herbal rectal implant or enema (I know, I know, but it beats a urologist's finger any day). This remedy is simple to prepare and is an excellent remedy for inflamed prostate and/or piles. To prepare this herbal implant, boil (for 10 minutes) 2 ounces of ground Flaxseed in a quart of distilled water. Strain, cool this mixture to the degree that you can comfortably leave your finger in it for ten seconds, and squeeze out all the mucilage and oil. To this mucilaginous, oily liquid add 1/4 teaspoon of Lavender aromatherapy grade, pure, steam distilled essential oil (never use synthetic essential oils, for you will not get the medicinal actions that you want). Place in a tightly closed container and shake these together vigorously. Always be sure to shake this mixture well before using. Employing the use of a small rubber bulb (baby syringe), lie down on your side and inject anywhere from a teacup to a pint of this decoction into the rectum. Retain the herbal implant as long as possible. Repeat 2 to 3 times a day. Refrigerate and keep the remaining unused mixture tightly capped to prevent loss of the Lavender essential (volatile) oil. Warm the mixture before using. Use this preparation within 72 hours.

The following anti-inflammatory aromatherapy grade essential oils can give pleasant relief from the stress of prostate inflammation (and the inflammation and swelling of hernias). Use a 5% dilution of aromatherapy grade essential oils of Blue Camomile, Lavender and/or *Eucalyptus polybractea.* To make a 5% dilution mix 50 drops total of any one or a combination of these essential oils in 50 ml (Approximately 2 ounces) of any good quality fixed oil such as hazelnut, almond, wheat germ or olive oil. Rub this oil on the perineum (the area between the anus and the scrotum) as well as on the lower back and the lower abdomen. Repeat this 3 to 4 times a day. These essential oils provide soothing, anti-inflammatory, nervine and anti-microbial actions to the lower body. Essential oils penetrate the skin within minutes and are an excellent medium for getting plant nutrients to inflamed internal organs (see section on Aromatherapy).

The frequent use of alcohol, nicotine, caffeine and white sugar retards the action of these medicines and further irritates the organs.

One more thing

A concluding note of interest before we leave the area of the prostate gland is a theory regarding a potential contributor to chronic prostate enlargement. This has to do with the effects of a lifelong process of unexpressed or frequently unresolved arousal; titillation overload, so to speak. It is felt by certain practitioners, based on evidence gathered through observation and consultation with male patients, that this culture's popular involvement in the reading and viewing of sexually arousing materials along with passive participation as viewers of glossy magazine photos, billboard and common media imagery and strip-show-like erotic entertainment, etc., creates unreleased sexual energy in the male sexual organs, which over time can cause problems. Most high school male youths have appropriately descriptive terms ("lover's nuts," "blue balls") for the downright uncomfortable results of sexual arousal that are taken home on Friday and Saturday nights after an evening of promising and passionate, but disappointingly unconsummated foreplay with their lovers (An empathetic and compassionate note to you gentlemen: After taking the lady home, grab your car bumper (or other relatively immovable object) with both hands, and, using your leg muscles (not your back muscles) attempt to lift the car 3 consecutive times, relaxing about 5 seconds between lifts. This exercise spends residual frustration and opens the venous flow. Engorged blood will circulate back into the pelvis, and genital discomfort will disappear like a fading fantasy. Certainly a few weekends of high school or college campus sexual frustration won't hurt you (makes a man out of you, right?); however, a lifelong input of various forms of unmoved arousal does appear to have an effect on the prostate gland which ultimately reacts by expansion and consequent inflammation. It appears that regularly moving out this stimulated energy is necessary to help prevent enlarged, inflamed prostate. Warm, fulfilling sexual relationships are high on the list of preferred methods to accomplish this, but if no relationship is happening, masturbation (lonely as it can be) is also on the list of preventive measures.

Chinese medicine places great value in retaining sperm and seminal fluid or at least expending it in moderation. This oriental system of health-care often recommends non-ejaculatory sex. This technique is suggested in the context of maintaining balance between the intake and outflow of energy and body nutrients. Generating sperm requires large amounts of nutrients and vital energy. For the sake of male health and vitality this unique male commodity should not be casually dispensed. According to Traditional Chinese Medicine (TCM) sperm is the physical manifestation of "jing." Jing is translated to be "essence." To understand jing deeply is to understand that principal which imbues the body with a true sense of being alive. This is more easily explained by describing the experiences of embodying adequate jing. When there is abundant jing the individual's energy is exuberant, the hair is luxurious, the eyes sparkle and glisten, there is spring in the person's gait and all the senses are sharp, and a long and healthy life ensues. The major causes of jing depletion are "overwork" and excessive "ejaculatory sex."

Time between ejaculations must be taken into account so that the body can take in the appropriate nutrients to reproduce the ejected sperm and seminal fluid (maintain jing). Age is a factor in determining how much time is required to efficiently replace these nutrients. It is recommended that a man take his present age and multiply it by two-tenths (.2) to efficiently determine how many days to let pass between ejaculations (a 30 year old man would best space his ejaculations a minimum of 6 days apart [30 X .2 = 6]). According to this Chinese system of male health-care, if sexual relations make themselves irresistibly available before this minimum period of time has passed since the last ejaculation, non-ejaculatory sex is recommended.

The Eastern system of Tantra Yoga recommends transmuting seminal fluid and moving this energy up the chakra system, rather than ejaculation of the fluid out of the body. (For information about this system of sexual yoga refer to the publications: *Tantra the Art of Conscious Loving*, Charles & Caroline Muir, Mercury House Inc. San Francisco, 1989. *The Art of Sexual Ecstasy: The Path of Sacred Sexuality for Western Lovers*, Margo

Anand, Jeremy P. Tarcher, Inc., Los Angeles, 1989.)

The important idea to bear in mind is, if you are going to generate the energy of sexual arousal, it is in your best interest to somehow move it as well. Retaining it in a stagnate state evolves potential prostate problems.

The Penis

That notorious organ that no one trusts. TV's perennially censored flesh; Hollywood's most unphotogenic performer; the surgeon's first male target; one of a male's most vulnerable possessions; *Phallus officinalis*; (in some circles, *Phallus vulgaris*); shaker and mover; the great stimulator of whispers, wonder and lengthy guesses.

The penis consists of three cylindrical bodies of erectile tissue held together by connective tissue and skin. Two of these bodies lie side by side on the top of the penis, while the third body, which is significantly smaller, lies below and between the other two. Like everything else, both of the two larger bodies have been given an official Latin name which is *Corpora cavernosa penis* and the little lower body is referred to fondly as *Corpus spongiosum penis* (it also has an alias, *Corpus cavernosum urethrae*). Passing through C. spongiosum is the penile section of the urethra which extends from the bladder through the prostate. A covering of skin, devoid of fat, is loosely applied about the three bodies of the penis. The corpora are capped at the end by the *glans penis* (the head), which is normally cozily tucked into and covered by a protective fold of skin called the *prepuce* (foreskin). In circumcision the prepuse is cut off, so the glans is forever thereafter exposed. The penis has a less constant relation to general male body size than any other organ. 125 pound male authors like to include that sort of information.

Anatomy of an erection

Each of the three bodies of the penis is sponge like and contains blood. When the arteries that bring blood to the penis dilate, bringing more blood to it, and, simultaneously, the veins that carry blood from the penis constrict, so that less blood leaves, engorgement is produced and the penis becomes erect. This entire phenomenon comes under the involuntary control of the autonomic nervous system and may (or may not) occur at any time from psychological as well as physical stimulation. The external male sexual apparatus exists as a relatively vulnerable organic design, and its normally active abilities can be easily thwarted.

115

According to the *British Medical Journal*, 4-89; 298:1072 a man who rides on a narrow, hard bicycle seat over long distances can temporarily impair the efficiency of the arteries and nerves which service the penis. This damage can cause problems such as numbness, temporary and long term erection loss and impairment. Although it may not be in fashion at the Tour de France, the use of a soft seat is a much kinder foundation for the male sex organs to sit on while biking and will possibly help enhance any intimate post-event celebrations.

Circumcision — Common form of disregard for men's rights

In the United States, a new parent's mandatory first question in male child-care is still, "Should we leave him intact?"

Other questions parents possibly ask at this time are: Do we want our boy to look different in the locker room? After all, shouldn't he look like his dad or his brothers? Why does he have a foreskin anyway? What does it do there? Is having a foreskin clean or healthy? Won't it hurt my son to have part of his penis cut off? But questions all too seldom asked are: Why do they strap the baby's arms and legs to a board to perform this "painless" surgery? Aren't there inherent risks with genital surgery like there are in all other kinds of surgery; risks such as hemorrhage, major infection, possibly a child left with a deformed glans or a deformed meatus (opening) which is left too small? Might circumcision possibly hinder my boy's adult sexuality and his feelings about the safety of life and treatment by other human beings?

As I write this section, I feel anger rising inside. Anger at the system that intimidated my parents to proceed with this, in my opinion, senseless and risky mutilation. I feel indignant displeasure (another way of saying resentment) for the collusion of physicians and my (ill informed) parents which made that decision for me, abusing my rights and destroying my birthright with irreversible genital surgery. I do know that if I had been asked at the time of my birth (or any time thereafter), if I wanted my foreskin removed, and I had arrived from the womb fluent in the language the adults were speaking, I would have firmly crossed my chubby little legs and said without any hesitation, "You must be joking, forget it! Get me out of this hospital!"

The rich history of infection of the penis in the western world stems from the not too distant past when our European ancestors believed that bathing was bad for the health; consequently the foreskin created a perfect environment for breeding infection. Today the infection rate is reported to be 14% in the uncircumcised male and 8% in the circumcised. Obviously, we all need to wash regularly, and we need to teach little boys and their parents how to wash a penis, but really moms and dads, it's not necessary to cut parts of it off.

In (western) history, male genital surgery began in the English speaking countries in the late 1800s to prevent male masturbation, which the elders of the day had agreed caused blindness and disease. This initial cultural ignorance has perpetuated the practice of circumcision via the western medical profession ever since. Today the U.S. holds the bizarre status as the only nation left on the globe which still practices routine non-religious, non-medical circumcision. It's my guess that it is probably a lucrative surgical practice, or it would have been removed from the hospital routine long ago. The annual cost of circumcision in the U.S. is estimated at $200 million, but the tides are changing, and third-party payers have begun to reclassify circumcision as cosmetic surgery and are refusing to pay for it. It's looking like insurance companies and accountants will ultimately keep males intact.

Every generation of doctor has found a new excuse for circumcision. Today's foremost speculation that routine circumcision could reduce urinary-tract infection, veneral disease or prevent infection due to the AIDS virus is absurd. More than 95% of male children never experience urinary-tract infection regardless of the presence or absence of a foreskin, and 60% to 90% of the men in Los Angeles, Miami, San Francisco and New York infected with AIDS were circumcised at birth. The state of mind that suggests routine circumcision on baby males as a non-religious ritual to avoid possible infection might also consider removing a young girl's (or an adult woman's) clitoris, labia or later her breasts so that she will never have any trouble with them, or it might suggest pulling out the teeth so they won't decay . . . Obviously it's not that simple. Why cut off a male's foreskin based on a similar rationale?

Approximately 80% of the world's male population remains intact, not circumcised. Due to enlightened, self-educated parents who question the need to subject their sons to the pain of the surgical procedure, the circumcision rate in the U.S. is consistently decreasing. By 1986 about 45% of newborn males left American hospitals whole and intact. This means that about half of the males in high school locker rooms will look different than the other half. So, an intact foreskin is no longer a young boy's psychological/

social problem.

The steps involved in male genital hospital surgery go as follows:
- The baby is removed from the parents.
- The male baby's arms and legs are strapped to a board to prevent movement.
- The genitals are scrubbed in preparation for surgery.
- The foreskin (the *prepuce*) is torn from the glans (head) of the penis to which it is normally attached to protect this internal organ (the glans) from feces, urine and diaper irritation (later from burns, fingernails, dirt, fly-zippers, jungle and forest undergrowth, etc.).
- After tearing the foreskin from the glans it is slit lengthwise, allowing insertion of the circumcision instrument which cuts off the foreskin.
- This is usually done without anesthesia due to the physiological risk of anesthetics to the baby. Historically, those same elders (the masturbation authorities) conveniently decided that babies felt no pain due to their immature nervous systems. I assume this is similar to the pain they also wouldn't feel if they were abused somewhere outside the operating room. Parents and scientific studies have soundly disproved this theory and have proven this traumatic procedure is undeniably physically painful and psychologically stressful to the newborn boy.

A relatively more humane home circumcision ritual, the Brith Milah, is practiced in the Jewish tradition. I'm told that the infant is given a cloth to suck on, which has been soaked in sweet wine, probably experiencing his first high since floating in the womb. The baby is held on his father's lap and the cutting is done in the presence of loved ones and friends with a celebration afterwards. I'm also told the baby barely cries, if at all, but I find that difficult to imagine.

It might be of interest to us "normal" males who have been circumcised, to learn that the foreskin is (was) laden with sensitive nerve endings which enhance the sexual experience. Furthermore, this foreskin is intended to protect the delicate glans (designed to be an internal organ with a protective hood) which is extremely high in nerve endings, keeping it warm and moist, so that the glans won't become dry, thick and hard, thereby losing some sensitivity for sexual experience.

During one of my seminars on male health-care, a female nurse who had observed a number of circumcisions shared a story with us. She noted that frequently, while a female nurse scrubbed and prepared male infants' genitals for surgery, the babies' penises became erect. It dawned on her that, "I was observing the young infants having a sexual experience." And that soon following this erotic experience and fondling by female hands the male child experienced sudden traumatic pain and psychological stress. Her question was, "What effect might this have on the male's ability to feel trust and spontaneity with females in future sexual experiences and intimate relationships?" Who knows? I'd venture a personal guess that it doesn't help much. In studies of neo-natal and birth-time consciousness it is found that babies possess a high degree of awareness. So when, after the profound experience of birth, a male child's penis is handled by a nurse preparing him for genital surgery, soon after which he experiences severe pain, the juxtaposition of these programs may have direct relation to some circumcised men's general lack of trust in any relationship and specific anxiety in sexual relationship with women.

For those who would like to know more about the divinely inspired function of intact foreskin in male lives, I must tell you, it is very difficult to find any insightful, in-depth information about the anatomy and physiology of male organs. The brightest, most informative source of information on this issue that I have located is the National Organization of Circumcision Information Resource Centers, P.O. Box 2512, San Anselmo, CA 94960, (415) 488-9883. This is a health group organized by health professionals and physicians to provide parents with information on the benefits of "intactness." They make available newsletters, video tapes and other publications on neonatal circumcision and penis health-care.

Penis/Foreskin inflammation

The penises of those baby boys who escape the hospital with foreskin intact are not home safe yet. The head of the penis and the foreskin develop as one structure. What is physiologically normal in boy infancy is for the foreskin to adhere to the glans of the penis. This design keeps the urine, feces and various other diaper debris and rashes off of the glans. It, in fact, protects the penis from infection and keeps the opening of the penis adequate. That's why we have our little prepuces given to us at such a young age. If left alone, the foreskin comes loose on its own and then for the rest of our lives protects our glans from a variety of predators and mishaps. The ill-advised (most doctors in the U.S. tell parents to pull back the foreskin and wash the penis daily) attempts to draw the foreskin back before it is ready to come loose causes it to tear from the glans, causing pain, irritation and possible infection.

Health-care of an intact penis

Gentle knowledgeable care of a brand new intact penis is that special, extra little task parents of a new boy are asked to perform. The following insights and guidelines for this loving parental duty are quoted directly from literature which is compassionately distributed by the National Organization of Circumcision Resource Centers:

"The foreskin of an infant should *never* be retracted because it is attached to the glans. Separation of these two structures occurs gradually during childhood and the age at which a boy will be able to retract his foreskin is different for each child. This process should never be hurried! Forcing the foreskin to retract will cause pain, bleeding and possibly infection and adhesion.

"Phimosis is the name given to an unretractable foreskin. This normally exists in almost all newborn babies and in some men throughout adulthood. It rarely causes problems. However, should painful erection occur, gentle stretching of the foreskin opening will, in time, allow for retractability. To remove the important protective foreskin with circumcision is seldom necessary to correct phimosis.

"The natural shedding of the skin cells from the foreskin lining and the glans helps in the process of separation of these two structures. The cells which have been shed form a substance known as infant smegma. The baby's body effectively discharges this harmless material which can then be wiped from the tip of the foreskin during the bath. External washing with a very mild soap and water is all that is required to maintain adequate hygiene.

"During puberty, sebaceous glands begin to function, secreting an oily substance. This additional product in adult smegma protects and lubricates the glans. At this time a male simply retracts the foreskin and cleans to prevent accumulation of smegma."

If your little boy's prepuce is prematurely torn from the glans and irritation or infection occurs in this area, or if irritation occurs in this area on any male child (or adult), sprinkle on a mixture of powdered Golden Seal, Comfrey and Slippery Elm. Use equal parts of each herb. Distribute some of this mixture in the diaper (or jockey shorts) as well. It will be very helpful to wash the infected area frequently with a tea made of the same herbs, using 2 parts Comfrey, 1 part Golden Seal, 1 part Slippery Elm. If the infection lingers, give a tincture or tea of:

Echinacea	3 parts (anti-microbial/immune enhancing)
Marshmallow root	2 parts (soothing demulcent/healing)
Catnip	1 part (fever cooling/nervine)
Fennel	1 part (assists digestion/relaxing/ pleasant flavor)
Golden Seal	1/2 part (anti-microbial)

This will help relax him and help his natural immune system eliminate the infection.

Following are two remedies (taken from *The New Healing Yourself* by Joy Gardner) which are also effective for treating an irritated or infected foreskin.

Cornstarch Soak. Dilute 1 tablespoon of cornstarch in 1/4 cup warm water. Soak a small clean white cotton cloth in this solution. (I suggest adding 1 drop of Lavender essential oil to this mixture). Apply gently to the foreskin for 1 to 2 minutes. Repeat this 3 times a day. The swelling should diminish the first day and should disappear completely in a day or two.

Cider Vinegar. Dilute 1/2 teaspoon apple cider vinegar in 1/4 cup warm water (with 1 drop Lavender essential oil) and apply as above.

Penis Soaks — The P.S. of couples' mutual health-care

This technique for male hygiene and external herbal therapy was originated and is strongly suggested by a clinical herbal therapist named Cascade Anderson-Geller. One can think of this as a male (reverse) douche to be used if you itch, after making love, or any other time you suspect a problem. It is also a practical method for administering herbal washes to a little boy who is troubled by irritation of the penis or foreskin, if you can get him to quit giggling about the process long enough to do it. Without question, it is most important for a man whose female partner may have a vaginal malady to use these penis soaks. Many of these vaginal/uterine infections such as gardnerella (also called hemophilus), trichomonas, monilia (yeast or candida infections), chlamydia, venereal warts and cystitis or urethritis are transmitted or reinfected by the male member during sexual intercourse. The micro-organisms are passed back and forth between partners to the chagrin of both, especially the female. Most often the male, because he doesn't offer as perfect a breeding arena, doesn't experience the symptoms as intensely and uncomfortably as the female. At the same time, both partners must work to bolster their immune systems.

To perform a penis soak simply hold a (tall, medium or short) drinking glass filled with a strong infusion or decoction of appropriate herbs and hang in there for about 5-10 minutes. (If your foreskin has not already been sent to prepuce heaven, retract the foreskin throughout the soak). The tea should be as warm as possible. It is helpful to include the testicles in the soak too, so you might graduate to a vase or a jar as a container. An alternative method is the common sitz bath, filling a small basin or plastic tub with the warm herb tea and sitting in it. This is probably more trouble to prepare, but it is comfortable and frees both hands, so you can read a magazine, shave or adjust the VCR while you're sitting there.

In general, I recommend using combinations of the strong aromatic herbs for this male herbal soak, such as equal parts of Yarrow, Sage, Lavender and Chaparral. If you use pure essential oils for health-care, you can include in the soak 1 to 2 drops of one or a combination of the following essential oils: Tea Tree (*Melaleuca alternifolia*), Lavender (*Lavendula vera*) and Bergamot (*Citrus bergamia*). Disperse the oils well, soak for 5-10 minutes at least once, but preferably 2 to 3 times a day. I know that the thought of hanging into a vessel of herb tea does not immediately strike one with the most manly of images. I can relate to your resistance and appreciate the visual hilarity of the adventure. However, when communicable infection is involved between caring lovers, each partner has a responsibility to the mutual cure. No matter how absurd the image of this therapy strikes you, in times when your female partner is stressed with reoccurring vaginal infection, discomfort and pain, the most chivalrous act is a daily hygienic penis soak until the cycle of reinfection has been stopped. Keep in mind that this will not only help your female partner, but it will also enhance your relationship and ultimately hasten and improve your sexual reunion. Words of love are merely promises.

Non-Specific Infection

When doctors aren't sure what specific name to give to a woman's vaginal infection, they call it "non-specific vaginitis," and they usually prescribe some brand of antibiotic. After this doesn't work, and often as a result, a yeast bloom has manifested to accompany the original infection, many women seek the help of an herbalist. I give this female douche formula to you because it is helpful for the male partner to use it for a penis soak or in a sitz bath concurrently with the female's self-care. It will help you both become more comfortable and much happier, sooner. For this male consideration (exceeded only by shaving before making love) your female partner will bless you. This douche recipe has given blessed relief:

Chaparral	2 parts (anti-oxidant/anti-microbial)
Oak bark	2 parts (astringent)
Marshmallow root	1 part (soothing demulcent)
Periwinkle, fresh if available	4 parts (tonic/astringent)
Yarrow	1 part (anti-microbial)

Strain the tea through cotton muslin cloth and douche (penis soak) 2-3 times a day. Hot tea reduces the itching, so make the douche as hot as is comfortable. As we are all learning, it always takes two to solve problems between partners.

Genital Warts

While addressing the unusual subject of penis soaks in the context of partner mutual health-care, I want to include some relevant information on HPV (human papilloma virus). This is a virus that can be passed from person to person through sexual intercourse. It can contribute to the cause of genital (venereal) warts and according to the medical profession can cause cancer of the cervix and less often, cancer of the vagina, vulva, uterus and in men, cancer of the penis. The warts caused are initially too small to be seen by an untrained eye, and, in women, these warts are often too far up inside the genital tract to be visible. As the warts grow they begin to appear as hard raised skin and eventually take on the classic cauliflower-like warty appearance. Genital warts occur on a man toward the tip of the penis, occasionally under an existing foreskin, or on the scrotum. Diagnosing these genital warts in the female (normally through an examination called a colposcopy) is expensive, but a male can find out if he has HVP very easily by using, you guessed it, a 'diagnostic' penis soak. Submerge your penis and scrotum in a container of diluted 10% vinegar (1 part vinegar to 9 parts water) for six minutes (good opportunity to practice your whistling). If you have genital warts, they, being very flat in the initial stage, will appear as white patches.

To treat this condition, it is important to work internally as well as externally. Take herbs which have an anti-viral, immune enhancing action

123

with herbs that nourish, cleanse and build the liver, along with a diet that includes increased vitamin C and zinc. A suggested herbal formula for this purpose is:

Milk Thistle	3 parts (liver tonic)
Calendula	2 parts (Vulnerary, anti-inflammatory, anti-viral)
Scullcap or Wild Oat	1 part (nerve nutrient)

Take as a tea, 1 cup 3 times a day or as a tincture 25 drops 3 times a day.

Externally, the use of pure essential oils to treat this condition can be very helpful. Combine :

Lemon	4 drops
Patchouli	4 drops
Tea tree	4 drops
Cinnamon leaf	1 drop

Apply this combination with a q-tip to the warts only. Avoid the skin around the warts as much as possible. I would not suggest this combination for women treating internal vaginal warts as it would be very difficult to control the application of this oil combination, and it can cause irritation of the surrounding tissue. Another combination that is easily prepared is: 1 ounce of vegetable or castor oil (mixed half and half with an oil infusion of St. John's Wort, if available) to which is added 3 capsules vitamin E oil (800 IU each) and 15 drops of Thuja essential oil. Shake this well to disperse the essential oils. Apply this mixture to the warts twice a day, rubbing it in well. This may tingle and feel warm. Wash hands well before and after application.

I suggest you also consult an allopathic physician to find out what treatment is suggested in their system of medicine. I believe they use caustic solutions, cauterization, freezing and/or surgery. If you do choose these allopathic techniques, follow up by nourishing yourself with the suggested herbs to promote healing and to help prevent recurrence. It is obviously important to determine your situation with regards to this virus for your own health and for the health of your sexual partner(s).

Genital Herpes

Herpes genitalis, a virus, gets the bug's share of the blame for causing genital herpes; however, it requires a receptive human host to develop an outbreak of the herpes blisters. The first herpes outbreak is usually the most potent, and it is often accompanied by swollen glands and fever, as the body's immune system rallies to deal with the acute infection.

Some individuals feel weak and sick at this time, and rest is most helpful. A cluster of painful blisters appears suddenly below the waist, usually in the pubic or anal area, in men they can also appear anywhere from the base to the tip of the penis shaft. The blisters rupture after 1 to 3 days and slowly heal in another 3 to 5 days. A second outbreak can occur within a month. Subsequent recurrences are milder due to the herpatic antibodies that have been created, and, if the underlying stresses are resolved, recurrences taper off as the years go by. Herpes is generally spread from partner to partner when the sores are present, so be kind and avoid sex during outbreaks. During this outbreak stage the herpes virus can also be transferred to a new location on the body. There are simple procedures that will minimalize this risk of accidental transfer.

- Don't touch the sores.
- Wash your hands if you do touch the sores.
- Upon waking up wash your hands before rubbing your eyes. The eyes are particularly vulnerable.
- If you wear contact lenses, always wash your hands before inserting the lenses.

Despite disappearance of the outward signs of infection (blisters), the herpes virus does not leave the body. It remains in a dormant state, in nerve tissue near the site of infection. There are two important factors that appear to be related to viral reactivation— general health and stress. Both factors lower resistance. For those individuals who have herpes, a recurrence of herpes blisters is often a nerve response to anger, general stress, sexual stress and/or chronic fatigue. Some practitioners believe that the outbreaks are influenced by a person's reaction to the moon phases. Make note on your calender or appointment book and see if your outbreaks regularly coincide with a particular phase of the lunar cycle, unless, of course you are absolutely sure, without a shadow of doubt that your body and spirit are not effected by the moon's body and its reflection of nighttime sunlight. If you can establish a lunar connection, you can prepare and alter your lifestyle activities to be more self-nourishing during those cyclic times. A flare up of herpes blisters is a practical barometer of one's current emotional environment. Review your immediate situation and feelings and make appropriate amends. It is probably time to be more kind to yourself. Time to pull back and be more internal for a while. Frequently, prior to the actual outbreak of genital herpes blisters, if you pay close attention to your body's messages, a precursory symptom (a warning sign of nerve agitation) will present itself. This symptom can appear as a rheumatic pain in a toe joint or in a knee joint, or a hypersensitive patch will manifest along a nerve meridian somewhere on the surface of the skin of the lower body. These symptoms can be the harbingers of coming dermal outbreaks. This is when you take stock of your current emotional lot and learn more about your ways. This is a time to contain your energy and limit any excesses such as over work or excessive sex, actions that might expend too much energy. Drink a cup of White Sage tea. This herb is tempering and helps one to reduce appetites of all kinds. It will assist you to return your energy and attention to yourself. To help you avoid potentially debilitating, energy draining conditions, use the combination of Chamomile and Scullcap to gently sedate your sympathetic nervous system (that part of the autonomic nervous system that relates to the outside world). Spend some time in creative solitude, abstain for the time being, meditate and rest up.

Genital herpes is a sexually transmitted disease. Many people who have herpes are also experiencing conflict about their sexuality, or they are involved in a relationship that is not healthy for them. These personal imbalances create stress that can predispose one to experience herpes attacks. It is helpful to take nourishing herbs such as Saw Palmetto and Ashweganda to generally build and tone the nervous system and the reproductive organs. Seeking out the source of this stress and dealing with it in a positive way will help you ward off recurring outbreaks and will bolster your body's receptivity to herbal treatment.

To help relieve the acute phases of this condition, make a preparation consisting of:

Calendula flower tincture	3 parts
Oregon Grape root tincture	1 part
Gumweed bud and flower tincture	1 part
Cleavers tincture	1 part
Burdock root tincture	1 part
Black Haw tincture	1 part

Think of this as a "herb-pes" formula. Take 30 drops 2 to 3 times a day internally and apply the same compound topically on the first sign of dermal irritation. David Winston, herbal practitioner and teacher in New Jersey suggests making a Licorice tea wash and applying this to herpes blisters. He has found that this heals them quickly. He recommends (at the first signs of outbreak before the eruption of blisters) applying ice on the area for as long as possible, 3 to 4 times a day. This will often prevent the eruption of blisters.

Avoid all foods that are high in sugar and all foods high in arginine amino-acid (all nuts, peanuts, peanut butter, chocolate, carob, coconut, grains, raisins, coffee) and increase your intake of lysine foods (milk, cheese, beans, nutritional yeasts, eggs), also take 3 to 5 (500 mg), L-lysine tablets a day as a preventive measure. Increase this to 3 (500 mg) tablets, 2 to 3 times a day during an outbreak. Avoid meat, fried foods, cooked tomatoes and citrus. Herpes is a fiery irritant to the nervous system and skin, so avoid any peripheral circulatory stimulants such as Cayenne, Ginger, curry, coffee and spicy foods like Mexican or East Indian food. Emphasize foods rich in calcium and B-vitamins such as nutritional yeasts, yogurt, miso and green leafy vegetables. This herbal and dietary control will help you, but introspection, increased self-insight and appropriate physical/emotional/mental modifications will give you the most healing service.

Aromatherapy treatment employs the anti-viral plant essential oils of Tea Tree (*Melaleuca alternifolia*) which is immune enhancing as well, Bergamot (*Citrus bergamia*) which also inhibits herpes simplex 1, Geranium (*Pelargonium Asperum*) and Eucalyptus (*Eucalyptus globulus*). Combine 1 drop of each with 5 ml (1 tsp.) Aloe vera gel. Mix this blend well and apply to outbreak 3-4 times a day. To make a larger quantity, use 5 drops of each essential oil in 1 oz. Aloe vera.

Note: The essential oil of Bergamot can cause photosensitivity. This is not a problem with genital application (unless you sun bathe in the nude), but if you are applying this remedy to a cold sore on the face, it's best to avoid the sun.

Safe Sex Alert

A cautionary note to tag on the practice of safe sex. Some individuals have found that the mysterious lubricants and spermicides which are found in and on condoms can cause rashes, glans-urethral rawness and may stimulate genital herpes eruptions. These lubricants might affect the vaginal canal of the female partner as well. So, if you are having troubles in these areas and nothing else appears to be the cause, you might consider changing your brand. Is nothing simple anymore?

Testicles, Testosterone and Sperm

The testicle is the primary organ of sex in the male. Like its counterpart, the ovary, the testicle has two distinct functions. It forms the

127

male germ cells (sperm), and it is also an endocrine gland, secreting sex hormones into the blood stream.

As a male fetus develops inside its mother's uterus, its testes begin to secrete testosterone when it is only 4 weeks old. This testosterone then assists the fetus to develop the formation of a penis, scrotum, prostate, seminal vesicles, vas deferens and other male sexual organs.

Testosterone secretion by the fetal testes is caused by a hormone called chorionic gonadotropin, that is formed in the placenta during pregnancy. Immediately after his birth, the male child disconnects from the placenta, removing this stimulatory effect. The testes become dormant, and the sexual characteristics remain at a standstill until puberty. At puberty the reinstitution of testosterone secretion causes the male sex organs to begin growing again. The testes, scrotum and penis then enlarge about ten-fold.

In addition to the effects on the genital organs, testosterone exerts other general effects throughout the body to give the adult male his distinctive characteristics. It promotes growth of hair on his face, along the middle of his abdomen, on his pubis, and on his chest. On the other hand, it causes baldness on male individuals who have a hereditary predisposition to male pattern baldness (see section: Hair Loss). It increases the growth of the larynx so that the male, after puberty, develops a deeper pitch to his voice. It causes an increase in the deposition of protein in his muscles, bones, skin and other parts of his body, so that the male adolescent becomes generally larger and more muscular than the female.

In order to produce spermatozoa, the testes must be at least 1 degree C. less than the central body temperature, so the testes in most mammals must descend into the scrotal sac. Testosterone causes the testes to descend from the abdominal cavity into the scrotum. When the production of testosterone by the fetus is insufficient, the testes fail to descend, remaining in the abdominal cavity in the same manner that the ovaries remain in the abdominal cavity of the female. If the descent of the testis is stopped while the gland is still in the abdomen the condition is called *cryptorchism* (hidden testis).

If the testes do not descend into the scrotum there will be a poor germinal epithelium (tissue that forms sperm cells) and poor spermatogenisis (the process of formation, development and maturation of sperm). Occasionally a male baby is born with a testicle that has failed to descend to the scrotum. Generally an undescended testicle will not produce live sperm, but unless it is also congenitally abnormal, its output of hormones is usually not impaired. As explained above, the testes usually descend before birth, but about 10% of boys are born with one or both still on the way. In most of these children the undescended testicle(s) arrives within a few weeks. If this does not occur, sometimes a doctor can bring down an undescended testicle by manual manipulation and gentle pressure providing there is no mechanical obstruction or adhesions. Practitioners of Oriental medicine will employ moxa (applying heat) and needling of specific points of the lower body that will give a downward motion to the gland. About 3% of boys are still cryptorchid at puberty, but spontaneous descent of the testicle often occurs at this age (sometimes even at the eighteenth year) from the increased hormonal levels developed at that time. Some doctors will recommend surgery or hormonal therapy to bring the testis down. Hormone therapy will cause descent in not more than 10 to 20% of cases, and it is probably safe to say that if this treatment is successful, the testis would have descended spontaneously at puberty. Some research indicates that the need to perform surgery is doubtful, although current medical opinion has it that the undescended testicle has a significantly higher danger of malignancy than a testicle that has normally descended. The highest rate of malignancy of a displaced testis occurs at ages 28 to 32 years. Displaced testes, if not placed in the scrotum by the age of five or six years, will lose their spermatogenic activities, so if both testicles remain undescended then sterility is almost inevitable and corrective therapy should be considered.

If there is any problem with the development of a young boy's gonads, it will be helpful to supply him with nutrients that assist his young body to adjust and normalize this condition. An excellent gonad gland tonic herb is the Saw Palmetto berry. Prepare a mixture of:

Saw Palmetto	3 parts (nutritive/gonad tonic)
Corn Silk	1 part (demulcent/genito-urinary tonic)
Catnip	1 part (gentle nervine/astringent)
Alfalfa seed & leaf	1 part (high vitamin/mineral content)
Fennel seed	1(+) part (digestive/flavor)

Keep in mind that Saw Palmetto is not a great tasting herb, so go as heavy on the Fennel as required to make the brew more flavorful. This formula could be made as a tea, a tincture or as a glycerine extract, whichever form is most practical to administer to the child. Give a half a cup of tea or 25 drops of tincture 1 to 2 times a day.

Orchitis

Orchitis is an inflammation of a testis. The acute condition is marked by fever, pain, swelling and a feeling of weight in the testicle. Orchitis usually occurs in an adolescent as a complication of mumps; it can, however, accompany any other acute infection. Inflammation of the testicle (occasionally both testicles are affected) due to mumps develops in about 25% of males who are past puberty. Swelling of the testis usually begins about 5 to 7 days after the appearance of enlargement of the salivary glands. Involvement of the testicle is preceded by headache, increased feeling of uneasiness, a rise in temperature and occasionally nausea and vomiting. The swollen testicle can become 2 or 3 times its normal size, will be very sensitive to touch and will be quite painful. The swelling usually disappears within 7 to 10 days. If the gland shows a decrease in its normal size after the swelling subsides, atrophy is indicated. Sterility results only if both testicles are involved, and both have subsequently atrophied; however, this is normally not accompanied by loss of hormonal function. Therapy consists of bed rest, some form of scrotal support, placing an ice pack on the testicle, and, of course, treatment of the primary infection. The use of Dong Quai as a sexual organ tonic is very helpful for this condition. Also include Crampbark, Black Haw and Roman Chamomile, for these herbs will help tremendously to relieve the pain of this condition. They are anti-spasmodic, anti-inflammatory, relaxing nervines which have a strong affinity for the genital organs.

Testicular Self-Examination

It's well known by all males that the testicles are tender, delicate and sensitive organs. They can be injured easily and are vulnerable to various pathologies. It is important for men to be familiar with their bodies and to perform simple testicular self-examination (TSE) monthly starting at about age 15. If you feel any abnormalities, it is advisable to see a health practitioner. TSE only takes about 3 minutes and is easiest done in the shower or bath. The heat causes the scrotal skin to relax and soapy fingers increase sensitivity to touch. The technique is as follows:

1. Hold your scrotum in the palm of your hands. Then, roll one testicle gently between the thumb and fingers of both hands. There should be no hard lumps or nodules.

2. Examine the epididymis, the comma-shaped cord found behind the testicles, where sperm is stored and transported; it is the location of most

non-cancerous problems.

3. Examine the vas deferens, the sperm-carrying tube that lies directly under the skin and runs up from the epididymis. Normally, the vas feels like a firm, movable smooth cord. This is the easily accessible tube that is sealed by the surgeon to cause sterility.

4. Repeat the exam on the other testicle.

It's interesting to study and learn about your male parts from an anatomy text book (a collection of body maps) and from a text on human physiology. A textbook of general urology is also highly informative. I'm truly amazed at how ignorant about our own bodies most of us manage to remain throughout our lives.

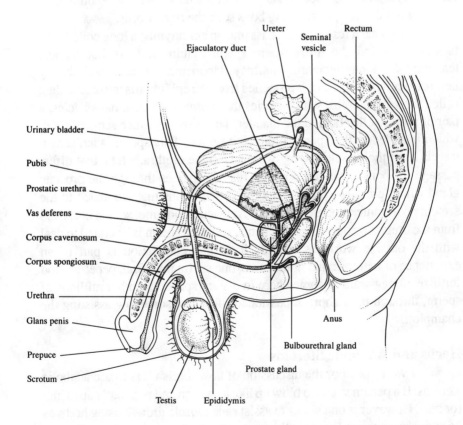

The male scrotum and contents: *the epididymis, vas deferens and testis.*

Sperm Trek

As most of us know, we men father sperm in our testicles, the male nursery organs. We devote a lot of time and vital energy to this paternal task producing sperm at an alarming rate, creating up to 400 million of these little genetic cloners in each brood. With all the androgenic hormones flowing around this area, these energetically mobile male sperm cells are highly motivated to leave home and seek adventure; and the vital adult male is usually similarly motivated to assist them. That's one of the reasons why men are so special.

The woman's nursery organ, the ovary, only makes available one egg a month, which assumes a more passive posture awaiting with patient anticipation the massive attention it hopes to soon receive. This is one of the reasons women are so special. As T. Elder Sachs would say, "Young girls listen for a voice to speak; young boys seek the right words."

From each testis, sperm pass into an epididymis, a long coiled tube tucked in behind the testis where sperm mature and are housed and tempered for their impending journey. Upon male arousal and shortly before ejaculation, sperm are propelled from the epididymis into a long duct called the vas deferens, which carries the sperm to the seminal vesicles, a pair of sacs that lies behind the bladder. These sacs produce seminal fluid, which is added to the sperm, producing semen. This sperm laden semen travels from the vesicles along two ducts to the urethra, a tube that offers passage for both urine and semen. This tube passes through the prostate gland which produces further supportive secretions that are added to the semen; no organic expense is spared. At ejaculation time, semen is ejected from the urethra through the erect penis, and each sperm is liberated to deal with the outside world as it finds it. If this ejaculation is part of an experience of heterosexual intercourse, one sperm may find, penetrate and fertilize an egg waiting somewhere in distant space, the other millions of sperm, through their short impassioned lifespans, somehow assisting the champion.

Herbs and Anabolic Steroids

I won't belabor the discussion of how foolish it is to use anabolic steroids. If a person wants to blow up like a balloon and pop that's up to him (or her). However if one wants to assist sane muscle growth using herbs as hormonal precursors for anabolic growth, I can offer some information and assistance. *There is no plant that gives anabolic steroids*. A number of plants supply steroidal saponins which are anabolic steroid precursors that the body can use to manufacture for itself the desired growth hormones to build itself naturally and healthily. These plant (steroid precursor) constituents are not actively anabolic themselves, they are building blocks that the body can use to build its own anabolic steroids. These plant steroidal precursors will never push the body beyond its normal limits. The fact that nature won't do this might illustrate that too much macho is not healthy in any game. Using 'roids is like aggressively overharvesting the forests, or shooting all the elephants and grizzly. They are all macho disconnectors that lead to internal and external ill health. Plants that provide anabolic steroidal precursors are Wild Yam, Sarsaparilla, Licorice, Damiana, Yucca and Saw Palmetto. Saw Palmetto is actually more of a sexual organ tonic so it is used more to support male testosterone production. Ginseng also has the steroidal saponins, but it is quite expensive, and the steroidal saponins in the less expensive Wild Yam and Sarsaparilla have a closer chemical construction to the anabolic steroids. Each of these plants can be taken individually or in combination, as teas or as tinctures. Take 1 cup of tea or 15 to 25 drops of tincture in the morning and evening.

Prolonged use of anabolic steroids severely damages the liver which is responsible for metabolizing testosterone. Testosterone that is formed in the testes can only be used by the body's receptors after it is metabolized by the liver. Consequently as the liver disintegrates so does the libido. It has been reported in an FDA Drug Bulletin (October 1987) that in males, some of the additional side effects of anabolic steroid use includes: enlarged prostate, breast enlargement and testicular atrophy with subsequent sterility or significantly decreased sperm count.

Another herb also commercially offered as an herbal alternative for anabolic steroids is Yohimbe, a West African stimulating aphrodisiac whose actions have a direct effect on the sexual centers of the spinal cord increasing tonicity, possibly stimulating male potency. It is proven to cause penile erection giving relief of impaired sexual function, also giving increased sexual appetite. Impotence of functional origin is directly influenced by it. Yohimbe is possibly a mildly toxic plant and should not be used unreservedly until we learn more about it. No evidence shows it to be anabolic, merely stimulating. It is frequently adulterated in commercial products, with some other plant used in its place. Siberian Ginseng, an adaptogenic herb which helps the body adapt positively to stress and has a deep immune system enhancing action, is a prostatic tonic which is known to boost physical energy. But beware, it is also frequently adulterated, with other plants used in its stead. Bee pollen, a highly nutritious food, is a bee product utilizing the male germ which propagates life in the plant kingdom. It contains all known water soluble vitamins and also contains a gonadotropic hormone which stimulates sex glands supporting the production of testosterone and growth hormones.

Each of the steroid precursor herbs I have discussed will provide excellent support to your workout and growth program. It is important that you purchase these herbs from a reliable and knowledgeable herbalist who can assure high quality herbs and accurate identification of the desired plant, so you get the results you pay for.

Virility, Fertility and Longevity
Impotence — the absence of arousal in a man's life

What is impotence? The concept communicated by the term "impotent" is often a rash judgement. In most cases, the absence of arousal is the more accurate issue at hand. In regards to impotence or low sexual energy, I see individuals living lifestyles that are highly conducive to the onset of low blood-sugar and sluggish adrenal function. They exist day-to-day in routine jobs and sedentary domestic life that neither stimulate their creative capacity nor arouse their life-force. Eventually, along with the chronic experience of this daily dis-motivating occupational and/or domestic environment, come the physical symptoms of low blood-sugar: diminished circulation, low immune strength and low adrenal and procreative force. When a male individual's life does not stimulate and arouse his male spirit, how can he expect a sexual partner to wade through the emotional and physical barriers to stimulate sexual arousal? The body's central organ of sexual response is the brain. An individual needs to be self-aroused by the joy, power and creative stimulation of his own life first; physical arousal will follow, spontaneously enhancing performance in other arenas.

I don't think that in most sexual relationships, it is either the man or the woman who is at fault if all isn't going well. The mutual relationship is expressing impotence. Each sexual relationship develops its own sexual and emotional patterns, and both partners contribute to and are responsible for this evolution. If either or both partners don't enjoy the experiences of this mutually generated sexual energy, then dissatisfaction needs to be communicated, suggestions made and the pattern changed to once again arouse the participants.

Sometimes a man can become sexually impotent because he has made sexuality and sexual activity *too* important in his life. "Impotence," in this instance, may be a plea for balance, an expression of the other aspects of the wise Inner Being demanding equal time for development.

There are many herbs and exercises that can assist a couple to stoke the fires of expressive love, reducing impotence to an ash. See the list of exotic herbal formulas at the end on this chapter and refer to the books in the Resource section, *Taoist Secrets of Love: Cultivating Male Sexual Energy* and *Healing Love Through the Tao: Cultivating Female Sexual Energy* by Mantak & Maneewan Chia. Also, *ESO, Extended Sexual Orgasm* by Alan & Donna Brauer and *Conscious Conception: Elemental Journey Through the Labyrinth of Sexuality* by Parvati & Baker.

Drugs: Licit and Illicit

At one time, nine out of ten cases of impotence were blamed on emotional problems, but today it is being shown that half the causes are actually physical, due directly to disease symptoms (such as diabetes which causes poor circulation) and life-style habits, with the highest risk factor being . . . smoking. I hate to expose a real man while he's down, but there appears to be a convincing battery of evidence recently released which shows that tobacco smoking significantly increases the risk of impotence. Well, Marlboro man, at least that's still one heck of a horse you're ridin'. It has been found that almost two thirds of impotent men smoke, and that they smoke nearly two times as much as the smoking rate of the general male population. If you're having trouble in bed and you're a smoker, seriously consider snuffing the cigarettes out for life. That gesture alone may very well restore your potency. Being a non-smoker myself, I may be exposing my naivete; I guess it's possible that smoking a cigarette is better than sex. Or is it that sex is better with a cigarette?

Anyway, it appears that smoking and sex for many men are terrible bed partners. Physiologically, it requires good blood flow to the extremities to produce and sustain a useful erection. It has been found that one smoker in four has poor circulation to the penis, whereas only one in twelve non-smokers has this problem. Translating this into statistic-speak, it means that the link between smoking and damage to penile circulation is over 90% substantiated. Later in this chapter I am going to suggest some herbs that help improve a man's sexual potency, but continued tobacco smoking will probably antidote them. According to a newsletter titled, "Sex Over Forty," published by PHE Inc., P.O. Box 1600, Chapel Hill, N.C. 27515, "only one or two cigarettes can cause an immediate impairment of sexual function."

But indulgence in tobacco alkaloids is not the only drug risk to male potency. While nicotine constricts blood vessels, alcohol works as a depressant that dulls impulses of the central nervous system, including those that stimulate the penis. Chronic heavy drinking impairs the male body's supply of testosterone and increases the amount of estrogen. Chronic beer drinking causes even worse symptoms than chronic drinking of wine or hard liquor, possibly due to the chemical additives or fermentative impurities commonly used in present day brewery "cheating" which is necessary in order to quick-age the beer rather than letting "time" do the aging. Low body water levels can lead to temporary impotence. Alcoholic beverages cause net body water loss. Drinking abundant clean water can restore function.

Marijuana alters the perception of time and may appear to prolong pleasurable feelings. This plant can help some individuals relax when necessary and focus their attention on feelings rather than on distracting thoughts, in which case moderate use might enhance one's lovemaking. However, frequent use of Marijuana has been shown to lower the level of androgen that a man can produce. Androgens are the main hormones in both men and women that determine the level of ones sex drive, the libido thermostat controls. Low androgens in men diminish interest in sex as well as adversely affecting erection.

Cocaine and amphetamines are parasympathetic blocking agents, but concurrently they are sympathetic stimulants. Sexual contact, arousal and erection is a parasympathetic nervous system event, while ejaculation is controlled by the sympathetic nervous system. Consequently, a man using these drugs can produce a quick ejaculation, usually premature, but cannot usually sustain arousal and an erection for any length of time. Although there are many users who rapidly deny these effects.

Next on the list of problem drugs are medicines, both prescription and over-the-counter (OTC). The high-blood-pressure drugs called sympathetic blockers, such as *Aldomet*, *Catapres* and *Ismelin* are reportedly the most troublesome. If you are having trouble with high blood pressure, see the section in this book on hypertension for information about herbal non-drug remedies. Use of these herbs does not contribute to male impotence. The widely prescribed anti-ulcer drug, *Tagamet*, also causes impotence in many male users. As discussed in the section on treating ulcers, Marshmallow root and leaf are superior botanical agents for soothing and healing ulcers as well as other wounds, and they do not contribute to impotence. Antihistamines, used to control symptoms of allergies and colds, and decongestants, which constrict blood vessels, are OTC drugs that can cause temporary impotence. And the highly popular drug "overwork" can and commonly does impair potency. It inhibits male potency the same as does fatigue caused by insufficient sleep, emotional tension and depression.

Diabetes

Adult-onset diabetes is said to be the cause of nearly half of all male impotence due to the stress of high blood sugar, which also predisposes a man toward clogged arteries inhibiting circulation. Often a man who is troubled by experiences of impotence is not aware that he has manifested this underlying diabetic condition which affects men in their mid forties or early fifties. There are basically two types of diabetes: (A) an insulin dependent form in which it is assumed that the person's pancreas is no longer creating insulin wherein his blood sugar level needs to be constantly monitored and (B) a non-insulin dependent form of diabetes in which the pancreas is capable of creating insulin but something else is interfering with the overall regulation of blood sugar.

Treating form (A) insulin dependent diabetes requires the attention of an individual well trained in monitoring the blood sugar and insulin levels. This is tricky and should be left to a competent technician. Herbs are best used here to treat the primary complications or accompanying symptoms of this degree of diabetes. Cardiovascular complications are treated well by use of Hawthorn berries, Horsechestnut and Ginkgo. Common bladder infection due to the excess sugar in the diabetic urine are treated well with genito-urinary anti-microbials and tonics such as Echinacea, Uva Ursi, Yarrow, Buchu and Garlic. Stress due to the experience of impotence and high blood sugar is treated well with Siberian Ginseng and Suma which at the same time help the body deal with the overall stress of all these physical problems. Suma is reported by some herbalists to be (amongst many other applications) a pancreatic tonic that regenerates pancreatic cells. Although it has deep folkloric roots in South American cultures, its use is very recent here, and we have a lot to learn about its actions.

Form (B) non-insulin dependent diabetes can be treated more directly by using bitters to stimulate the pancreatic secretions and excretions; Gentian, Yarrow and Fringe Tree bark are excellent bitters, and Fringe Tree has a particular affinity for the pancreas. To help lower blood sugar levels the use of hypoglycemic herbs are indicated. These herbs are pancreatic tonics and their hypoglycemic action helps reduce sugar content in blood by increasing the efficiency of insulin (there is no evidence that these herbs increase insulin production). Herbs having hypoglycemic action are: Devil's Club, Goat's Rue, Burdock, Nettles, Sweet Potato, Pea, Fenugreek, Olive leaves, Mulberry leaves and Garlic. To treat the accompanying symptoms of diabetes, supporting the cardio-vascular system is a major priority. Of course here we will use the cardio-vascular herbs Hawthorn berries, Ginkgo, Yarrow and Garlic. Male impotence resulting from this condition is dealt with by using the hypoglycemics discussed above, along with Wild Yam, Sarsaparilla and Siberian Ginseng, for all these herbs help normalize the hormonal problem that is also affecting the sexual functions of the male organs. Sexual dysfunction related to poor blood circulation is treated by the cardio-vascular herbs just listed. In addition, the adaptogenic herbs Siberian Ginseng and Suma deal with the overall stress inherent in these conditions.

And lastly, appropriate diet plays a major role in managing blood sugar levels for all diabetics. Detailed information on this subject can be found in the *Merck Manual*, a medical reference text that is important to have in any domestic and professional health library.

Hypoglycemia

Hypoglycemia can be considered the functional opposite condition to diabetes in that it is a condition of low blood sugar brought on by the appearance of too much insulin secretion. This condition is one of the predisposing factors that triggers, in time, the onset of diabetes. Diet control plays a major role in regulating this condition, and to help better understand the dynamics of diet for healing this condition I recommend a book titled, *Hypoglycemia: A Better Approach* by Paavo Airola, Ph.D. The nutritional approach outlined in this book for managing a low blood sugar condition is well researched, sound and effective. Some foods and herbs that are helpful in stabilizing both low or high blood-sugar are: Onions and Garlic, Horseradish, Cranberry, Oats, Sunflower seeds, Bitters, Nettles, Suma, Celery, Barley, Spinach, Carrot, Cashews. Tomatillo, Artichoke, Jerusalem Artichoke, Broccoli, Cauliflower, Blueberry fruit and leaves, Olive oil and leaf, Burdock root, Dandelion and Mugwort.

Kegel exercises

Kegel exercises contribute directly to male sexual health and potency. Routine practice of these exercises strengthens the entire sexual apparatus. The Kegel exercises are discussed at length in this book in the section on the prostate.

Oriental Insight

Oriental science teaches a strategy for treating impotence which is to be used while toning the genital system with herbs. It suggests having no sex and no masturbating (and not even thinking of sex as much as possible) for 100 consecutive days. This way you can build up male sexual potential. You do not waste each little bit that is built by getting a little edge then losing it. Oriental practitioners direct one to build up a reservoir to draw from instead of continually emptying and depleting the male cauldron.

Herbs to Use

Herbs that are particularly appropriate for treating impotence, helping to refill the cauldron, are:

Ashwagandha — An East Indian sexual tonic herb long regarded as promoting fertility and sexual potency. It is a specific for this condition and is impressively effective. It is a primary strengthening tonic used in Ayurvedic science. It is safe, non-irritating and will not overstimulate sexual energy.

Garlic — According to oriental science, 7 to 8 cloves a day will balance systemic yin and yang. It might be a little difficult to get a date with this kind of breath however.

Ginkgo — Being a reliable peripheral vasodilator, Ginkgo has been shown to be an excellent agent for treating arterial erectile dysfunction. It has a direct effect on endothelial cells which enhance blood flow of both penile arteries and veins without any change in systemic blood pressure. The first signs of improved blood supply and regained potency can be seen after 6 to 8 weeks. Continue treatment up to 6 months.

Epimedium — The Chinese name is *Yin Yang Huo*. It is indicated for impotence, stimulating sexual activity and sperm production. Should not be used for prolonged periods of time.

Yohimbe — For short term acute need. Use small amounts infrequently (see the Male Herbal section), just before making love. Gives a increased sense of well being and a sense of openness. Use of this herb can help get one through some difficult times, but its use is not a cure for poor relationships or for the effects of an unwholesome lifestyle.

Saw Palmetto, Ginseng, Sarsaparilla and Wild Yam. (See "The Male Herbal" section for specific information about these herbs.)

Combine these specific herbs in a wholistic formula that also supports other conditions that may be present in an individual's symptom picture (e.g. Nervous system tonics such as Wild Oat and Scullcap and adaptogenic and adrenal gland tonic herbs such as Ginseng, Licorice, Siberian Ginseng and Suma to deal with stress; Ginkgo with Hawthorn to help insure adequate peripheral penile circulation).

Infertility

A couple is judged infertile by clinical standards if conception does not occur after twelve months of adequate cohabitation. About 10% of heterosexual relationships are barren; spermatogenic (development of mature sperm) deficiencies in the male are responsible in at least 40% of these.

Clinically, the most obvious contributors to male spermatogenic deficiency are:

- low sperm count or deficiencies in maturation of germ cells in the semen (which may be a secondary effect caused by hypogonadism (deficient activity of the testis) or hypopituitarism (diminished activity of the pituitary gland)
- low percentage of motile sperm (sperm capable of spontaneous movement)
- short duration of sperm motility
- low percentage of normally formed sperm

Other contributors to male infertility, though rare, are:

- obstruction of the conduction system and
- hypothyroidism (a state produced by deficient secretion of the thyroid gland)

The cause of the above conditions is not usually so obvious. Stress, nervous anxiety and/or an underlying low state of health are three major possibilities. Survival stress due to burn-out can result in a man having no interest in anything other than personal survival issues; his body expressing this in multiple ways.

Creating appropriate combinations of herbs based on the specific needs of the individual man will build a strong nutritional base for a program to help reverse male infertility.

- The adaptogenic herbs, Siberian Ginseng, Ginseng, Suma and Licorice, greatly assist a man to deal with all forms of stress and anxiety. They are excellent tonic herbs to help build the state of health and adaptation to stress necessary to produce adequate sperm count and the libido to deliver it.
- System tonics that build underlying vitality to help reverse infertility and low adrenal energy are: Damiana which is a specific for this purpose. It is a nerve tonic with a strong affinity for the sexual organs. Hawthorn and Ginkgo work to increase cardiovascular power, improving circulation.
- Gentian, Mugwort, Yarrow and Golden Seal are bitter herbs having a secondary affinity for the sexual organs. They stimulate appetite, digestion and assimilation necessary for improving health and increasing energy.
- Sarsparilla, Licorice, Wild Yam and Ginseng provide hormone precursors to help enhance hormonal health.
- Saw Palmetto and Ho show wu are herbs noted to help increase sperm count and improve sperm motility.
- Herbs having alterative action improve the condition of the blood and facilitate overall improvement of health. Alterative herbs that are also specific for the reproductive system supply primary nourishment for eliminating infertility. These herbs are: Sarsaparilla, Red Raspberry leaves, Burdock root and Saw Palmetto berries.

Aromatherapy treatment

Receiving therapeutic body massage on a regular basis, using 5 to 10 drops of pure Rose essential oil added to one ounce of sweet almond oil as a massage oil, is specific to treat infertility, for Rose essential oil appears to increase sperm cell count. The deep relaxation of the massages alone will do wonders for the adrenal and nervous systems. It is helpful to also take Rose oil internally for this condition (one drop of pure Rose oil taken once a day in a little honey and water for two weeks, rest a week, then repeat). In spite of its cost, in the sphere of reproduction and sexuality, Rose is the plant of choice. It has long been renowned as an aphrodisiac. It has a powerful tonic effect on the circulation, digestion, liver and nervous system and probably most important is its effect on the mental and emotional levels. Rose is a gentle but potent anti-depressant, relieving anger and fear, and it is a specific for treating a hangover. True Rose essential oil is very expensive. If you find any for less than $20 a milliliter it is probably not real Rose oil. There are many adulterants in the market place.

When infertility per say is a problem, it is a couple's problem. Sexual technique of the couple needs to be considered, awareness of the "fertile" period in the menstrual cycle taken into serious consideration and exploited. Ejaculation should be avoided for at least three or four days before this time in order that the male can deliver the best quantity and quality of semen. The general health of both members of the couple should be systematically improved by these methods:

- Regulate diet and exercise.
- Vitamin B complex foods and supplements should be insured, especially in the man's diet, so normal inactivation of estrogens by the liver is insured.
- Eradicate any infection, in the male particularly of the prostate.
- Alcoholic, tobacco and other drug excesses need to be curbed, best eliminated altogether.

A cervical cap (a device ordinarily used to block semen from entering the cervix) containing fresh semen placed over the cervix may improve the chances of conception.

Male Contraception

It is important for a male and a female to feel whole, healthy and fertile. Conceiving, birthing and raising children is a sacred event in our lives ... the spirit of a perfect kiss is a happy child (T.E.S.). However at this particular time in the history of our species each of us must take a close look at the impact our expressed fertility will have upon the welfare of our global human family and upon the potential quality of life that will be created for our wonderful children. Mother Earth's environment is showing stretch marks from the explosive swelling of our human population. It is not up to someone else to ultimately control population growth. The fact that the total population of human beings on this planet is racing toward 7 billion explains why we are simultaneously evolving a "naked planet" in an attempt to feed, clothe and house each of us. Like a blanket of hungry locusts, we are consuming Earth's natural animal, vegetable and mineral resources at an alarming rate and casually depositing waste materials in our wake in order to sustain our increasing numbers. At this rate of population increase and absence of recycling procedures, we are simply not journeying into a bountiful, ecologically sound future for our loved offspring to experience. Human population control is an issue that is far more urgent and timely than many of us are presently aware, especially we who live in the still remotely populated land mass of the U.S. and Canada.

Current plant research in Mexico and the Far Eastern countries for developing "new," safe and effective tools for population control is looking seriously at a number of reversible anti-fertility plants which have ancient histories of female and male contraceptive action. The best reversible anti-fertility plant is probably residing in one of our planet's remaining rainforests. It is important that our western family unit of the human species support and contribute to this time-critical research. Our children will honor us for this insight and wisdom.

If excessive sexual drive is a difficulty-factor in one's attempt to moderate one's male-seed sowing there are a couple plant seeds (actually one is a pit) that can possibly help. According to one of my most astute herbalist colleagues, Ed Smith, date pits and pomegranate seeds contain human estrogen (probably why dates and pomegranates are both so delicious). Eating these plant parts (be sure to powder the date pits first) can help decrease excessive sex drive. But, disallowing "decrease" to have the last word, I'll share with you that for another herbalist friend of mine, whose name shall remain confidential by request, Raspberry leaf (organic), taken as a tea, has acted as a reliable aphrodisiac.

> a moment's contemplation,
> what mild bitter-pleasure moves timidly
> within my tiny bowl of tea?

Longevity

Being realistic about longevity, we can underpin a plan for life extension on three well-substantiated axioms of gerontology. These axioms have been researched and published by Dr. Ernst Jokl, a clinical professor of sports medicine and neurology at the University of Kentucky Medical School. They are:

- Sustained exercise and training inhibits the decline of physique which normally comes as a man ages.
- Sustained exercise and training inhibits the decline of physical fitness which normally comes as a man ages.
- Sustained exercise and training inhibits the decline of mental functions which normally comes as a man ages.

143

As Dr. Jokl states, "old athletes up to age 80 are as fit or fitter than nonathletes half their age." You don't have to be a full-time athlete to remain fit, but you do have to exercise regularly to remain youthful and healthy. You have no control of your chronological aging, but you do control your biological aging. It is known for sure that what we used to call natural and inevitable aging is not inevitable and is not natural. It is simply the usual pattern we see, because the majority of people exhibit similar degenerative disorders.

The body is a marvelously adaptive organism. If one performs regular aerobic activities cardiovascular capacity increases; lift weights, and the muscles, bones and connective tissues get stronger; stretch regularly, and flexibility improves; manage stress, eat a sensible nutritious diet and get sufficient rest, and vital energy magnifies; drink sufficient water and protect the skin from harsh elements and the skin and hair age more slowly. All of these activities are well within each person's power to initiate and pursue. Each individual can expand his own longevity by adopting a longevity lifestyle. Play in an occupation that you love, experiencing warm friendships, and when all these factors that are in your control are in place, getting older will be a stimulating, non-enfeebling process of remaining healthy, enjoying life on this beautiful planet and realizing more wisdom. I believe this is what longevity is all about.

As a man ages he experiences a natural polarity reversal. His testosterone hormone production decreases and the estrogenic side of his whole being becomes subtly more expressive. The male being becomes less aggressive, more gentle, his interests turning more inward for the continuation of his spiritual evolution. A woman experiences a similar reversal with estrogen decline interacting more confrontingly and firmly. These are normally smooth transitions, and they facilitate the continual development of subtle maturing awareness. Men become more lovers than pursuers. It is important for boys and men of all ages to be aware of natural male-energy changes and to understand and honor this phenomenon.

For herbal assistance the most obvious combination that comes to mind is regular intake of Hawthorn flowers and berries and Ginkgo. These two tonic herbs work exceptionally well together to tone and strengthen the heart and brain. Include a few more herbs that are well known to improve memory and central nervous system function and that neutralize free radicals (high energy molecular fragments that can run amuck in the body contributing to some diseases and to the aging process), and you have an excellent longevity plant-ally at hand. I suggest the following combination as a basic herbal formula for longevity enhancement:

Hawthorn	4 parts
Ginkgo	4 parts
Siberian ginseng	3 parts
Gotu Kola	2 parts
Ho shou wu (often erroneously called Fo-Ti)	2 parts
Rosemary	1 part
Skullcap	1 part

Note: Whenever you boil water for herbal preparations, or for any other eating purposes, avoid the use of aluminum pots and cookware. Health sciences strongly suspect a dietary link between Alzhemier's disease and unnatural aluminum deposits found in the cerebral cortex of the brain. Alzhemier's disease disrupts the cognitive functions of aging people. This disease places a tremendous burden on longevity to say the least. The use of aluminum is also suspected of greatly irritating arthritic conditions (the aluminum industry criticizes these suspicions as flawed research). If you inspect the inside surface of any well used aluminum pot, you will find it extensively pitted. Aluminum particles have left the cooking utensil and mixed with the liquid solvents (especially the acidic and salty ones) which, unfortunately, were most likely the breakfasts, lunches, hot beverages, snacks and dinners of the user. Aluminum also enters the body through impure drinking water, commercial baking powder, aluminum wrap, aluminum cans, aluminum anti-perspirants, analgesic and antacid OTC medicines and through many current medical vaccines in which alum and aluminum phosphate are included as preservatives.

Longevity Foods
Ms. Bee

If I were asked to select the world's most skilled herbalist and to find the five most excellent potency and longevity enhancers produced on this planet, I'd go directly to Honey Bee turf. The Honey Bee is the Master Herbalist of our planet. She extracts from her local flora and processes through her unique mastership five of the most precious substances found on Earth: honey, royal jelly, pollen, propolis and beeswax. Her skills offer male and female human beings a highly sophisticated menu of foods for nurturing their hormonal systems and improving the quality and length of their lives.

145

I feel that the honey bee is also one of this planet's most exploited animals. I sincerely hope that the reader of this book, who decides to use bee foods will obtain them from beekeepers who work in compassionate symbiotic balance with their apiarian commercial partners.

Dr. Paavo Airola, in his books *Rejuvenation Secrets From Around The World—That Work* and *Everywoman's Book*, reports that Dr. Nicolai Tsitsin, a famed Russian biologist and experimental botanist, spent many years seeking ways to extend life. He sent letters to 200 of the oldest human beings on the planet asking them how they had earned their living and what had been their principle food. 75% of these folks replied. All of them, without exception, stated that one of their principle foods had been honey, a large number of them also being bee keepers. Further investigation by Dr. Tsitsin found that what these people had actually eaten was the residue at the bottom of the bee hives, having sold the pure honey at the market. Laboratory studies showed this residue to be pure pollen that had fallen off the bees' legs as they deposited their honey. A secret of these centenarians was a diet of pollen-rich, natural, unfiltered and unprocessed honey.

Other studies, independent of Dr. Tsitsin's, isolated five other factors also shared by centenarians. They all lived in high altitudes, held positions of responsibility in their community, were vigorously active all their life, had relatively unvarying, set routines and ate a wide variety of unprocessed foods.

The rejuvenating property of pollen rich honey is attributed to the fact that pollen is a direct propagator of life. It is the male germ of the plant kingdom. It is gathered by bees from flower blossoms, mixed with the bee's own digestive enzymes and flown back to the hive. Pollen contains all the known essential nutrients necessary to sustain life, all known water-soluble vitamins (including B_{12}), a rich supply of minerals, trace elements, proteins, carbohydrates, fats, enzymes, steroidal hormone substances and also a gonadotropic hormone (a hormone which is similar to the pituitary hormone, *gonadotropin*, which stimulates sex glands). Both honey and pollen have undergone extensive research, mostly in Russia and Sweden. Both have been found to increase the immunological mechanism and stimulate and rejuvenate glandular activity thereby improving general health.

According to Airola and other sources, pollen is reputed to:
• Increase calcium retention
• Increase hemoglobin count
• Have a beneficial effect on the healing process in conditions such

as weak heart, liver and kidney disorders, constipation, colds, poor circulation, arthritis and insomnia

- Rich in aspartic acid, an amino acid involved in the rejuvenation process especially in the rejuvenation of the sex glands
- Improve energy, endurance and stamina levels due to its rich nutrient composition
- Act as a digestive aid
- Relieve allergy symptoms (see my note below) and bronchial disorders
- Improve prostate problems
- Combat the side effects of chemotherapy treatments
- Used as a skin rejuvenator and
- Has mild aphrodisiac properties

Note: A word of caution regarding the eating of bee pollen. Pollen is collected from a wide variety of flowers. Each batch you purchase or collect is usually composed of different pollens. Be sure to sample a small amount of the raw pollen from the batch that you have chosen to use. On occasion an individual will find that he or she is allergic to certain ones. I get a mild reaction to any pollen samples that include Chamomile pollen. Also, keep in mind that pollen, honey, propolis and royal jelly are highly concentrated nutrients. You require only small amounts to receive their full nutritional benefits. Honey is a concentrated sugar. It is truly a royal sweet and is produced by the bees for their own survival. They produce a lot of it, and I believe in consciously harvesting abundance, but always leaving abundance remaining. Eat small amounts of honey, leaving most of the bees' production to the bee colony. I recommend that honey be eaten as a concentrated nutrient, not merely as a sweet. If you feel you are craving sweets, recognize this as a dietary symptom and take a dose of bitter herb extract to balance out the sweet flavor craving you're experiencing. (See Green's Hypothesis #2)

Following are two basic herbal formulas incorporating bee pollen, designed specifically for male care. Alter them to suit specific symptom pictures.

1. For male adrenal gland nourishment:

Irish Moss	4 parts	Wild Oat	2 parts
Bladderwrack	4 parts	Cayenne	1/2 part
Licorice root	2 parts	Bee Pollen	3 parts
Sarsaparilla	2 parts	Ginger root	2 parts

Siberian Ginseng	2 parts	Ho shou wu	2 parts

Mix and powder these seaweeds, herbs and bee pollen and put into size #00 capsules. Take 1 to 2 capsules, twice a day, or take 1/2 teaspoon of the powder 2 times a day. Exercise regularly.

2. For impotence and/or prostate problems:

Bladderwrack	3 parts	Bee Pollen	3 parts
Gota Kola	2 parts	Wild Oat	2 parts
Saw Palmetto	2 parts		

Prepare and take as formula #1 above.

Royal Jelly is a food produced by the bee herbalists to feed the queen bee. It enables the queen to live 20 times longer than the other bees even though she is producing over 2,000 eggs a day which is a weight greater than her own body weight. Royal Jelly is high in mineral content and is a prolific source of the anti-stress vitamin, pantothenic acid as well as all the other B vitamins, including B_{12}. It is 13% protein, among which are 18 amino acids including all 8 essential amino acids. Studies reported by Dr. Airola show that royal jelly:

- Increases resistance to disease.
- Has an anti-viral and anti-bacterial action, particularly with streptococcus and staphylococcus.
- Lowers cholesterol in human studies.
- Accelerates the healing of wounds when applied topically.
- Accelerates the formation of bone tissue.

Other sources indicate that it appears to work on the nervous system, helping one to feel calmer, and has a beneficial effect on warding off the symptoms of arthritis.

Like other nutrient rich whole foods, Royal Jelly falls into the category of tonic and rejuvenator. As it is non-toxic and there are no known ill-effects from its use, it offers a superior alternative to other pick-me-ups like sugar, alcohol and caffeine, which tend to have a drop-off effect a few hours after use. Royal Jelly's concentration of stable nutrients and its complete list of essential amino acids make it an exceptional supplement for vegetarians and other individuals who are cutting down on meat and dairy. As with all natural supplements, a regular regime is important. The full benefits of using this food emerge after 4 to 6 weeks of regular use.

Propolis is made by bees from tree resins which have anti-microbial actions to protect the tree. This resin is collected by the bees and remetabolized with their own secretions to be used as glue in building and repairing their hives. It is anti-bacterial and anti-viral. The bees also use it to disinfect their hives, placing it around the entrance and around any intruder they have killed to disinfect its carcass. Propolis contains a complex of biologically active enzymes, vitamins, minerals and a special combination of flavonoids which act as cell building components.

Propolis can be chewed as it comes from the hive or it can be made into a liquid extract to treat sore throats and other internal infections. These properties work to raise the body's natural resistance to disease by stimulating and rejuvenating the body's own immune system. Individuals in my family chew a piece of raw propolis (approximately the size of a kernel of corn) whenever they feel a sore throat or any upper respiratory symptoms coming on. While chewing the raw propolis the saliva becomes activated by the resins, and as the saliva is continually swallowed it efficiently distributes the anti-microbial components of the propolis throughout the throat and adjacent areas. After a while, your saliva will actually begin to gently sting your mouth. You can take the propolis out of your mouth for about a half hour and then return it again. Eventually it breaks down as you chew it, and you can swallow the remainder. Ray Hill, the man who is credited with re-introducing the use of propolis to the western cultures, says in his book, *Propolis — The Natural Antibiotic*, that propolis "offers the same immediate action as laboratory produced antibiotics, but without toxic or other side effects." When my daughters were children they enjoyed chewing propolis, so we found it to be a practical and effective medicine for children. I am impressed with its action and keep it on hand in our home and first-aid travel kits. For other internal infections, we take 15 to 30 drops 3 to 4 times a day from a propolis tincture that we make from the raw propolis. When chewing raw propolis, be forewarned that bees have not felt the need to standardize the consistency and stickiness of their product, so when chewing certain (not all, mind you) pieces of propolis, you will find that they readily and tenaciously stick to your teeth. It is advisable to chew raw propolis quite gingerly at first to test it out; if you find it to be relatively soft and sticky, suck on it instead and sort of knead it against the roof of your mouth with your tongue for a while rather than chewing it. It can be a healthy challenge in oral gymnastics, but the health-promoting results are well worth the experience.

Some Exotic Herbal Formulas & Recipes
Designed Specifically to Nourish the Male System

I want to credit my friend and companion herbalist, Rosemary Gladstar, with the following four exotic herbal recipes. Rosemary gives these formulas freely to all who attend her classes, but I suspect that only those individuals who embody the soul of a connoisseur actually prepare them. These herbal preparations make excellent gifts for the man who has everything and intends to use it.

1. The following recipe manifests a collection of ingredients that help provide a man with a continual store of energy. It contains nutrients that are supportive for the male "yang" energy, and is formulated to nourish and tone the male reproductive system over a period of time.
Combine the following *powders* in a bowl:

2 tablespoons	Siberian Ginseng powder
2 tablespoons	Ginseng powder
1 tablespoon	Ginger powder
4 tablespoons	Bee Pollen
6 tablespoons	Pumpkin seeds (ground)
1 tablespoon	Sesame seeds (ground)
1 to 2 tablespoons	Spirulina (a fresh water algae)

Combine in another bowl:
> 3/4 cup of sesame seed butter, almond butter or peanut butter
> 1/4 cup honey

Gradually add the first mixture to the second and knead into a paste. Add roasted carob powder and, if you like, a lightly roasted shredded coconut to sweeten and flavor. Roll into balls and each day eat 1 before and 1 after your daily exercises.

2. Rosemary's Long Life Elixir given next is a male system tonic. Its flavor and culinary presence brings to mind words such as "exquisite" and "for the Gods." It is an herbal tonic which builds strength and vitality, formulated to be taken over a long period of time.

Ingredients:

Ginseng roots	1 to 3 whole roots (restorative tonic/ adaptogen)
Saw Palmetto	1/2 part (reproductive system tonic)
Sarsaparilla	1 part (prostate/glandular tonic)

Wild Yam	2 parts (hormone precursors/tonic)
Sassafras root bark	1 part (alterative/tonic)
Siberian Ginseng	1 part (general tonic/adaptogen)
Ginger	2 parts (circulatory stimulant)
Damiana	1 part (prostate tonic/sexual vitality)
Licorice	2 parts (adrenal gland food/harmonizer)
Ho Shou Wu	2 parts (CNS nutrients/builds male chi)
Astragalus	2 parts (deep immune system support)
Star Anise	1 part (warming stimulant)

Place all the herbs in a quart size glass jar and cover them with a quality brandy. Put the lid on tight and let the extract sit for 6 to 8 weeks in a warm, shaded area. After the weeks have passed, strain the ingredients, discard the spent herbs, but save the whole Ginseng root(s). To each cup of herbal extract add 1/2 cup of black cherry or some other kind of fruit concentrate available in a natural food store (DO NOT USE A FRUIT JUICE, for this will spoil the elixir). Place the Ginseng root(s) back into the elixir. Sip 1 to 2 tablespoons of the elixir daily, storing the rest of it in a refrigerator.

3. An aromatic Long Life Wine that is served as an herbal tonic. If this doesn't, in fact, lengthen one's life, it will certainly help make it a more romantic life. Drink this herbal wine daily in moderate tablespoon doses or take a wineglass full once or twice a week.

Ingredients:

Ginseng	1 root
Damiana	1/4 oz.
Astragalus	1/4 oz.
Coriander seed or pods	1/4 oz.
Star Anise	1/4 oz.

Place herbs in a jar, warm a bottle of red or white wine and pour it over the herbs. Cap herbed wine and let it sit 1 to 2 weeks. Strain the herbal wine, pour it back into the original wine bottle and add back the Ginseng root.

4. An Herbal Fertility Formula designed to help increase sexual potency and vitality in men. 1 to 4 tablespoons should be taken daily, over a period of 3 to 6 months.

Ingredients for group Ω :

| Ginseng root | 1 root |
| Saw Palmetto berries | 1/2 oz. |

Yellow Dock root	1 oz.
Wild Yam root	1/2 oz.
Damiana leaf	1 oz.

Ingredients for group π :

Strawberry leaf	1/4 oz.
Raspberry leaf	1/4 oz.
Nettle leaf	1/4 oz.
Comfrey leaf	1/4 oz.

Simmer the herbs in group Ω in one quart of water over a low heat for 45 minutes. Remove this decoction from the heat and add to it the leaves of group π, stir, cover and let it all sit over night. The next day, strain all herbs from the tea. Place this tea on a very low fire and slowly reduce the herbal liquid to 1/2 quart (1 pint). To each cup of this concentrated liquid, add 1/2 cup honey and 4 tablespoons brandy (the brandy is optional). Store this liquid formula in a refrigerator.

Thank you, Rosemary.

I want to credit one of my other herbalist colleagues, Amanda McQuade Crawford, MNIMH, with the next two life-inflaming herbal recipes, introducing them in Amanda's words, "Aphrodisiacs are named for Aphrodite, Goddess of Love. Here are recipes for wild potions, tonics for women and for men. Remember that love cannot be forced, but it can be created. Use these potions with happiness and goodness."

5. Tried and True Tonic for Men

Ingredients:

Prickly Ash	1 oz.	Licorice	1/2 oz.
Orange Peel	1/2 oz.	Thyme	1/2 oz.
Sarsaparilla	1 oz.	Saw Palmetto	1 oz.
Cinnamon	1/2 oz.	Yohimbe	1/8 oz. (optional)
Valerian	1/2 oz.	Ginseng	1/2 oz. or more

Cover the herbs with 80 proof alcohol (e.g. brandy, vodka) and store in a cool, dark place for 2 weeks. Shake the mixture daily. Then strain and add to taste: honey or barley malt. Replace the Ginseng root(s) in the bottle and leave them indefinitely. Take 1 tablespoonful daily.

6. Red-to-Orange Chakra Express: an herbed red wine

Ingredients:

Allspice	1/2 oz.	Ginger	1 oz.
Cloves	1/8 oz.	Fennel	1/2 oz.

Cinnamon	1/2 oz.	Star Anise	1/2 oz.
Astragalus	1 oz.	Bay leaves	1/2 oz.
Nutmeg	1/2 oz.	Guarana	1/8 oz. (optional: contains caffeine)

Use leaves, seeds, barks and roots as whole as possible. Put into large, see-through bottle, tightly stoppered. Cover liberally with good beaujolais or burgundy wine. Allow two weeks before straining. Warm to room temperature or low heat before sipping slowly. Will store in refrigerator for 2-3 years.

Thank you, Amanda.

And here's one more:

7. Green's Male Song Tea designed to fill the Male Spirit with even more pizzazz.

Sassafras root bark	2 parts
Licorice root	1 part
Ginger root	2 parts
Orange Peel	1 part
Marshmallow root	2 parts
Sarsaparilla root	1 part
Ginseng root or little rootlets	1 part
Cinnamon bark	2 parts

Combine all ingredients with water and simmer over low fire (1 full teaspoon of herb mixture per cup of water). This decocts into a deliciously "yang" male brew. Alter the parts and add whatever to suit your taste.

9

General Health-Care

Human Immunity

Personal hygiene, both external and internal, coupled with regular exercise and a strong functioning immune system is a human being's finest health insurance and the most sophisticated defense against disease. Biologically, each of us is equipped to function as a whole and independent being, quite able to resist invasion of our body tissues by foreign organisms. Wholistically, however, if we allow our nervous system and immune system to become overloaded and over stressed, we seriously wound ourselves and invite ill-health into our life experience.

For a little over a hundred years now, we Westerners have believed that disease attacks us indiscriminately from outside ourselves, and that we live our lives as victims at the whim and pleasure of invisible germs against which we have little defense except the external magic of Western science and the mystique of commercial medical/pharmaceutical technology.

This pervasive cultural belief system has a history that reaches back to the 17th century; to a Cartesian-Newtonian, mechanical, reductionist view of the human body and of humanity's relationship with the universe. This reductionist approach to investigating and understanding the body and its relationship with health and disease divides the body into as many parts as possible, then analyzes each of these parts separately (medical specialization) in the belief that the whole human being will eventually be understood, a little like studying and labelling the pieces of a clock in hopes of eventually understanding time. Some 19th and 20th century beliefs that can be traced directly to these 17th century assumptions about health and illness are:

  • There is an "in here" inside my body and an "out there" outside
    my body that are separate and quite distinct from each other.

154

- The human body is merely a biological machine.
- Disease is a thing in itself, a foreign and hostile entity separate from myself, that is capable of entering and damaging my body.
- Illness is a calamity that strikes from outside of me and must be endured with the help of palliative medications.
- Health is merely the absence of disease symptoms.
- Healing (like disease) occurs independently of the mind, emotions and human consciousness.
- The level of health depends on the quality of medicine.
- Health (healing) results from what someone or something does for us or to us, rather than what we do for ourselves.

In the 1800s our Western cultural science still perceived the human body as a collection of parts that existed as mostly separate from the spirit, mind and emotions. Hand in hand with this perception, Western civilization began to embrace the belief — which has evolved into nearly a religious belief — that our Western science and its particular scientific method is a uniquely objective, dispassionate, direct line of sight into truth and reality.

It must be pointed out that "science" is merely a cultural way of knowing, and nothing more. Science is not absolute, but is relative to already existing cultural beliefs. A culture's science is a subjective, deeply conditioned, cultural attitude toward the world, which has taken shape in the collective consciousness of the culture over centuries. The Oriental-Asian sciences, the shamanic science of the Mexican Huichol Indians, the Haitian Voodoo science, etc., are each vastly different but equally valid ways of knowing and experiencing reality. Each of these sciences evolved from a different cultural perception of reality, but each of these sciences is no less real or unreal than our own. We live what we know. If we believe the universe and ourselves to be mechanical and vulnerable to attack by micro-organisms, we will live mechanically and give overwhelming power to the local micro-organisms. Norman Cousins discusses this phenomenon: "The greatest force in the human body is the natural drive of the body to heal itself, but that force is not independent of the belief system, which can translate expectations into physiological change. Nothing is more wondrous about the fifteen billion neurons in the human brain than their ability to convert thoughts, hopes, ideas and attitudes into chemical substances. Everything begins, therefore, with belief. What we believe is the most powerful option of all."

We Westerners believe that germs cause disease. Few of us question this "fact" of life. Looking at the cause of human disease through the eyes of a germ-theory which sees microbes as the *primary* cause of disease is much like viewing life in general through the eyes of Hollywood film makers. In fact, we have been doing both for about the same amount of time. Like all Hollywood plots and celluloid illusions, the infamous "germ theory" as initially proposed by Louis Pasteur and Robert Koch in the late 1800s is over-simplified, inaccurate and tragically misleading when applied to daily life. But it reigns as the cornerstone and foundation of our culture's common concept and understanding of the cause and cure of human disease.

The overwhelming rapidity with which the germ theory of disease became accepted by the Western allopathic medical profession was a spectacular historical phenomenon. And although I'm sure today's allopathic physicians no longer believe that germs are the sole cause of disease, there has been very little public educational information to the contrary promoted and sponsored by this influential group of health authorities, and there has been equally little informed, insightful media coverage that would help educate the lay population to believe otherwise. This is not meant to demean the persistent, informed efforts of the allopathic general practitioners and family doctors who spend the bulk of their professional time imploring their patients to change lifestyle habits so their patients will quit killing themselves with self-destructive diet, drink and smoke.

The historic one-germ-one-disease theory initially put forth by Pasteur and Koch in 1881 basically postulated that each type of germ is responsible for invading an unsuspecting individual and producing a specific type of illness. In their historic "Doctrine of Specificity," they postulated that "certain microscopic entities whose appearance in space and time correlates well with other physical manifestations of illness are causative of illness." This Doctrine of Specificity, Pasteur's original theory that germs were the primary cause of disease, was quickly refuted and disproven by a number of his contemporaries, most notably Claude Bernard and I.M. Setchenov.

In spite of the published research findings of Pasteur's and Koch's contemporaries, demonstrating the profound limitations in Pasteur's conclusion, Pasteur's initial theory was dynamically reinforced by the actions of the current university trained allopathic physicians (at that time referred to as the "regular" doctors). These regular doctors were desperately seeking a nucleus around which to build some sort of "science" so as to move into a form of prominence as a healing profession, setting themselves apart from the other diverse systems of health-care that were co-existing. Historically, this came at a time when the regular doctors' heroic use of bleeding, leeches, and mercury was killing their patients. The initial postulates of Pasteur and his co-proponent Robert Koch unintentionally provided the regulars an eagerly adopted scientific nucleus.

Little notice was taken when in 1882 Pasteur restated his theory describing germs as a secondary rather than primary cause of disease; the debilitated terrain came first. The linear events and politics of the misinterpretation and rise into prominence of his initial theory of disease and the succeeding medical practices thereof makes interesting reading. It illustrates how belief systems based on certain assumptions — which are marketed as a science, though not necessarily based on irrefutable evidence — can move and design the collective consciousness of an entire culture.

What I believe is more relevant and significant for the laymen of today is the unsung work of Pasteur's fellow contemporary research scientists. They clearly demonstrated in rebuttal to Pasteur's doctrine of specific etiology that:

- Disease micro-organisms seek their natural habitats: diseased tissue.
- Germs vary their fermentative effect in conformity with the medium in which they find themselves (I suggest referring to the role of germs in disease more accurately as the Germ Banquet Theory).
- The host has to be in a certain state of debility before germs can settle into body tissue or cause disease.
- The disease process is dependent on the terrain, the underlying health of the body.

Our cultural belief system needs to dispel its exaggerated, misleading fear of germs and replace this conditioned response with a positive attitude toward nourishing and maintaining a spontaneously disease-resistant condition of health. Whether or not we fall prey to the natural activities of microbes depends much more on the ecological state of our communities, our bodies and our diets than on the presence of bacteria and viruses. We breathe in and swallow many thousands of microbes every hour without any ill effects. In fact, human beings in good health harbor many potentially pathogenic microbes such as diptheria, meningitis, polio virus and staphylococci bacilli, and sometimes disease symptoms are present without specific "causative" germs. As Lewis Thomas lucidly points out in his work, *The Lives of a Cell,* "Most bacteria are totally preoccupied with browsing, altering the configurations of organic molecules so that they become usable for the energy needs of other forms of life. In real life, even in our worst circumstances, we [humans] have always been a relatively minor interest of the vast microbial world. Pathogenicity is not the rule. Indeed, it occurs so infrequently and involves such a relatively small number of species, considering the huge population of bacteria on the earth, that it has a freakish aspect. Disease usually results from inconclusive negotiations for symbiosis, an overstepping of the line by one side or the other, a biologic misinterpretation of borders."

Mind you, if a body's underlying health is low and its tissues have been adversely affected by microorganisms, the body will usually need help to diminish the microorganism population, strengthen the affected tissue and bring about a healing. At this point of crisis, a change in nutrition without the concurrent use of more concentrated preparations will often be insufficient. Timely use of concentrated (herbal or chemical) medicine is appropriate and often necessary. Herbal teas and other concentrated herbal extracts are vitally active nutritional medicines; the most concentrated herbal agents being the pure plant essential oils (see "Aromatherapy" section). After a crisis has subsided, change in general nutrition and lifestyle is appropriate and probably essential to rebuild and strengthen the body's terrain and enhance its immune system.

Nature is a truly balanced economy. When the chemistry of the body is thrown out of balance by factors (which are basically in our control) such as faulty nutrition, routine pig-outs, overwork, lack of exercise, overstress, lack of cleanliness, environmental pollution, negative thought patterns, suppressed feelings, radiation, accidents, etc. toxins accumulate and the entire organism marshals its healing forces in an effort to meet the emergency and make adjustments. This effort is expressed in many ways: fever, disturbed breathing, accelerated circulation (swelling/inflammation), intensified bowel elimination (diarrhea), swelling of lymphatic glands, pain (indicating presence of irritants), eruptions and/or mucous discharge to expel poisons and/or catarrh. These are actually symptoms of the body's spontaneous self-healing process. They are signs that the body is taking care of business.

Other factors that may increase our susceptibility to microbial infection are extremely poor living conditions such as widespread famine or the introduction of infectious agents with which we have not had any experience — which is the principle behind bacteriological warfare (or the giving of pox-infected blankets as gifts). These last two factors create potentially life-threatening situations, but they do not constitute the main problem of disease in ordinary life where human beings, animals and microbes establish an equilibrium endemic to the community.

Germs are companion species to all living beings on this planet. They are an essential and normal part of our internal and external environment. They assist us in maintaining a balanced and efficient biological economy. When we allow our bodies to reach a saturation point of accumulated morbid matter, germs proliferate and set up a dynamic process in the body, frequently referred to by non-medical practitioners as a cleansing or healing crisis, i.e., fever, expulsion of mucous during a cold or flu, etc. Healthy tissue is resistant to microbial invasion and proliferation. It isn't until body tissue develops a malnourished disease condition or a poorly attended wound that a weakening of its defenses occurs and infection is allowed to spread. We have come to associate microbes with various disorders that occur during these times of proliferation and we regard them as causes rather than symptoms.

Experiments have shown that bacteria can change their form by altering their medium and environment (i.e., a pneumococcus to a streptococcus and a streptococcus to a staphylococcus). As Florence Nightingale stated after years of studied observation and intimate experience with hospital patients, "There are no specific diseases; just specific disease conditions."

It has been suggested that some of these disease conditions might be sown by the geography of our mind. Some medical researchers theorize that chronic negative thought causes the separation of micro-organismal genetic material from normal cells and this replicates independently in the environment of toxic tissue. An overgrowth of micro-organisms is seen as the result of disease rather than the cause, with disease (and health) occurring in humans partially due to how they think. The mind is a powerful creator.

Recent evidence from brain and consciousness research, anthropology, microbiology, neurophysiology and elemental physics conflicts with current orthodox medical science. These research disciplines reveal that body, mind and consciousness are inseparable, an indivisible whole, a dynamic continuum. The universe, so long thought to consist of innumerable separate parts, appears at its primary level as an unbroken wholeness, a single dimension independent of Time and Space in which the apparently (to the senses) separate parts are not in the least separated, but are (Divinely?) intimately connected.

Evidence that clearly challenges the Cartesian theory of mind-body separation comes primarily from investigation of the structure, chemistry and function of the human brain and nervous system and from studies of the neurophysiology of stress, of split-brain patients, biofeedback, meditation and the vast windows that have been opened by the evolving insights of quantum physics. Our universe is being perceived and experienced as four dimensional, with Time as the fourth dimension. An unbroken wholeness is the newly evolved understanding of the order of reality, an order in which all things—space, time, matter and energy—are immediately and intimately connected at the most fundamental level of reality. These data represent strong supportive evidence for the wholistic assumption about the nature of man and of man's interaction with the world in relation to health. Health is equated with an individual's experience of this harmony of the oneness of man and cosmos. Nature is not a force over which we must triumph, but is the ultimately compassionate medium of our transformation. Illness is seen as a guide, a teacher; possibly our life's most profound teacher. The symptoms of our condition are dynamic attention-getters which contain clear metaphors for what is missing, what is excessive or what is otherwise out-of-balance in our lives. Once we learn to make sense of rather than merely suppress or palliate our symptoms and begin to see more clearly their immediate appropriateness in our life, the next steps in our healing process become more obvious, and consequently we know and understand ourselves better.

Unfortunately, many practitioners of "modern" medicine and the general consciousness of our lay population have not joined this culture's scientific/spiritual revolution that is replacing the mechanistic Newtonian view of the world with quantum physics, recognizing and marvelling at the magnificent interrelatedness of all things.

Quantum mechanics strongly recognizes that the conscious observation of the patient by the therapist and laying of hands on the patient alters the state of the patient faster than the speed of light (There is a mysterious and wonderful power that one human being can have on another through the simple act of caring). This discovery brought into focus for us by Mr. Einstein and his contemporary visionaries proved that an "observer effect" happens instantaneously when the human mind is applied or directed to a physical experiment or to another living being. This is a profound discovery, significant in the history of medicine and healing, and it serves as a bedrock on which chiropractics, homeopathy, shamanic and other forms of biocybernetic medicines can further build their health-care sciences. Modern techniques are frequently merely variations of ancient ones. It is to be hoped that conventional medicine will not continue to look the other way while the nonmedical sciences confirm the validity of the alternate therapies which western mainstream medical science has continually denied. Clearly these alternate therapies do not bolster orthodox medicine's obsolete social prestige and profit motivation, but from my recent professional relationship with young inspired allopathic physicians, it is obvious to me that the consciousness of allopathic medicine is being forcibly uplifted (rather than allowing itself to be abandoned by its progressively more enlightened patients) by these bright, sincere allopathic healers who refuse to continue looking the other way.

Like the dynamic function of disease and tragedy in each of our personal lives, the highly visible ARC/AIDS epidemic is functioning in our culture as a crisis, bringing about cataclysmic though ultimately positive change and revolutionary alteration of stagnant beliefs. The ARC/AIDS disease process is spotlighting a sizeable, though not yet popularly perceived, crack in the teaching of the sacrosanct Doctrine of Specificity. The continual inability to ignore this fissure arises from the layman's deeply conditioned attempt to (understand) fit ARC/AIDS into the one-disease-one-cause bag. As is customary, most of us are passively waiting for the magic bullet vaccine to be manifested by some medical miracle worker. Yet, almost every month new viruses other than the HIV virus are discovered that are associated with the disease process. The ARC/AIDS disease process is found to be a host of diseases which have a host of tissue pathologies and attending micro-organisms.

Today there is a relatively new medical concept called *Co-factors*. Co-factors are agents (chemical, germ, diet, behavior, stress or lifestyle habits) which have been demonstrated to be part of the cause of a disease process, that influence health and make it possible for disease to occur. The "unorthodox" wholistic health-care practitioners have been teaching this concept for years. In cancer research the word "Promotor" (synthetic chemicals) is used instead. But there cannot be stated a one-promotor-one-cancer theory either, because a single promotor can be related to several types of cancer or in some cases it causes no cancer at all.

Now that ARC/AIDS and cancer are opening the bag, it's merely a matter of time before the cat steps out. And sooner or later the public will catch on to the implications of this for all disease. The implications line up as follows:

- The onset of disease processes is not a stroke of bad luck, the attack of a germ or a simple matter of being in the wrong place at the wrong time.
- There is no single cause for disease. Disease is the result of many different factors unique to each person's life.
- For the most part, these factors are within the range of choices made by the person who develops the disease.
- The patient is not a victim, the doctor (or any other health practitioner) is not the savior.
- There is no "fix-it" or "magic bullet" system of health-care, be it allopathic, homeopathic, chiropractic, naturopathic or herbal.
- Disease is ultimately under the control of the person, not the doctor. The state of one's health does not depend on the state of medicine.
- It is what we choose to do in our life that makes the difference.

The tragedy of the past hundred years of popular belief in the one-germ-one-disease theory is that we lay people have come to fear and blame germs as the cause of our disease, and we have willingly transferred responsibility for our health from ourselves to the doctors or to any other practitioner who offers us a "magic bullet" or an "I'll fix you" cure.

It remains that normal, well-nourished, well-exercised human tissue functioning in a reasonably hygienic environment, motivated by healthy thought and emotions is not successfully overwhelmed by other organisms. It is the inability of a human being's natural resistance to adapt to external forces and maintain the body's physical integrity that promotes disease by developing debilitated, diseased tissue. This allows competing micro-organisms a tactical advantage and a fertile environment for growth.

Returning to the concept that "science is a cultural way of knowing the universe," I would like to share some insights presented in a book which was reviewed in *Newsweek* magazine (Sept. 19, 1988 issue) titled *Medicine & Culture* written by a medical journalist named Lynn Payer. Lynn Payer has found in her eight years as a medical journalist that the way doctors view disease and deal with their patient's ailments is determined predominantly by the doctor's national, cultural heritage. Medicine as practiced in the U.S. is quite aggressive, having evolved from the "can do" spirit of the frontier. Wanting to do as much as possible, American doctors order more diagnostic tests and focus more on the role of external agents, including micro-organisms as a cause of disease than do their European colleagues. They also prescribe drugs more frequently, whenever possible resort to surgery, view disease as an enemy to be conquered, are quick to prescribe massive doses of antibiotics for most any infection and expect their patients to be equally as aggressive in their efforts to "beat" the disease. Compared to this manner of practicing medicine, British medicine appears to be considerably more benign. English doctors don't regard the body as a machine, don't suggest regular checkups and order only half as many X-rays as American doctors do. English doctors, when in doubt about a patient's condition, will choose to not treat the symptoms (granted this probably has much to do with economic necessity). French doctors are very respectful of body aesthetics. They use surgery as infrequently as possible; have great respect for a woman's childbearing ability; perform hysterectomies only for extremely serious conditions and believe that the patient's constitution and bodily terrain plays a major part in disease, prescribing nutritional supplements to enhance the terrain more often than prescribing drugs to kill germs. (Note: French physicians employ the use of essential oils with well-documented success in promoting health and treating disease. Consequently aromatherapy is so highly respected in France that it is covered by the French socialized medical plan including the cost of prescribed essential oils.)

Lynn Payer's most salient conclusion is that the physician's choice of diagnoses and treatments is more an art, clearly (like a culture's science) a reflection of the culture from which it comes.

Community Immunity

Over 140 years ago, a medical researcher named Robert Virchow published a statement that remains a cornerstone for social and community health. Following his studies of a number of epidemic outbreaks, he pointed out that: "History has shown more than once that the fates of the greatest empires have been decided by the health of their peoples or of their armies, and there is no longer any doubt that the history of epidemic disease must form an inseparable part of the cultural history of mankind. Epidemics correspond to large signs of warning which tell the true statesman that a disturbance has occurred in the development of his people which even a policy of unconcern can no longer overlook."

This lovely little planet is our celestial turf, and at present, our species needs to work on cleaning up the yard. Today, human-made global pollution and accompanying stress (our universal co-factors) appear to be skewing planetary living conditions via our human bodies, in favor of the micro-organisms (especially the viruses). Herpes and AIDS with the human papilloma virus (HPV) rapidly gaining in prominence are presently our civilization's most visible warnings.

It appears to me that the nervous systems and the immune systems of our human bodies are systematically depleting themselves as they respond to the necessity of continually detoxifying the body's intake of our excessive manufacturing of environmental pollutants. We are once again contending with a lesson on practical hygiene. Historically, this is not our species' first bout with widespread, contagious, fatal community diseases sponsored by poor hygiene. Due to the extremely poor living conditions and pathetic personal hygiene of the 15th century European lifestyle, the collective human immune system in the European cultures fell below the threshold of successful resistance to the Pasteurella pestis bacteria, creating a continental arena for the bubonic plague. Today, due to poor internal and external environmental conditions developed by our modern civilization and commerce, once again our collective nervous and immune system is falling below a threshold of successful resistance. The waters that flow within our body mirror those that flow in our environment. When we dump and spill toxic waste into the oceans, rivers and lakes and underground streams, we dump the identical waste into our bodies' blood streams, and our immune systems have to clean it up. We can't escape this dynamic inner/outer connection. Nothing can ever be "thrown away." There is no "away." It all stays right here on our planet, in our bodies, which are everywhere and in every way interconnected. Pollute the air outside our lungs with exhaust fumes or toxic sprays and the same toxic air is taken into our bodies. Our bodies are not somehow insulated, apart from the surrounding environment. Our immune systems are designed to efficiently filter this external environment as it comes within, but each individual's immune system has its limits. Ultimately, we process internally what we create externally. Cancer, chronic infections, Auto-Immune Deficiency Syndromes, etc. have arrived here *with* our environmental pollutants. These disease conditions appearing in our bodies are not separate from the disease conditions we are creating on our planet's surface. Spray our crops with poisons and we eat poisonous foods. "Germs" are not attacking us, causing illness in us. They are thriving, according to the design of Nature, in our internal system which is becoming less and less able to expel them with its preoccupied, overstressed, depleted natural resistance. They are living efficiently on the internal toxic waste that is accumulating within humankind; it is the same waste that mankind is spreading on the planet and eating, dumping in the water and drinking, diffusing into the air and breathing. All the elements of our environment flow through our bodies like water and sand through a fine sieve. In our body, if these elements are pure and natural, they nourish and invigorate; if not, they stress and burden our immune systems. Male (and female) health depends on male (and female) care of our planet. A conclusion regarding human resistance to disease drawn by anthropologists James Downs and Hermann Bleibtreu in their text book, *Human Variation* (Glencoe Press, 1972) reads as follows: "differential rates of disease occurrence between populations cannot be safely assumed to be the consequence of inherited racial traits. To date, the preponderance of evidence suggests that the contrary is most likely true and that disease has more to do with the way a population lives than with the susceptibility of its ancestors."

We are seeing another page of history being filled by the saga of humankind's bout with a highly contagious, highly fatal, community disease sponsored by poor hygiene. This time it is named the AIDS (or cancer or whatever) plague. On one level, our personal hygiene and living quarters sanitation has improved greatly due to what was learned about what was required to rise above the plague bacteria of the Middle Ages. Now we must learn to clean up our global air, waterways and earth surface to rebuild our resistance to the present day plagues. We'll never kill off the viruses; it's not necessary (15th century's Pasteurella pestis bacteria still exist in great quantity). We'll again have to learn how to restore a hygienic environment, enhance our immune systems and successfully rise above lethal viral infection. The virus will continue to exist as a companion species, but with a restored nourishing environment, the human species will no longer be so vulnerable. We will become wiser as a result, and our political and economical structures will have been forced to evolve in order for our species to survive.

Take care of the Earth; it's good medicine.

Perceiving the cause, prevention and cure of disease in a new light as discussed above, humankind might begin to accept more direct responsibility for its own doing and undoing and quit trying to blame the primary cause of its illnesses on "germs." Western medicine's commitment to a germ theory of disease has repeatedly failed to eradicate or even reduce overall disease in spite of spending billions on technological research, seeking more ways to kill more germs. There is just more to it than that. Though immune suppressant antibiotics have helped to stem acute infection, they rank a weak second in disease prevention to simple immune system supporting, personal and environmental hygiene and nutrition for fostering individual and community health. And these over-prescribed germ-killing antibiotics are now proving powerless against many of today's new strains of antibiotic-resistant germs that have taken on mankind and its medicines (See "Aromatherapy" section).

As I see it, no modern drug can heal deeply stressed, toxin-bombarded human bodies. It can only act chemically and can merely suppress symptoms for a while. Drugs have no curative power. We have to go back to the basics, relearn and again practice simple nutrition and hygiene. However, this time we have little choice but to tend first to local, national and global environmental hygiene.

Our planet Earth, that is our total global and immediate environment, has to be cured of humankind's "sanitary," but environmentally toxic, throw-a-ways. There is no drug or chemical that will suppress or remove this unprecedented environmental condition or that will magically rid our homelands of our own (not some germ's) crude pollution; just as there is no drug or serum that will magically cure a human being of cancer, arthritis, AIDS or any other chronic condition of ill health. We have to change our lifestyle, embracing fundamental hygiene, the medical profession's greatest medical discovery. I believe there is no other practical answer to the health issues we face today.

It is concerning the cleaning up and elimination of toxic waste that the current overt power structure must pause in its irrationally avid pursuit of progress and hear the wisdom of wholistic herbalism. As herbalism teaches, it is first, our symbiotic relationship with the plants, the animals and the minerals that begets wellness and greatness and true prosperity. We world-wide bosses, politicians, corporate chairmen and military generals, the fathers, the brothers, the sons, all, must soon comprehend what is causing today's plagues; what is causing disease in our lives and our family member's lives. But, lest this becomes a finger pointing solely at the male gender and not simultaneously at the female, it must be noted that today women are substantial stockholders of this nation's corporate structure. As investors women are demanding progress, profit and routine dividends. Males may presently be the *overt* corporate and political powers, but the females are the *covert* powers contributing equally to the western corporate and political responsibility (and/or irresponsibility) that is creating a major proportion of our global environmental conditions. The intelligence and wisdom of the current global human power structure is being challenged (pressured) by disease to support the cleansing and healing of our planet. If I may renovate a timely vision: Ask not what your country can do for you, ask what you and your country can do for our planet and its inhabitants. This will I hope, in time, evolve the concepts of corporate-responsibility, political-integrity and military-intelligence out of the category of oxymoron.

It would be tremendous public relations and healing for a business/corporation (as it sincerely invests in the significant control and elimination of its environmentally hazardous practices and technology) to simultaneously caretake (adopt) a threatened or endangered animal or plant species and invest significantly in this species's preservation. You can bet that I will support and use the products of a corporation that is sincerely cleaning up its own act and also shows the heart and consciousness to invest its energy helping me save the elephant, or the grizzly, or the spotted owl, the dorcas gazelle, the redwoods, the golden seal herb, the tiger, the tiny kangaroo rat, the dwarf wedge mussel, the black-necked crane, the Asian river turtle, the wild ducks, the tiger salamander, the frogs, the . . .

Rx: To enhance your immune system: Do something on the job, at school and at home to help clean up our planet (we can all use the exercise). Eat whole, unadulterated, high complex carbohydrate, low fat, quality-protein foods, chew well; take time for adequate bowel movements; incorporate into your diet immune supporting herbs such as Echinacea, Calendula, Yarrow, Astragalus, Siberian Ginseng, Yerba Manza, Horseradish, Garlic & fresh Basil (think, pesto), Usnea, Thyme, Nasturtium and Osha root to name a few. Exercise and stretch regularly; have fun with your life and strive to meticulously avoid chemical food additives and medicines unless absolutely necessary.

An immune supporting life-style includes: Therapeutic body massage for stress reduction, laughter & kindness (see *The Healing Brain:*

Medical Discoveries about How the Brain Manages Health by Ornstein & Sobel), regular vigorous exercise with adequate rest and sleep, growing a vegetable/flower garden and planting more trees; avoiding prolonged excesses and developing the ability to comfortably say "no" when feeling "no." Taking care of one's self and one's precious community. As James E. Lovelock, geochemist and author of the book, *Gaia, A New Look at Life on Earth* told an interviewer on KNBR radio, "We'll never knock off the planet; it can take care if itself. We may knock off ourselves as a species, but life will go on. You have to do something personally. Don't expect government to do it."

Aromatherapy

At the beginning of this herbal I briefly discussed the contrasts between what I called "allopathic" and "alternative" medicines. Working with aromatherapy, we find a unique blend of these two general approaches to health-care. Like Apollo and Artemis working together again, at last. We have the availability of extensive medical research regarding the pharmacological activity of essential oils, and we have the immediate sensual, experiential effects of fragrance on our personal human psyche.

Aromatherapy, the use of pure essential oils to enhance health, beauty and psychological well-being, possesses the unique aesthetic dimension of aroma to add to its potent medicinal energy. Everyone, man, woman and child can enjoy using aroma. Presently and throughout history, selecting aromas for one's personal use is an act in which both males and females indulge with equal care, enthusiasm and enjoyment. This choice of aromas is intuitive and completely personal. Using fragrances takes advantage of our nose's direct hookup with the limbic system, that part of the brain connected with memory and emotions; the part of our brain that stays in touch with our most ancient roots and with the saga of our evolution as a species. A special feature of this scent-triggered memory is that, not only do we relive the memory evoked by a scent, but we re-feel the emotions that went with it. By tapping into the limbic brain, a direct key to which is scent, using the sensual aromas of plant's essential oils we can regain awareness and the feelings of our genetic, vital connection with the Earth (the elements), with the other animals and with the plants. This can profoundly change one's perspective to things. All things. The aroma of essential oils has the therapeutic, healing ability to change a human being's feelings (in a different fashion, but as gently and benignly as the Bach Flower Essences do). Aside from the scent, the physical properties, herbal actions and pharmacological effects are complementary therapeutic elements of the energy of essential oils. These elements are more Apollonesian, so to speak, and understood more by some through the language of medical research.

The olfactory nerve cells are unique in the human nervous system. They are the only nerve cells that regenerate themselves. Also, unlike the cells of other sensory systems, one neural cell both receives and transmits impulses to the brain. This is the body's two way communication system to the rest of nature. This is how the aroma of flowers and pheremones speak to our soul.

It is often a difficult task to adopt lifestyle techniques that one is not familiar with, especially when it comes to the emotion triggering issues of diet and health-care. In order to initiate an understanding and belief system that allows experimentation with an unfamiliar technique, one has to perceive introductory information through a trusted and familiar language. The rational language of science or the language of mainstream medical research appears to me to be the language most trusted and understood by the majority of males rather than the more illusive language of intuition. The medicinal use of natural plant essential oils, while being extremely primal, sensual and intuitive, is at the same time backed by an impressive battery of scientific, phytomedical research and literature published by French allopathic physicians practicing aromatherapy and phytotherapy. But there is a limit to what one can communicate about a plant using only this technical language. Science is often unable to explain why plant remedies work. Western scientific method very often inhibits a true understanding of the action of herbs, because the entire plant (or essential oil) is rarely, if ever, tested. Only a component of the plant (or of the oil) is tested and usually only on its effects on disease (rather than disease prevention and health maintenance) and usually on non-human animal systems rather than on humans suffering from illness (however, the French phytomedical literature is based heavily on empirical research, derived from treating sick folks). Evidence accumulated from scientific research into the action of essential oils establishes a means of dialogue that can help bridge the gap for some individuals between empirical and rational investigation.

I offer this particular introduction to aromatherapy to men (and women) who appreciate the availability of scientific medical research for paving their inroad to a new concept for alternative health-care. European phytomedical research has unintentionally scribed quite a unique bonding circle around the allopathic and the alternative approaches to health-care. As expressed by Dr. Kurt Schnaubelt, author of *Aromatherapy Course*, "With regard to aromatherapy these research studies are interesting, even though they usually fail to recognize the greater concept. Their value lies in the fact that, by using a format and terminology acceptable to mainstream medicine, they serve to overcome doubts. Another aspect is that these studies usually lack an understanding of the nature of a whole essential oil. Often the objective is to prove the efficiency of a single component. Quite interestingly, such studies often report that a complete essential oil is more effective than could be accounted for by the sum of the effects of its components. Such unintentional proof of a wholistic viewpoint is quite frequent in medicinal plant research."

The purpose of this brief introduction to aromatherapy for male health-care is not to explain how to use essential oils or to discuss the materia medica of this system of phytotherapy. For a source of that information, you are well advised to subscribe to Dr. Schnaubelt's "Aromatherapy Correspondence Course" or attend in-depth workshops in "Aromatherapy Training" taught by my wife, Mindy Green, at the California School of Herbal Studies. I do, however, want to present a brief explanation of the antimicrobial action of essential oils. And though I'm more inclined to discuss the powerful immune enhancing qualities of many essential oils, I find it very interesting how these essential oils at the same time fatally perplex the local micro-organisms. I'm convinced that they do it much more cleverly than the medical antibiotics to which micro-organisms are developing an alarming natural resistance. I understand that there are now in existence certain strains of micro-organisms that are even antibiotic dependent; they cannot exist without regular servings of pharmaceutical antibiotics.

The antimicrobial action of essential oils is the property of these aromatic oils that has been known by humankind for the longest time. Consequently, essential oils have been used as preservatives for foods and cosmetics and as medicines in most all human cultures. Modern science has been studying this effect since the late 1800s, but only recently has research been published that partially explains how the cellular and molecular mechanism of essential oils manifests this antimicrobial action.

The molecules that construct essential oils are quite small, penetrating the skin 100 times more effectively than water and 10,000 times more effectively than salt. A consequence of this characteristic is that essential oils have the inherent ability to dissolve in and easily penetrate lipid skin tissue. This ability to penetrate the skin is extremely high compared to other substances. Applying diluted essential oils to the skin is as therapeutically efficient (probably even more effective) than taking them orally. It's been found that essential oils (being lipid soluble) will dissolve in biological membranes. The cell walls of bacteria are such membranes, and in these cell walls most of the breathing and consequent formation of ATP (an important energy source of the living cell) takes place. It has also been found that essential oils contain terpenoid compounds, and that low concentrations of different terpenoid compounds can significantly inhibit oxygen intake (cellular breathing) and the formation of ATP in the cell walls. The terpenoid compounds that are known to have the strongest antibacterial effects, such as thymol and carvacrol can completely block oxygen intake in cell membranes (this is all discussed in Kurt's correspondence course and Mindy's classes).

The plant genius of essential oils' particular method of "doing in" aerobic bacteria resides in the fact that they block oxygen intake, and the microbe simply cannot adapt to impaired breathing. If the essential oils were to interfere with only a specific aspect of bacterial living, like pharmaceutical antibiotics do, it is likely that resistance would be developed. Pharmaceutical antibiotics interfere with a very specific metabolic function that certain individual bacteria within a strain have resisted and adapted to, reproducing and creating a mutant strain that is completely resistant to (sometimes dependent on) that particular antibiotic. This adaptation by micro-organisms does not occur with essential oils. Essential oils likewise have a direct effect on *anaerobic* bacteria like tetanus and clostridium. The action of the essential oils fatally interferes with the ATP energy metabolism of these anaerobic bacteria.

As outlined by Pierre Franchomme in his Phytoguide No. 1 titled *Aromatherapy: Advanced Therapy of Infections*: "Essential oils are most certainly the best remedy known against infections. They act directly to neutralize pathogenic germs and, simultaneously but indirectly, to correct the humoral terrain and regulate the immune system. They can therefore be qualified as "EUBIOTICS" because they favor life, as opposed to antibiotics (meaning "anti-life") which are principally destroyers of anaerobic flora. Aromatherapy is a serious alternative to anti-biotherapy." One of the biggest advantages of using essential oils as antibiotic substitutes is that they do not disrupt or harm beneficial intestinal flora. They are effective in a wholistic program against pathogenic bacteria, parasites, fungus and yeast, but most exciting is their effectiveness against virus. Aromatherapy supports the body's own immune system.

External applications of mild essential oils used for skin care in massage oils or bath oils and bath salts are efficient agents for routine use to reduce the likelihood of bacterial infection because of their antimicrobial properties and the ease with which they penetrate the skin (see section on Skin-Care). Also, as nutritional supplements, some essential oils are highly efficacious. Essential oil of Rose, for example, increases the production of healthy sperm. Concurrently, and equally important, essential oils smell exquisite, instantly inducing olfactory and emotional aesthetics into one's immediate environment.

I want to make one final note in regards to the use of essential oils. Pure essential oils are 70 times more concentrated than the herbs they are extracted from. This increases their healing powers but also increases their toxicity level. They can be very irritating to the skin if applied undiluted. It is necessary to dilute (to a 2% to 10% solution) essential oils with a fixed oil such as hazelnut oil, sweet almond or wheat germ oil or in water before using them therapeutically or cosmetically. An example of a 2% dilution is 10-12 drops of essential oil in 1 oz. of carrier fixed oil. There are some exceptions to using undiluted (neat) essential oils: Lavender and Tea Tree can be safely used neat on bites, burns, scrapes, etc. with no burning or irritation. Please consult an aromatherapy book for more information. If one wants to take essential oils orally, do so *only* with the supervision or advice of a skilled aromatherapist. When prepared and administered correctly (which is not difficult to learn, but requires knowledge) pure plant essential oils are powerful healers.

I foresee Aromatherapy as the branch of phytotherapy that will gracefully pierce the medical/pharmaceutical shield and become a widely embraced system of natural healing. I sincerely recommend pursuing the study of this phyto-art and science (see list of aromatherapy texts in Herbal Resources section).

Diet

The quality of the food we eat determines the quality our body becomes, and this determines the quality of our performance. There are hundreds of so-called scientific and/or miracle diets floating around in the health literature and media. Presently the American Dietitian's Association

(ADA) is even trying to cook up a little California state bureaucratic monopoly for their "university-trained expertise." If they succeed, these nutritional scholars who have brought us such culinary marvels as hospital food, military, prison and public school cafeteria foods will then be the only legal advisers on nutrition and diet in the state (and most all the other states if all goes as they have planned). It will be technically illegal for me or any other non-ADAer to give you our "layman's" opinion and experience regarding nutrition. So, before that malnourished possibility occurs, I'd like to put in a few words for delicious, well-chewed, whole, wild or organically cultivated, unadulterated, high in natural fiber, low oil and fat, low salt, non-synthetic-chemically-free-with-no-toxic-preservatives-or-colorings, complex carbohydrate meals, eaten in an aesthetic, relaxed environment. Thank you.

And for even more robust health, routinely compliment this whole-some eating with equally relaxed and unrushed time to respond to bowel movements *whenever* nature calls you to eliminate. Squatting on the toilet seat or elevating your feet by resting them on a box while sitting on the toilet is far more supportive of healthy bowel movements than the customary sitting position.

Vitamin/Mineral Supplements

Supplements cannot fill in for the nutritional debt created by poor diet and poor eating habits. Today's high-tech vitamin/mineral pills and powders will never duplicate whole foods. Vitamin and mineral supplements work well with good nutrition, if these supplements are not over-consumed. I see people consuming them like drugs . . . using far too much and often paying drug-like prices. These people would do much better nutritionally and economically if they knew that regular consumption of sea vegetables would satisfy *all* their mineral needs. Sea vegetables such as Kombu, Hiziki, Nori, Kelp and Dulse can be purchased at most health food stores. These need to be rinsed and soaked then added to soup stock or used with rice. Kombu is especially good when cooked with beans.

To help determine your need for vitamin/mineral supplementation, take a close look at the wholeness of the foods you're eating, the extent of the pollution in your environment and your level of stress. If you are eating quality foods, live in a clean environment and know how to mellow out regularly, that's probably all you need. If you live or work in a polluted environment, this external environment needs to be detoxified as it comes into your body as food, drink or in-breath. Supplementary vitamins and

173

minerals can help your immune system perform this task. If you choose to eat adulterated, unwhole, chemically treated food products, then again supplements are helpful (probably essential) to supply some of the nutrients that have been lost or destroyed during the adulterating, refining, "convenience fooding" processes, but even with these supplements, don't expect optimal health. Nothing can replace chewing and assimilating delicious, simply prepared, organically grown, whole foods.

All vitamins and minerals are essential for maintaining good health. This is common knowledge, and I will leave discussion of the full range of these micro-nutrients to other authors such as Richard Passwater, Earl Mindell and Paavlo Airola (see resource section of this book). I will discuss a few supplements that I feel are especially relevant to male nutrition.

Vitamin A
This vitamin is essential for the overall health of male reproductive organs, affecting specifically the production of sperm. Supplementing with vitamins A and E has helped some males build their sperm counts back to normal. I recommend taking at the same time herbs that help the body nourish and balance its hormonal system. Herbs such as Sarsaparilla, Wild Yam, Ginseng and California Spikenard (*Aralia Californica*) contain testosterone-like phytosteroids which the body can transmute into hormones. Marked deficiency of vitamin A has been studied as a cause of reproductive organ atrophy. Vitamin A, which is given in free abundance by fresh young Dandelion greens and other wild and bitter greens, is also easily obtained from green or yellow fruits and vegetables, dairy products, apricots, green leafy vegetables and carrots. When grown in soil that is fertilized with chemicals, these foods are found to contain significantly less vitamin A and minerals. If you chose to take vitamin A supplements, follow the recommended dosage. Beta-carotene, the best-known member of the carotenoid family of which 40-50 have vitamin A activity, is in my opinion a superior, more nourishing source of vitamin A supplementation. Carotenoids are converted into vitamin A molecules in the small intestine and act as a provitamin (a precursor of vitamin A). They are found in high concentration in the adrenal glands, the reproductive organs, the spleen, pancreas and retina of the eye. 99% of the beta-carotene sold in the U.S.A. and Canada is synthetic. The best natural sources of the full carotenoid spectrum are spirulina algae; organically grown yellow-orange vegetables such as carrots,

pumpkins, squash, sweet potatoes and yams; some red vegie-fruits such as tomatoes and red peppers; dark green vegetables like asparagus, broccoli, kale, collards, spinach, lettuce and fresh young *Dandelion* greens which also add a wild touch of bitter to your daily salads. Some fruits rich in beta-carotene are sour cherries, nectarines, papayas, peaches, apricots, cantaloupe and prune plums.

Zinc

This mineral is found in sea vegetables, organically grown pumpkin seeds, sunflower seeds, brewer's yeast, garlic, spinach, mushrooms, sensitive sea animals (especially oysters) and soybeans. The male hormone is not produced without zinc. Zinc is required by males to normalize testosterone production and to maintain healthy reproductive organs. Men with chronic prostatitis often have low zinc levels in both prostate fluid and semen, and patients with prostate cancer also appear to have low zinc stores. Boys need zinc to mature sexually, and men need zinc to help prevent prostate problems and impotence. Zinc is necessary for healthy skin and hair growth. Zinc promotes the healing of heart damage. Its deficiency is indicated as a causative factor in atherosclerosis and is implicated with hypertension. Pregnant mothers are best advised to get adequate zinc in their diets or as supplements. This will greatly assist their male children to develop properly.

It's my belief that zinc is lacking significantly in the commercial, supermarket-bought foods. The agricultural and commercial food processing technology loses the nutritional zinc somewhere in between the germination of the seeds and the dinner plate. I don't have much faith in store-bought mushrooms either. They are a product of heavy chemical fertilization and toxic fungicides. Wild mushrooms when accurately identified and eaten like any wild food are excellent, but only a few of us eccentric folks eat wild foods anymore, so supplementary zinc should be seriously considered. Dosage varies from 10 to 40 mg. daily to 50 mg. three times a day, depending on the severity of the symptoms of zinc deficiency (such as enlarged prostate, hesitancy on urination, decreased force of urinary stream and/or excess night time urination). Some research suggests that as a food supplement, zinc picolinate is best absorbed; amino-acid chelated zinc, zinc gluconate or zinc orotate in this order testing next best. Small amounts of zinc may boost the body's immune system, but excessively high amounts may impede the body's defenses. People who smoke heavily and those who share the same air require more dietary zinc due to the toxic cadmium content of smoke which interferes with the body's metabolism of zinc.

When using zinc supplements therapeutically, the relative role of copper becomes an issue, because both minerals compete for the same absorption sites in the intestines. Yet zinc requires the presence of a little copper to be usable by the body. To further complicate the mathematics of recommended dosages of each, it is a fact that considerable amounts of zinc are lost in sweat, while only a small amounts of copper leaves the sweating body. These facts, like so many such technical details, illustrate the major problem I see when individuals attempt to supplement their diet with laboratory designed and manufactured pills. Everything one plans to accomplish with a pill-full of some nutrient requires a complex list of rules and precautions that seem unending. This is one reason I put my faith in the biological familiarity that exists between plants and my body. Unadulterated, unrefined plants have all these rules and precautions pre-computed in their ancient genetic micro-chips. Only 2 to 3 milligrams of copper a day will compensate for even very large doses of zinc. Eating a diet that provides at least 2 milligrams of copper will suffice for those taking additional zinc. This is not difficult for many foods rich in zinc are also rich in copper, but not excessively rich; what did I tell ya? Foods such as raisins, nuts, avocados, green vegetables, mushrooms, beans and peas will provide adequate daily copper. Beware, however, of refined foods, such as white flour products, canned soups, margarine etc. for these have been rendered very low in copper.

Important zinc allies for preventing and treating prostate problems are the vegetable oils containing essential fatty acids. Essential fatty acid/ prostate studies have used flaxseed oil in their research. This oil is commercially available, but it goes rancid quickly. Unrefined, organic sesame oil, sunflower seed oil, wheat germ oil or safflower seed oil are all high in essential fatty acids.

Magnesium

This mineral plays an important role in the production of sex hormones. Men with prostate problems may find magnesium helpful. And since the prostate produces part of the seminal fluid, it is possible that magnesium can contribute to correcting sterility. Natural food sources of magnesium are nuts, wheat, soy, buckwheat, milk products, Parsley and Mustard.

Selenium

This is a micro-nutrient that men appear to need more than women as the testes hold a concentrated amount of this nutrient which is believed important for sperm production. Some information suggests that selenium in combination with zinc and vitamin E provides relief from enlarged prostate gland. Like iodine, selenium is not distributed uniformly in our soils, so it is often found lacking in our diets. Most densely populated areas of the U.S. have low to marginal amounts of selenium in the soil. According to research done by Richard Passwater, Ph.D., author of the books *Supernutrition* and *Supernutrition for Healthy Hearts*, selenium protects against heart disease, normalizes blood pressure, protects against plaque formation and, along with vitamin E, protects cellular membranes against attack by free radicals and chemical mutagens. Natural food sources of selenium (depending upon the extent of its presence in the soil) are: the bran and germ of cereals, and vegetables such as broccoli, onions and tomatoes.

Lecithin

This is one of the chief constituents of brain and nerve tissue. It is said that close to 20% of brain substance is made of lecithin. It is also present in abundance in the endocrine glands, especially the gonads, both male and female. The pituitary and pineal glands contain lecithin. It is an essential component of semen, and a sufficient supply is essential for normal semen production. Lecithin has been used successfully to treat male debility and glandular exhaustion, also to strengthen and rebuild the nerves. Some sources claim that lecithin improves virility and helps prevent impotence. Lecithin helps dissolve cholesterol deposits in the arteries, thus lessening the chance of heart disease. It is found in many animal tissues and plants, especially egg yolks, seeds, grains, nuts and soya beans. The lecithin is destroyed when these foods undergo commercial adulteration processes. Lecithin can be bought in any health food store in capsule, liquid, powder or granular form. If large doses of lecithin are taken, calcium should be added to the diet to balance the excess phosphorus obtained from the lecithin. Some excellent sources of calcium are nuts, sesame seeds, leafy greens and herbs such as Nettle and Oat straw.

Carnitine

Carnitine is an amino acid found in higher levels in males than in females. It appears to promote proper sperm motility. The body manufactures its own carnitine if given an adequate supply of the essential amino acids, but only if the body is allowed to digest and assimilate them properly. Protein (amino acid) digestion is initiated by the stomach acids. So, it makes sense to take a dose of bitters before meals to stimulate not only these stomach digestive juices, but also the pancreatic juices which are equally essential for protein digestion. Adequate pancreatic enzymes are also necessary for the male body to absorb zinc and essential fatty acids. Including simple, wild, fresh and free herbs such as young springtime Dandelion leaves in your diet helps everything work better.

Sweeteners

Speaking of dietary supplements and bitters brings to mind America's major food additive, sugar. I'm not interested in dwelling on the nutritional foolishness of eating refined white sugar or the synthetics, saccharin and aspartame (Nutrasweet). When our sweet lust is high, we are going to eat sugar (sweets), no matter who says what about it. So, until the common use of bitters (see Green's Hypothesis #2) starts to normalize our present sweet craving appetites, I would like to introduce to you an organic, unrefined sugar that is now commercially available, called Sucanat®. It is a 100% unrefined, evaporated cane juice complete with all its natural complex sugars and molasses. It is organically grown and certified to be free of chemical residue, with no additives and no preservatives. It's still a concentrated sweet, best not to be overused, but it contains all its quality nutrients, unremoved. It appears to be an important source of trace minerals, including essential chromium, in a natural balanced ratio. For detailed information about this sweetener, write the importers: Pronatec International, Inc., P.O. Box 193, Peterborough, NH 03458, or check with your local health food store. As a person who is convinced that the overuse of refined sugar is a major contributing cause of most of our current health problems, this organic cane (grass) juice used moderately looks pretty good to me.

Skin

(Also see aromatherapy section)
General Skin-Care for Males

Regular proper cleansing of the skin is essential and should be done each morning and evening. Since most men shave daily, effective skin cleansing is an easily added task. The following are suggestions for a simple cleansing routine. Splash the skin with warm water. The cleansing product you use should be pH balanced (4.5 to 5.5). Generally this type of product comes in a liquid form. Most bar soaps are very alkaline, which is hard on the skin and strips the skin of it's protective acid mantle. If you have a difficult time finding a good skin soap, you can use a good quality pH balanced hair shampoo. Lather the soap well and wash your entire face, including neck and close to the ears. Rinse well. Lather again, shave and rinse face. After washing the face, a toner/astringent should be used to close the pores and tone the skin. This product ideally should not contain alcohol, which is drying to the skin. Rose water and distilled Witch Hazel are good toners. If you use an electric razor, clean face, shave and apply the toner astringent. Next, moisturize with a lotion, cream or an essential oil blend specific to your skin type. (See below.)

Develop a habit of reading cosmetic labels and avoid products that contain synthetic perfumes, coloring agents and/or mineral oils. These are unnecessary ingredients, and they can irritate skin, clog pores and cause allergic reactions. Most health food stores carry good quality skin care products.

The use of a facial scrub once or twice a week is an important part of thorough cleansing of the skin, as it helps to slough off dead skin cells. Dead skin cells that are not regularly removed can: 1) make the skin look lifeless, 2) clog the pores, 3) lead to blackheads, 4) make the skin feel dry and 5) inhibit nutrients from penetrating and nourishing the epidermis. Shaving daily helps to remove these dead skin cells on the jawline and neck, but the scrub should be used especially on the nose, cheeks, temples and forehead to help remove dead cells and unclog the pores of these areas. Drink lots of pure water daily whether your skin is dry, oily, normal or otherwise.

Remember, many skin conditions will take several months to balance while others may right themselves in a matter of weeks.

Skin Care for specific skin conditions
Acne

Acne is quite a problem for a large number of males. Diet, of course, is a contributing factor, but it is seldom the only contributing factor. This condition is best treated internally as well as externally. For internal work support over-all elimination, employ herbs that give the following actions:

- Lymphatic: Cleavers, Echinacea and Calendula
- Alteratives which also give a secondary hepatic action: Burdock seed, Yellow Dock, Sarsaparilla (which is a helpful hormone

balancing herb as well) and Blue Flag (a remarkably helpful alterative herb for stimulating a sluggish liver. It is nearly a specific for acne, but it is a very strong herb, so use it carefully with children. Also Blue Flag does not store well. If it is over 8 months old, it will have very little activity left.)
- Diuretic: Cleavers and Nettle
- Anti-microbial: Garlic (to be included in the diet), Echinacea, Baptisia

Put together a formula which begins with:

Blue Flag	1 part
Cleaver	2 parts
Nettle	2 parts
Burdock seed	1 part
Sarsaparilla	2 parts
Echinacea	1 part

Use this for about a month (at which point increase the Blue Flag to 2 parts). If a person is quite upset about the skin condition add a nervine herb such as Black Cohosh, Valerian or Scullcap to help calm. Take approximately 30 drops of this liquid extract formula 3 times a day. You can take 1 cup of the tea 3 times a day, but if this is a teenager expecting him to drink 3 cups of herb tea a day is most likely unrealistic. Don't expect quick results. It takes time to alter the condition of the body, but perseverance renders excellent results.

Adolescent acne is primarily due to hormonal changes that occur in puberty; a condition which certain foods further aggravate. Following a cleansing diet that is abundant in fruits and vegetables with avoidance of acne aggravating foods (often difficult to metabolize foods) such as dairy products, oily foods, fried foods, sugars, soft drinks and junk food helps control the problem. Increase the amount of Sarsaparilla in the above formula to 4 parts to deal with the primary hormonal situation. Complementary external treatment is important, especially when treating acne. Cleaning the skin regularly and thoroughly is always the first and most important step. Calendula is an excellent external remedy for healing the skin. The most efficient preparation to use is an oil infusion (please refer to chapter titled Technology of Independence for making oil infusions). To a half ounce of Calendula oil infusion add 2 drops of each of the following pure plant essential oils: Chamomile, Spike Lavender and Juniper. Wash the skin and apply this skin oil to the problem area 3 times a day.

Normal to dry skin

A dry skin condition needs to be cleaned and exfoliated with a small luffah sponge or exfoliant scrub regularly to remove the dead cells which often contribute to a dull, dry feeling of the skin. This exfoliation allows the moisturizing therapeutic agents to penetrate the skin more easily. To a half ounce of a fixed oil such as almond, avocado or wheat germ add 2 drops of the following essential oils: Geranium, Sandalwood and Lavender. Wash the skin and apply this skin oil to the problem area 2 times a day. Dehydrated skin is often confused with dry skin and has more to do with lack of moisture in the skin than lack of oil. Drink lots of pure water throughout each day.

Normal to oily skin

Cleanse skin 2 to 3 times a day. To a half ounce of fixed oil add 2 drops each of the following essential oils: Lavender, Cypress and Lemon. Apply this oil 2 to 3 times a day to clean skin. Many people are reluctant to add an oil to an already oily complexion. Contrary to popular belief, applying essential oils in a fixed oil base onto oily skin does not increase the problem. In fact, putting a drying agent on the skin will make an oily skin condition worse, for the skin will interpret this dryness as a need for more oil, and the unctuous cycle will continue. The oils in this blend will help to regulate the sebaceous secretions of the skin. These essential oils with the carrier oil will send a signal to the skin that it need not produce additional sebum.

Sun damaged and mature skin

Treat these conditions the same as dry skin, except use the following essential oils in place of the dry skin oils: Lavender, Frankincense and Carrot Seed. If the skin is heavily damaged by extreme sun exposure or by exposure to any other damaging medium add to this mixture 2 drops of the essential oil *Helichrysum italicum*. This is a very expensive oil, but it works wonders regenerating new skin cells. I can relate a personal experience of using a mixture of these four oils on a condition of my skin which was diagnosed as a cancerous skin condition. I am thrilled with the results. Drink lots of pure water.

Bumps, bruises, cracks, nicks and cuts

Males who work a lot with tools frequently smash, bump, bruise or otherwise injure their limbs, especially their hands. In my experience one of the finest first-aid remedies is the application of an herbal oil compound which is easily made of equal parts of the olive oil infusion of Arnica, St. John's Wort and Calendula. Keep it in a small container in your tool box or pocket and when the need arises apply it immediately onto the injury. If there is an open wound, put the injury oil around the opening. The pain disappears and bruising is usually totally avoided. My wife never travels without a small bottle of it in her purse or pocket. We keep a bottle of this oil blend in our car and at our workplace.

Pure essential oil of Lavender (*Lavandula vera*) is the most versatile skin-care/first-aid package available. It is safe to apply to open wounds. It is antimicrobial, anti-inflammatory and can be safely used neat (directly to the skin without being diluted). It is an excellent remedy for burns, rashes, scrapes, scalds, nicks, cuts, punctures, bites and stings. Lavender essential oil smells delightful, and for all that it is capable of doing, it is inexpensive. It can be stored conveniently in places such as tool boxes, glove compartments, carpenter belts, desk drawers, etc. If it spills or its glass container breaks, the surrounding area will smell more beautiful for a few hours. Keep essential oils out of direct sunlight, and never store them in plastic containers.

Hands that do a considerable amount of construction work often get extremely dry and can develop painful cracks in the skin. To prevent or treat this skin condition purchase a good skin cream base. Choose one that is made with vegetable oils, not mineral oil. Mineral oil clogs the pores and is not moisturizing. To one cup of this cream base, add the following pure plant essential oils: Sandalwood - 5 drops, Geranium - 5 drops, Myrrh - 5 drops, Lavender - 10 drops and Blue Chamomile - 5 drops. Thoroughly blend in the plant essential oils. Apply this aromatic cream to the hands regularly. Keep the container tightly capped when not in use to prevent evaporation of the essential oils. Do not substitute synthetic essential oils or perfumes for these pure plant essential oils. The synthetics might smell somewhat like the plant essential oils, and they are less expensive, but they are a completely different entity, and they do nothing to nourish or balance the skin. There is much more chance of allergic reactions to synthetics than to pure plant essential oils.

Poultices of bruised (crushed or lightly chewed) fresh Plantain leaves applied regularly works wonders for healing dry, injured hands. Chemical burns and rashes also respond well to this herb. Of course, using rubber gloves when handling toxic substances and providing plenty of ventilation is fundamental preventive medicine.

Hair
About Hair Loss

In a culture preoccupied with the worship of youth and unwrinkled flesh and seemingly so ashamed of the physical symbols of age and life experience, it seems necessary to discuss the occurrence of hair loss in men and suggest a re-evaluation of its meaning. Receding hair line or male-pattern baldness is a sign of maturing maleness. It's great to be mature, well worth the loss of some hair. Hair loss is neither a symptom of slacking vitality and worth, nor of weakness, senility and loss of personal power. Why are so many of us men ashamed of and self-conscious about losing our hair? Possibly we are so conditioned to disrespect the process of aging and so prepared to dispose of our elders that any sign of approaching member-ship in this group fills us with despair and feelings of dispersing self-esteem? Via the mass media, our culture is giving the youth a monopoly on attractiveness, desirability and vitality — an unfortunate wasteful distrac-tion of mature creative humanity for those individuals who buy into this illusion. Male pattern baldness is a condition emanating from the effects of testosterone production — a feature of our male hormone. It is an integral part of being a man, nothing to be avoided, hidden or dreaded, merely to be re-evaluated and respected. A number of women have commented to me that they are attracted to men who have a high forehead, relating to it as a sign of intelligence. Personally, I'm most interested in the personal vision and consciousness occurring inside the head.

Keeping hair and scalp healthy is the object of this section, not the avoidance of a symptom of evolving male maturity.

Some time ago I found a little $2.00 book written by renowned nutritionist, Paavo Airola, entitled, *Stop Hair Loss*. It is published by Health Plus, P.O. Box 22001, Phoenix, Arizona 85028. I recommend it to any male who is disturbed and confused by his present hair loss or who anticipates a degree of baldness in his future. The information presented by Mr. Airola in the book is built around the work of Dr. Lars Engstrand, M.D., a famous Swedish scientist and professor at Karolinska Institute in Stockholm, ". . . who has presented conclusive evidence that his theory of the causes of baldness is a valid one."

According to Dr. Engstrand, baldness is caused by the pressure on the blood capillaries of the scalp affected by the tendinous membrane (or the galea) which is located on the crown of the head in both men and women. At the age of 15 years this membrane is paper thin and elastic on both sexes and remains so in most women throughout their life. However, on many men, starting at about 16-18 years of age, there is a considerable thickening of this membrane due to it being stimulated by the male sex hormones.

When the tendinous membrane becomes thick, it increases the pressure and tension on the scalp. This leads to an impaired blood circulation in the capillaries located above the membrane. These blood capillaries normally feed the hair follicles with nutrients necessary for hair growth. As a result, there is gradual diminishing of hair growth until the hair follicles are not able to produce any more hairs and the skin is left bare, creating what is termed "male pattern baldness." Approximately 90% of male baldness is due to the thickened tendinous membrane.

Hair Care

Certainly, heredity has a great deal to do with the condition of one's hair. However, no one is rendered powerless by genetics. There are many things one can do to condition the scalp and nourish and strengthen the hair.

- Experiments conducted in Sweden and the USA indicate that cutting down salt in the diet will keep hair more healthy and reduce hair loss.
- Iodine deficiency in the diet will cause dryness, thinness and poor growth of hair. Kelp, dried seaweed and seafoods are the richest natural source of iodine. Kelp and Dulse sea vegetables or tablets are also available in natural food stores.
- The micro-nutrients particularly essential for hair care are: Vitamin B complex, vitamin E, vitamin F (also called the essential fatty acids), vitamins A & D (the universally acknowledged vitamins for hair and skin to treat dandruff, dry, itchy and flaky scalp).
- All minerals, especially silica, magnesium, calcium, potassium, phosphorus, iodine and iron are needed.
- High quality protein, not necessarily high quantity (40-50 grams per day is normally sufficient) is essential for healthy hair and scalp.
- Emotional tension or prolonged mental stress and congestion cause constriction of the blood vessels of the scalp preventing the blood from coming to the hair roots, consequently over a lengthy period of time there can be noticeable hair loss.
- Traditional Chinese Medicine explains the basis of hair loss by

going back to the dynamic role of jing (previously discussed in the chapter titled "Specific Male Problems") in body sustenance. Jing originates and is housed in the kidneys. The kidneys rule male sexual reproduction and also the hair. Nurturing the kidneys with foods such as asparagus, artichoke, celery, aduki beans and the herbs Lovage, Parsley, Couchgrass and Yarrow and sustaining abundant jing by avoiding excessive ejaculation has a direct effect on hair health. The herb Ho shou wu strengthens jing and consequently helps prevent the hair from greying.

• Ayurvedic medical science sees graying and baldness as symptoms of stress and excessive thought which clogs the mind, producing excess heat in the head leading to hair loss, graying and insufficient sleep. An oil infusion of Gotu Kola using sesame oil for the fixed oil (this is called Brahmi Oil) is quite helpful to cool the scalp and brain, helping to stop graying and hair loss. Put a small amount of this oil on the finger tips and rub it on the scalp and hair at night before bed (wash it out in the morning). This is a cooling oil which cools the brain promoting mental alertness, clarity and improved memory. It also promotes sound sleep.

To stimulate hair growth and increase blood circulation in your scalp:

1. Finger massage the scalp at least twice a day. Place all 10 fingers firmly on your scalp and push the whole scalp in circular motions for 10 seconds (don't move the fingers, move the whole scalp). Then place your fingers in a new place and repeat until you have massaged the entire scalp.

2. Lie on a Slant Board or use any other contraption or position that reverses the gravity of the body forcing the blood to your head. This blood will penetrate into the capillaries of the scalp and feed the hair roots. Combine this position with the finger massage for 5 to 15 minutes twice a day. It will do wonders for your hair, your brain, your veins, your legs and your overall circulation. At the same time using a slant board 20 minutes 3 times a day is an excellent therapy for relieving (and preventing) painful prostate conditions.

3. You can combine the effects of the finger massage and slant board by massaging your scalp while leaning over with your head between your legs. The technique that works best for me is to stand with my feet about 18 inches apart. I bend over resting my elbows on my knees with my head down below my waist and the fingers of both hands on my scalp. I give

185

my scalp a good finger massage all over as described in #1 above. Believe me, it feels wonderful. Try it right now. One can do the same thing sitting on the edge of a chair or bed instead of standing. Sometimes, I put 30 drops of Rosemary essential oil into 1 ounce of Aloe vera juice and before bed massage a teaspoonful or so onto my scalp. As I sleep, hair follicles party and feast all hours of the night.

4. Regular hair and scalp brushing 2 to 3 minutes twice a day is a must. This cleans all sorts of debris from the surface of the scalp and at the same time deep massages the scalp. Don't be afraid of pulling out hairs. If they come out with brushing, they were coming out soon anyway. Brushing will stimulate the emptied follicles to grow new hairs. Place a very small amount of Rosemary essential oil in the palm of your hand and rub it onto the bristles of your hair brush. Brush this essential oil through your hair daily. Rosemary oil is an excellent conditioner for the hair shafts, and it is said to stimulate hair growth.

5. After washing your hair and body with a soap or shampoo rinse your hair and body with a quart container full of warm water, to which you have added 1 Tbsp. of apple cider vinegar (a 1 quart plastic yogurt container works great in the bath or shower). Leave this on for about a minute, then rinse. This vinegar rinse will re-establish your body, hair and scalp's natural protective acid mantle.

6. To a quart of apple cider vinegar (use white distilled vinegar, which is a petroleum distillate, only for cleaning windows and automobile parts, never on your body or in your food) add some Nettle, fresh Rosemary, Sage, Horsetail and/or Camomile (Approximately 1 ounce of herb to a cup of vinegar). Put the herbs into the container of vinegar and keep it close to your shower or bath. Use this herbal vinegar mixed with warm water as a daily hair and scalp rinse, and use it for that 1 tablespoon full mentioned in #4 above.

7. One can also apply the expressed juice of the Stinging Nettle to the scalp to stimulate hair growth.

Take good care of yourself; it's good medicine.

~*10*~

The Materia Medica Presented in this Herbal

When discussing an herb it is essential to make sure that we are talking about the same plant, so it is wise to use a plant's binomial name along with its common name for more accurate identification and communication. Country or common names are more poetic to my aesthetic sense and often give insightful clues to the plant's once common use by our ancestors. One can often feel from a common name a little of how this plant has been used traditionally by humans and by animals. Herbs have extensive history as practical medicine which is reflected in the common names. But using common names alone can be misleading. A single plant can be known by numerous common names, while a single common name is frequently used for a variety of different plants (plants that have some similar salient action).

Latin botanical names (in the poetic style of an innately unspoken language) can also reach into the folkloric history of the plant (eg., *Officinalis* means of the shop, from the office or store; an official medicine in popular use at one time by practitioners. *Vulgaris* means common, of the people, common home remedy). The word *botany* itself comes from the Greek word *Boskein* which means to eat, an indication of humankind's first purpose and use of plants as food and medicine. But Latin binomial names lean more toward describing the plant's botanical characteristics or applauding a botanist who published an official description of the plant. Latin names have a more universal (or at least global) perspective, and are understood equally throughout the world. *Ulmus* is an elm tree and *canis* is a dog in Ireland, Peru, Egypt, Viet Nam and the Soviet Union as well as in Canada and the United States. These binomial names are relatively more precise, but they are not carved in stone or hardwood, and they are occasionally changed as botanists learn more about the plant's botanical family affiliations.

    The following list of common and binomial names will help make it more clear exactly which plants I am recommending in this herbal.

Plants listed by common names

Agrimony	*Agrimonia eupatoria*
Alfalfa	*Medicago sativa*
Angelica	*Angelica archangelica*
Arnica	*Arnica montana*
Artichoke	*Cynara scolymus*
Ashwagandha	*Withania somnifera*
Astragalus	*Astragalus membranaceus*
Balm	*Melissa officinalis*
Basil	*Ocimum basilicum*
Bayberry	*Myrica cerifera*
Bearberry	*Arctostaphylos uva-ursi*
Black Cohosh	*Cimicifuga racemosa*
Blackberry	*Rubus villosus*
Bladderwrack	*Fucus vesiculosus*
Blessed Thistle	*Cnicus benedictus*
Blue Cohosh	*Caulophylum thalictroides*
Blue Flag	*Iris versicolor*
Bogbean	*Menyanthes trifoliata*
Boneset	*Eupatorium perfoliatum*
Buchu	*Agathosma betulina*
Burdock	*Arctium lappa*
Calendula	*Calendula officinalis*
California Poppy	*Eschscholzia californica*
California Spikenard	*Aralia californica*
Cascara Sagrada	*Rhamnus purshiana*
Catnip	*Nepeta cataria*
Cayenne	*Capsicum spp.*
Celery seed	*Apium graveolens*
Centaury	*Centaurium umbellatum*
Chamomile	*Matricaria chamomilla*
Chaparrel	*Larrea mexicana*

Chaste Tree	*Vitex agnus-castus*
Chicory	*Cichorium intybus*
Chickweed	*Stellaria media*
Cinnamon	*Cinnamomum zeylanicum*
Cleavers	*Galium aparine*
Coffee	*Coffea arabica*
Coltsfoot	*Tussilago farfara*
Comfrey	*Symphytum officinale*
Coriander	*Coriandrum sativum*
Corn Silk	*Zea mays*
Couch Grass	*Agropyron repens*
Cramp Bark	*Viburnum opulus*
Cranesbill	*Geranium maculatum*
Cubeb	*Piper cubeba*
Damiana	*Turnera diffusa*
Dandelion	*Taraxacum officinale*
Devil's Club	*Oplopanax horridus*
Dill	*Anethum graveolens*
Dong Quai	*Angelica sinensis*
Echinacea	*Echinacea purpurea*
	Echinacea angustifolia
	Echinacea pallida
Elder	*Sambucus nigra*
Elecampane	*Inula helenium*
Eucalyptus	*Eucalyptus globulus*
Eyebright	*Euphrasia officinalis*
False Unicorn	*Chamaelirium luteum*
Fennel	*Foeniculum vulgare*
Fenugreek	*Trigonella foenum-graecum*
Feverfew	*Tanacetum parthenium*
Fringetree	*Chionanthus virginica*
Flaxseed	*Linum usitatissimum*
Garlic	*Allium sativum*
Gentian	*Gentiana spp.*

Ginger	*Zingiber officinale*
Ginkgo	*Ginkgo biloba*
Ginseng	*Panax spp.*
Goat's Rue	*Galega officinalis*
Golden Rod	*Solidago virgauria*
Golden Seal	*Hydrastis canadensis*
Gotu Kola	*Centella asiatica*
Gravel Root	*Eupatorium purpureum*
Guarana	*Paullinia cupana*
Gumweed	*Grindelia spp.*
Hawthorn	*Crataegus spp.*
	Crataegus oxyacantha
Hops	*Humulus lupulus*
Horehound	*Marrubium vulgare*
Horsechestnut	*Aesculus hippocastanum*
Horseradish	*Armoracia rusticana*
Horsetail	*Equisetum arvense*
Ho shou wu	*Polygonum multiflorum*
Hydrangea	*Hydrangea arborescens*
Hyssop	*Hyssopus officinalis*
Irish Moss	*Chondrus crispus*
Kola	*Cola vera, C. acuminata*
Lady's Mantle	*Alchemilla vulgaris*
Lavender	*Lavandula officinalis*
Licorice	*Glycyrrhiza glabra*
Linden	*Tilia cordata*
Lobelia	*Lobelia inflata*
Ma Huang	*Ephedra sinica*
Marshmallow	*Althaea officinalis*
Meadowsweet	*Filipendula ulmaria*
Melilot	*Melilotus officinalis*
Milk Thistle	*Carduus marianum*
	(Silybum marianum)

Motherwort	*Leonurus cardiaca*
Mugwort	*Artemisia vulgaris*
Mullein	*Verbascum spp.*
Mulberry	*Morus spp.*
Myrrh	*Commiphora myrrha*
Nasturtium	*Tropaeolum majus*
Nettle	*Urtica spp.*
Oak Bark	*Quercus spp.*
Oat	*Avena Sativa*
Olive Leaf	*Olea europaea*
Orange	*Citrus aurantium*
Oregon Grape	*Berberis aquifolium Pursh.*
Osha	*Ligusticum porteri*
Parsley	*Petroselinum sativum*
Partridge berry	*Mitchella repens*
Pasque Flower	*Anenome pulsatilla*
Pau d'Arco	*Tabebuia spp.*
Passion Flower	*Passiflora incarnata*
Pennyroyal	*Mentha pulegium*
Peppermint	*Mentha piperata*
Periwinkle	*Vinca major (or Vinca minor)*
Pipsissewa	*Chimaphila umbellata*
Plantain	*Plantago lanceolata*
	Plantago major
Prickly Ash	*Xanthoxylum americanum*
Pumpkin	*Cucurbita pepo*
Raspberry	*Rubus spp.*
Red Clover	*Trifolium pratense*
Rosemary	*Rosmarinus officinalis*
Sage	*Salvia officinalis*
St. John's Wort	*Hypericum perforatum*
Sarsaparilla	*Smilax spp.*
Sassafras	*Sassafras albidum*

Saw Palmetto	*Serenoa serrulata*
Scullcap	*Scutellaria laterifolia*
Sheperd's Purse	*Capsella bursa-pastoris*
Siberian Ginseng	*Eleutherococcus senticosus*
Slippery Elm	*Ulmus fulva*
Sorrel	*Rumex spp.*
Southernwood	*Artemisia abrotanum*
Star Anise	*Illicium anisatum*
Strawberry	*Fragaria vesca*
Suma	*Pfaffia paniculata*
Tea Tree	*Melaleuca alternifolia*
Thuja	*Thuja occidentalis*
Thyme	*Thymus spp.*
Tumeric	*Curcuma longa*
Usnea	*Usnea spp.*
Uva Ursi	(see Bearberry)
Valerian	*Valeriana officinalis*
Vervain	*Verbena officinalis*
Wild Cherry	*Prunus serotina*
Wild Indigo	*Baptisia tinctoria*
Wild Lettuce	*Lactuca virosa*
Wild Oat	*Avena fatua*
Wild Yam	*Dioscorea villosa*
Willow Bark	*Salix spp.*
Witch Hazel	*Hamamelis virginiana*
Wormwood	*Artemisia absinthium*
Yarrow	*Achillea millefolium*
Yellow Dock	*Rumex crispus*
Yerba Manza	*Anemopsis californica*
Yerba Maté	*Ilex paraguensis*
Yohimbe	*Pausinystalia yohimba*
Yucca	*Yucca spp.*

❧11❧

The Male Herbal

Details about the actions and system affinities of most the herbs mentioned in this book are outlined below. It is most practical and helpful to have at least two or three herbals in your home library for reference. All the herbs mentioned in this herbal are eagerly discussed by other herbalists, and you will have no trouble finding reference to them in the herbals I have listed for you in the "Resource" section of this book. Please see the chapter titled, "Technology of Independence" for specific instructions on how to prepare these nutritional/medicinal plants as infusions, decoctions, tinctures, etc. for personal and family health-care.

Agrimony – *Agrimonia eupatoria*
Family: *Rosaceae*
Parts used: Aerial parts.
Actions and medical uses: Astringent, tonic, diuretic, vulnerary and cholagogue.
Systems affected: Digestive, genito-urinary, skin.
Specific indications: This herb appears to have been designed for the human digestive system. Its astringent action is strengthening to the stomach and intestines, and its bitter elements stimulate liver and digestive secretions, thus toning the digestive system. Agrimony is a specific for relieving childhood diarrhea, and is most useful in treating appendicitis. Agrimony is used to treat urinary incontinence and cystitis. It is beneficial in the relief of sore throats and laryngitis when used as a gargle. A salve made of this plant heals bruises and other wounds.
Combinations: Combines well with carminitive herbs such as Fennel or Cinnamon for relieving indigestion.

Preparations: *Infusion*: 1 cup, 3 times a day. *Tincture*: 15 to 30 drops in a little water 3 times a day.

Alfalfa (Buffalo Herb) – *Medicago sativa*
Family: Leguminosae
Parts used: Leaf, flower, seed and sprout.
Actions and medical uses: Nutrient, appetizer, diuretic, alterative and tonic.
Systems affected: Digestive, urinary, endocrine, overall body nutrient.
Specific indications: Avitaminosis of A, C, E, or K (Vitamin K is oil soluble, so it is not available by water infusion. Whole plant must be taken, as in tablet form). This clover-like plant is one of Nature's richest sources of easily assimilated protein, vitamins, minerals and trace elements. Used as a tonic beverage it also helps assimilate protein, calcium, potassium, iron and other nutrients. Also taken daily to improve appetite, improve the condition of the blood and relieve peptic ulcer condition. Relieves urinary and bowel problems and eliminates retained water.
Combinations: Works as a reliable tonic and nutrient adjunct with all other herbs. Combines with Slippery Elm for use in convalescent debility.
Preparations: *Infusion*: usually with a bit of Mint 1 cup, 1 to 3 times a day.
Precautions: None. Contains no unfriendly compounds; it's good for children, the elderly, pregnant and nursing mothers.
Other uses: Seeds commonly sprouted for use as fresh high vitamin/ mineral salad greens. An excellent forage plant, and a soil enricher due to nitrogen-fixing bacteria that live in swellings on the roots. Puts atmospheric nitrogen into the soil in the form of nitrates. Al-Fal-Fa, Arabic word for "Father of All Foods," has deep feeder roots that can penetrate the earth more than 60 feet seeking out minerals in the deep subsoil that are inaccessible to other plants.

Angelica – *Angelica archangelica*
Family: Umbelliferae
Parts used: Root, leaf and seed used medicinally; stalk used for confectionery.
Actions and medical uses: Carminative, stimulant, emmenagogue, anti-spasmodic, anti-rheumatic, antiseptic, expectorant, diuretic and diaphoretic.
Systems affected: Respiratory, circulatory, digestive, musculo-skeletal, genito-urinary.

Specific indications: Expectorant for bronchitis, coughs, pleurisy and most other lung conditions, especially when the condition is fluish or feverish or accompanying a cold. It induces sweating in fevers, cooling the skin. Angelica's warming properties and high carminative bitter essential oil content act as an antispasmodic to help relieve stomach and intestinal cramps (colic) and nausea as well as flatulence; aids digestion and promotes appetite; and it has an affinity for the urinary system as a urinary antiseptic for bladder and urethra inflammations. As it improves circulation and warms the body when taken internally and applied as a poultice or liniment, it has been used to ease cold rheumatic inflammation and peripheral vascular deficiency. Due to these warming circulatory properties, it also acts as a menstrual stimulant to help promote and regulate menstrual flow and as an antispasmodic to relieve menstrual cramps.

The Chinese herb, Dong Quai (Dong Kwai, Tang Kwei) is a processed, cured root derived from a particular species of Angelica (*A. sinensis*). *A. sinensis* possesses the actions of the other species, but is found to be more tonic. It is often referred to as the "Female's Ginseng" and is used with great success as a female sexual organ tonic and builder of the blood and circulation in the uterine area. It is equally useful as a male sexual organ tonic, especially in conditions such as prostatitis and orchitis (inflammation of the testicles which can be a painful complication of adult occurring mumps and gonorrhea).

Combinations: Angelica root is combined well with Coltsfoot for bronchial catarrh and with Camomile for dyspepsia; with Cramp Bark for genito-urinary cramping; Angelica leaf combines well with Camomile for digestive weakness.

Precautions: Angelica tends to increase the blood sugar level, so it should not be used by diabetics. It is a strong emmenagogue and is best not used by pregnant women or during excessive menstrual flow.

Preparations: *Infusion:* 1 teaspoon of herb steeped in a cup of water, take 1/2 cup 2-3 times a day; *tincture:* 1/4 to 1/2 teaspoon drunk in a cup of warm water; *poultice* or *liniment:* applied to chest or joints.

Other uses: Stalks are candied as a confectionery.

Arnica– *Arnica spp.*
Family: Compositae
Parts used: Whole plant.
Actions and medical uses: Anti-inflammatory, vulnerary.

Systems affected: Skin, musculo-skeletal.
Specific indications: External local use for treatment of sprains, bruises, sore muscles or wherever there is inflammation and pain on the skin. It is most effectively used wherever there has been damage to the blood-carrying tissues; where there has been blood escape from ruptured blood vessels due to sprains, strains or bruises also open bleeding (see precautions). Arnica treats inflammation of the veins or other inflammations of the skin region. This herb will also help relieve rheumatic pain and the symptoms of phlebitis. Arnica tincture applied externally helps restore circulation and relieve the burning, itching and swelling symptoms of unbroken chilblains.
Combinations: Excellent anti-inflammatory and vulnerary combined with Calendula and St. Johnswort as a compound oil infusion or compound tincture.
Precautions: Do not put directly onto an open wound or broken skin, rather put it around the opening. Arnica tea or tincture is very strong and should be taken internally only under the supervision of an experienced herbalist. It is safe and effective as a homeopathic preparation.
Preparations: Externally: prepare as an oil infusion or liniment, apply directly to irritated area. This liniment combines well with other water-alcohol preparations such as distilled Witch Hazel or Calendula tincture and essential oils for preparing a compound liniment or a soothing lotion.

Ashwagandha – *Withania somnifera*
Family: Solanaceae
Parts used: Root.
Actions and medical uses: Tonic, aphrodisiac, astringent, sedative.
Systems affected: Reproductive, nervous, musculo-skeletal.
Specific indications: This herb is popularly known as the Indian ginseng. It is used in Ayurvedic medicine to treat cerebral function deficits in the elderly, to enhance learning and memory retention in the normal population and to enhance anti-stress and immune response. An exceptionally efficient herb for treating male impotence and infertility. It is a specific strengthening tonic for countering poor growth in children as well as convalescence and the diseases of aging. Ashwagandha has an affinity with the nervous system improving strength of mind, treating wasting diseases, insomnia and neurasthenia. It shows an affinity with the musculo-skeletal system useful for treating joint and nerve pain as well as weaknesses in the knees and the

back. (M. Tierra)

Combinations: Combines well with Siberian Ginseng or Suma for preparing a highly nutritious adaptogenic tonic for the reproductive organs and the nervous system.

Precautions: None. This root is totally safe and effective for use with children, convalescent individuals of all ages and for nourishing the aged.

Preparations: Ayurvedic medicine traditionally infuses this root powder in boiled warm milk, taken 1 cup 2 times a day.

Astragalus – *Astragalus spp.*

Family: Leguminosaceae

Parts used: Root.

Actions and medical uses: Tonic, stimulant, diuretic.

Systems affected: Digestive, immune, respiratory, urinary.

Specific indications: Employed to enhance the overall immune system complex, treat chronic weakness of the lungs, and build general health. Astragalus strengthens digestion, sharpens metabolism by balancing the energy of the internal organs and increases energy; consequently it builds deep overall resistance to disease. Astragalus is a reliable tonic for the lungs and kidneys, being very effective for treating kidney infection especially when other diuretics fail to help. It acts directly to enhance the condition of the blood, being a specific for all wasting away and exhausting diseases. It promotes the healing of wounds.

Combinations: Well combined with other herbs to enhance their effects.

Precautions: None.

Preparations: *Decoction:* taken as a tonic beverage, also stewed as a food, decocted in the waters used for preparing rice, beans, soups or stews. *Tincture:* to be added to compounds to enhance the actions of the other herbs.

Bayberry– *Myrica cerifera*

Family: Myricaceae

Parts used: Root bark.

Actions and medical uses: Astringent, diaphoretic and stimulant.

Systems affected: Digestive, circulatory and skin.

Specific indications: Bayberry (which is not the same as Barberry — *Berberis vulgaris* or Bearberry — *Arctostaphylos uva-ursi*) is a circulatory stimulant, helpful in many conditions which are improved by increased circulation of blood and lymph. It is a reliable astringent for treating diarrhea and dysentery, and as a gargle it is helpful for sore throats. It is valuable for stopping hemorrhaging in the lungs and bowels.

Combinations: For digestive disorders it combines well with Agrimony. Combines with Cayenne to increase the circulation of blood and lymph, thereby stimulating more rapid healing of congested or infected mucous membranes.

Preparations: *Infusion:* 1 cup 3 times a day. *Tincture:* 15 to 30 drops 3 times a day. *Externally:* Bayberry is applied as a fomentation at night to relieve or help prevent varicose veins.

Bearberry (Uva-ursi) – *Arctostaphylos uva-ursi*
Family: Ericaceae
Parts used: Leaf.
Actions and medical uses: Diuretic, astringent, urinary antiseptic, demulcent, soothing tonic.
Systems affected: Genito-urinary.
Specific indications: Bearberry (also known as Kinnikinnick and Indian Tobacco) will influence all mucous membranes, showing a specific affinity with the genito-urinary system, giving an antiseptic, astringent and demulcent effect. It is extremely effective for treating chronic inflammation of the bladder and kidneys. It will soothe, tone and disinfect this system, and its tissue strengthening astringency can be helpful in treating prostate weakness and some forms of bed-wetting. Bearberry is used for treating catarrh of the bladder, leucorrhea, lingering gonorrhea and its associated symptoms. It will gradually diminish the discharge while it works to tone the tissue. The leaves of this herb relieve aching back caused by kidney trouble.
Combinations: Combines well with Marshmallow, Yarrow, Couchgrass, Buchu and Corn Silk to treat urethritis (infection in the tubes that carry urine away from the bladder), cystitis (urinary/bladder infection with frequent painful passage of urine) or pyelitis (infection and inflammation of the renal pelvis of the kidney, in males, often due to stagnant urine which has been blocked by enlarged prostate or stones in the kidney). Bearberry has a specific use for treating conditions where there are numerous small stones (gravel) or a calculus in the kidney or bladder. Combines well with Horsetail, Agrimony and Corn Silk to treat some forms of incontinence such as bed wetting.
Preparations: *Infusion:* 1/2 cup four times a day to treat infection. *Tincture:*

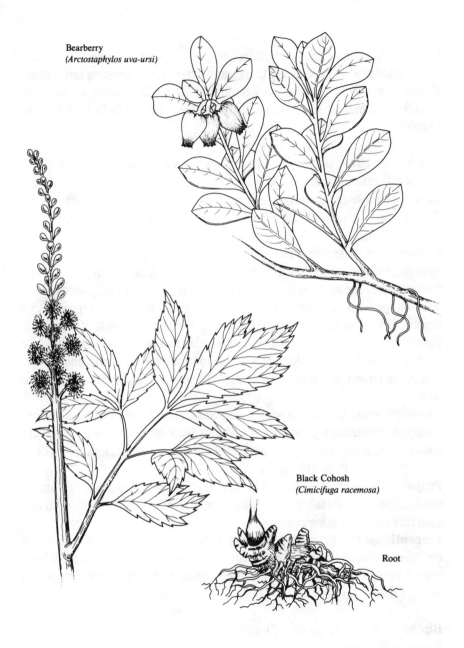

Bearberry
(Arctostaphylos uva-ursi)

Black Cohosh
(Cimicifuga racemosa)

Root

For treating urinary tract conditions, 60 drops in water as needed.
Precautions: Can be irritating to the stomach if used in frequent large doses.
Other uses: This herb is used singly or as an ingredient in smoking mixtures. It blends well with *Lobelia inflata* and Mullein leaf for this purpose.

Black Cohosh – *Cimicifuga racemosa (aka Actaea racemosa)*
Family: Ranunculaceae
Parts used: (dried) Root and rhizome.
Actions and medical uses: Anti-spasmodic sedative, alterative and emmenagogue.
Systems affected: Reproductive, muskular-skeletal, respiratory.
Specific indications: This herb is wisely used as a powerful relaxant and normalizer of the reproductive system. It is most appropriately used to help alleviate general pain and cramping pain in male and female reproductory organs. Likewise it is quite beneficial to use in the treatment of rheumatic pains, but also in relieving arthritic, muscular and neurological pains. As a respiratory anti-spasmodic, it can be use to treat intense symptoms such as whooping cough, and it relieves less severe upper-respiratory conditions as well.
Combinations: Combines with Yerba Santa, Gumweed and Elecampane for upper respiratory problems. Combines well with Yarrow, Crampbark and Saw Palmetto for treating sexual organ conditions and with Angelica root for treating rheumatic inflammation.
Preparations: *Infusion:* 1 cup 3 times a day. *Tincture:* 30 drops in water as needed. Small doses taken frequently throughout the day are more effective than less frequent large doses.
Precautions: Use dried (not fresh) plant parts of this herb. Most plants in the Ranunculaceae (Buttercup) family can be toxic when eaten in their fresh state. Drying the root and rhizome alters their organic chemistry, rendering Black Cohosh safe.

Buchu – *Agathosma betulina*
Family: Rutaceae
Parts used: Leaf.
Actions and medical uses: Diuretic, urinary antiseptic.
Systems affected: Urinary.
Specific indications: Buchu is one of our best diuretics, especially when

taken as a cool infusion. It is useful for treating water retention and urinary tract infection. Buchu is used to treat acute and chronic bladder and kidney and prostate infection. It is especially useful for relieving painful or burning urination. Taken as a hot tea, it acts as a stimulating diaphoretic, being useful in treating an enlarged prostate gland and accompanying irritated urethra.

Combinations: Combines well with Uva ursi for treating water retention and urinary tract infection. With Marshmallow or Corn Silk to treat burning or painful urination. With Couch Grass, Oregon Grape and Echinacea for treating infected prostate gland.

Preparations: *Infusion*: 1 cup 3 times a day. *Tincture*: 25 to 50 drops 3 times a day.

Burdock – *Arctium lappa*
Family: Compositae
Parts used: Root and seed.
Actions and medical uses: Alterative, hepatic, diuretic, bitter, diaphoretic, aphrodisiac.
Systems affected: Skin, blood, digestive, genito-urinary, musculo-skeletal.
Specific indications: Used over a long period of time, this plant is most valuable for treating, through internal action, chronic skin conditions such as acne, psoriasis and dry, scaly eczema. (Echinacea is better used to treat active acute toxicity that manifests as skin eruptions) Burdock contains essential oils which have diaphoretic action; taken internally, these volatile oils promote the elimination of wastes through sweating. This is most efficient for clearing conditions such as boils, styes, canker sores and other infections. Along with this diuretic action, Burdock seeds promote kidney function, helping the body to clear excessive blood acidity and kidney related toxemia. This works to help clear joint inflammation of the extremities. Burdock stimulates appetite and the flow of digestive juices, especially bile secretions, due to its bitter properties and hepatic actions. Over time, the alterative action of Burdock enhances metabolic processes and builds the body to a state of health, treating the surface indicators of poor health, such as skin disease, aching joints and sluggishness of the reproductive organs. Folk medicine considers Burdock preparations (taken internally and massaged into the scalp) effective against excess hair loss. It is also considered to be a strengthening aphrodisiac.
Combinations: Used internally with Sarsaparilla, Cleavers, Yellow Dock

and Red Clover for skin problems. Decocted with Comfrey root and taken internally for treating chronic persistent skin ulcers. Combines well with Damiana and Sarsaparilla for strengthening the male reproductive organs. **Preparations:** *Decoction and concentrate:* 1/2 cup 3 times a day for at least two weeks. If diuretic action is too great, drink last portion in late afternoon rather than evening. *Tincture:* Take up to 50 drops 3 times a day.

Calendula (Marigold) – *Calendula officinalis*
Family: Compositae
Parts used: Whole flower.
Actions and medical uses: Anti-inflammatory, astringent, vulnerary, styptic, antiseptic, anti-fungal, cholagogue, emmenagogue.
Systems affected: Skin, digestive, reproductive.
Specific indications: An excellent first-aid remedy. Used safely and effectively for all skin inflammations, be they due to injury or infection. Unlike Arnica, Calendula can be put directly onto an open wound. It is recommended to use this soothing flower on burns, external bleeding, bruises, slow healing wounds or skin ulcers. These same actions of Calendula are equally safe and effective for use on the internal skins of the digestive system. Use it for indigestion, digestive inflammation and peptic or duodenal ulcers, where it gives soothing anti-inflammatory action along with healing vulnerary and astringent actions. As a cholagogue, it gives relief in gall-bladder problems, aiding digestion. Calendula is reputed to be a normalizer of the female menstrual process. It helps balance the energy of male organs as well.
Combinations: Excellent anti-inflammatory and vulnerary combined with Arnica and St. Johnswort as a compound oil infusion or compound tincture, or with Garlic oil and Mullein flower oil for use as an ear oil. Combines well with Camomile and Marshmallow for nervous stomach and digestive problems. Combines well with Witch Hazel as a lotion for hemorrhoids and varicose veins, also with Goldenseal and Myrrh as an antiseptic application.
Preparations: *Infusion:* 1 cup 3 times a day. *Tincture:* 25 - 50 drops 3 times a day. *Externally:* Prepare as an oil infusion, lotion or tincture for skin conditions.
Other uses: A gorgeous uplifting yellow-orange dried flower for visual aesthetics in a potpourri.

California Poppy – *Eschscholzia californica*

Family: Papaveraceae
Parts used: Whole plant.
Actions and medical uses: Sedative, hypnotic, antispasmodic, anodyne.
Systems affected: Nervous, digestive.
Specific indications: This vibrant yellow-orange (California state flower) poppy is a cousin and non-addictive alternative to the Opium Poppy. It is far less powerful than the Opium Poppy and is most beneficial for use with children. Where there is a problem with excitability and sleeplessness it gives gentle sedative and hypnotic actions. It is useful for its anti-spasmodic action when needed. It is helpful for treating the pain of stomach and gallbladder colic.
Combinations: Combines well with Chamomile for restlessness, with Crampbark for pain or cramping.
Preparations: The green seed pods possess the strongest properties, but use the fresh whole plant including the roots. *Infusion:* 1 cup as needed. Taken at night it promotes restful sleep. *Tincture:* 15 to 25 drops as needed.

Cayenne (Red Pepper) – *Capsicum spp.*

Family: Solanaceae
Parts used: Fruit
Actions and medical uses: Stimulant, carminative, tonic, astringent, rubefacient, antiseptic.
Systems affected: Circulatory, nervous, digestive, respiratory, musculo-skeletal.
Specific indications: This is the purest and best stimulant known to phytotherapy, very prompt in its effects. Through the circulatory system its actions render an effect on the entire body. Cayenne affects the heart first, next the arteries, the capillaries and then the nerves. It is an efficient acute crisis herb taken as a first-aid remedy for all heart and circulation conditions, helping to prevent heart attack and stroke. Cayenne also stops bleeding in internal and external hemorrhaging, and is taken to treat insufficient peripheral circulation for relieving cold hands and feet. When used in hot foot baths for treating any apoplexies, the pressure is removed by equalizing the circulation. It is an excellent preventive or therapeutic remedy for colds, flu, debility, indigestion, headache, depression and arthritis. It is a specific tonic for the circulatory and digestive systems taken in small regular doses. Cayenne is useful in cramps, pain in the stomach and

bowels, and sometimes it will relieve constipation by warming the bowels, causing peristaltic action of parts which were previously contracted. Although quite hot, Cayenne does not burn the lining of the stomach, and uncooked Cayenne is not irritating.

Combinations: Combines well with Myrrh and Goldenseal for an excellent antiseptic wash.

Precautions: Cooked Cayenne can be irritating to the stomach as can many other cooked spices. Do not store this powder in paper or plastic containers. The paper absorbs Cayenne's essential oils, and these oils will melt plastic.

Preparations: *Infusion:* 1 tablespoon (of a strong infusion) is mixed with hot water, as needed. For warding off heart attack in an emergency, use a rounded teaspoon of *Cayenne* powder to a cup of hot water. *Tincture:* 3 to 10 drops in a little hot water as needed. *Externally:* rub Cayenne tincture on inflamed joints and wrap with cotton flannel overnight for sprains and arthritic pains. Powdered Cayenne placed directly on cuts will hurt, but it will efficiently stop the bleeding.

Other uses: Sprinkle a little (not too much) powder in shoes or socks to warm cold feet.

Chamomile – *Matricaria chamomilla* (German Chamomile)
Anthemis nobilis (Roman Chamomile)

Family: Compositae

Parts used: Flower. (*Matricaria chamomilla* is preferable for flavor.)

Actions and medical uses: Anti-spasmodic, carminative, anti-inflammatory, antiseptic, vulnerary, analgesic, anti-catarrhal.

Systems affected: Nervous, digestive, urinary, musculo-skeletal, skin.

Specific indications: A mild sedative, excellent for children as well as adults and the elderly. Chamomile is calming to the nervous system, most useful for treating insomnia, restlessness, nervous irritability in children, anxiety, nervous indigestion, flatulence, travel sickness, nasal catarrh and other forms of inflammation. The flowers prove to be an excellent treatment for stomach and intestinal complaints which are characterized by cramps or gas pains. The infusion (tea) of these flowers has a soothing effect on cramps or other painful symptoms in the kidney and bladder region. Chamomile is an excellent anti-inflammatory for mucous membranes, joints, muscles, wounds and skin irritation used internally and externally.

Combinations: Combines with Hops and Valerian for nervous restlessness, with Marshmallow and Hops for nervous indigestion.

Preparations: *Infusion:* 1 cup 3 times a day. Also used as a mouth wash. *Tincture:* 20 to 50 drops 3 times a day. *Externally:* As an eye wash for sore, inflamed eyes. As a soothing healing poultice or fomentation or for washing and treating the inflammation and pain of festering wounds.

Chaparral (Creosote Bush) – *Larrea mexicana* (*aka L. tridentata*)
Family: Zygophyllaceae
Parts used: Leaf and stem.
Actions and medical uses: Alterative, antiseptic, antibiotic, diuretic, expectorant.
Systems affected: Digestive, skin, circulatory, eliminative, respiratory, genito-urinary.
Specific indications: This intense flavored desert plant is a potent healing aid to the entire body. As Dr. Christopher says, "It is very bitter, but to the needy and courageous, it works fast for difficult conditions. It tones systems and rebuilds the tissue. It cleanses the lower bowel and tones peristaltic muscles. It is used to treat arthritis, rheumatism, stony deposits, stomach disorders, bladder problems, kidney troubles, hemorrhoids and inflammation of wounds." Chaparral has shown itself to be a free-radical inhibitor, helping to protect the liver and lungs from these destructive agents. It is a strong anti-oxident, useful in preserving oils and fats in skin oils, massage oils, salves and lotions. It is applied to all nature of wounds and skin conditions as an antiseptic and healer.
Combinations: Chaparral's flavor can be improved to some extent by combining it with Licorice. Chaparral combines well for internal and external use with other antimicrobial herbs such as Echinacea, Oregon Grape or Golden Seal. Combines well with Milk Thistle and Oregon Grape to protect the liver, with Elecampane, Yerba Santa and Gumweed for protecting the lungs. Combine with Angelica root, Black Cohosh and Wild Yam for relieving joint pains, rheumatic and arthritic conditions. Combine with Golden Seal, Myrrh and Calendula for an effective antimicrobial skin application.
Preparations: *Tincture:* Begin with 15 to 30 drops 3 times a day, for difficult conditions build up to 1 teaspoon per dose. *Capsules:* 2-#00 capsules, 3 times a day as a normal dose. *Decoction:* Drinking this herb as an infusion or decoction is almost incomprehensible to those who have tasted Chaparral tea; however, 1/2 cup 3 times a day is the dose for the needy and the courageous. *External:* Applied as a liniment, salve or tincture. Used for

first aid or long term applications. Apply to wounds or skin conditions as needed.

Chaste Tree – *Vitex agnus–castus*
Family: Verbenaceae
Parts used: Ripe berry.
Actions and medical uses: Tonic.
Systems affected: Genito–urinary.
Specific indications: Historically this plant was used as a male herb to help reduce male libido, being especially useful for cloistered monks and those gents entering the priesthood, consequently the common name Chasteberry. It later acquired the reputation as a woman's herb, and is predominantly used to treat women's hormone related health problems. Chaste Tree berry is a hormone balancing herb. Its actions are normalizing, assisting the body to do what is most appropriate. It stimulates and normalizes pituitary gland function, especially the progesterone function of this gland. The most common use of the Chaste Tree berries is to normalize the activity of progesterone and estrogen, the female sex hormones. It is indicated for disorders related to hormone dysfunction, such as premenstrual stress and menopausal changes in women; however, it is also helpful for men who are experiencing difficulty with their mid-life changes to adjust to this important transition. Herbalist Christopher Hobbs, in his excellent booklet, *Vitex! The Female Herb*, points to studies which indicate that this herb can help control acne in both male and female teenagers. Weiss mentions that it gives a good response in cases of premenstrual herpes on the lips.
Preparations: *Infusion:* 1 cup 3 times a day. *Tincture:* 20 to 40 drops 3 times a day. *External:* John Gerard speaks to making a salve of the Chaste Tree leaf and applying it to the scrotum to help reduce swelling of the testicles (see orchitis).

Cleavers – *Galium aparine*
Family: Rubiaceae
Parts used: Whole aerial part.
Actions and medical uses: Diuretic, alterative, anti-inflammatory, tonic, astringent.
Systems affected: Lymphatic, urinary.
Specific indications: Our finest lymphatic tonic. Along with its alterative and diuretic actions, this lymphatic herb is ideal for treating all problems where the

lymphatic system is involved, such as enlarged lymph nodes (tonsils, adenoids, etc.), skin diseases and eruptions, and ulcers and tumors that are the result of poor lymph drainage. Used to treat kidney and bladder inflammations including stones and gravel obstructions, scalding urine and irritation at the neck of the bladder. Cleavers also has a mild action upon the bowels.

Combinations: Combines well with Calendula and Echinacea for lymphatic problems. Combines with Marshmallow and Uva-Ursi for treating bladder or kidney inflammation.

Preparations: Fresh plant juice is most effective. 2 to 3 teaspoons in a little water taken 3 times a day. *Infusion:* 1 cup 3 times a day. *Tincture:* 30 to 60 drops 3 times a day.

Comfrey – *Symphytum officinale*
Family: Boraginaceae
Parts used: Root and leaf.
Actions and medical uses: Astringent, demulcent, nutritive, vulnerary, expectorant.
Systems affected: Digestive, respiratory, musculo-skeletal, urinary, skin.
Specific indications: Traditional names based on empirical herbal science range from Knitbone, Knitback and Healing Herb to Bruisewort and Boneset which partially indicates what Comfrey has been successfully used for centuries. It is the classic folkloric remedy for human ailments. Comfrey stimulates cell proliferation, magnifying both internal and external wound-healing. Its astringent action helps alleviate hemorrhaging wherever it occurs, be it in the stomach, lungs, bowels, kidneys or rectum. Its demulcent components soothe bronchitis and irritating cough and acts as an expectorant. The highly demulcent mucilage inherent in Comfrey heals gastric, duodenal and external ulcers.
Combinations: Combines well with Marshmallow and/or Meadowsweet for treating gastric or duodenal ulcer. Combines with Horehound and Elecampane for respiratory problems. Use in combination with Marshmallow, St. Johnswort and Calendula as a soothing, healing salve.
Precautions: See toxicity section below. This does not apply to external use of Comfrey as a poultice, fomentation or salve.
Preparations: *Infusion:* 1/2 cup 3 times a day. For internal bleeding, use 1 cup every two hours until bleeding has stopped. *Tincture:* 15 to 40 drops 3 times a day. *Externally:* leaf is applied topically as a poultice or fomentation on bruises, sprains, athlete's foot, wounds and ulcers; root is applied

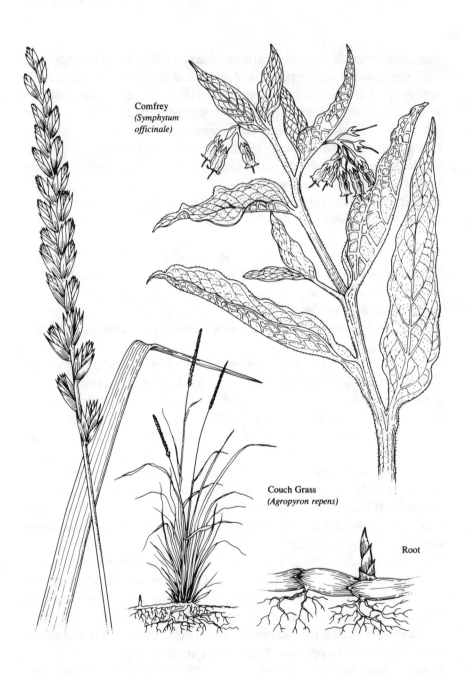

Comfrey
(Symphytum officinale)

Couch Grass
(Agropyron repens)

Root

topically as a fresh root preparation for wounds, ulcers, fractures, hernia and for the promotion of the suppuration of boils. Note: Some wounds and/or ulcerations need to drain prior to healing on the surface. Also deep wounds need to heal the deeper tissue prior to healing over the surface tissue. Before applying Comfrey externally to a wound, which will rapidly heal the surface tissue, make sure deeper tissue is appropriately healed. This is hastened by taking Comfrey internally.

Toxicity: Pharmacologists have revved up a high powered-bandwagon concerning potential liver-toxicity from long term internal use of Comfrey due to "pyrrolizidine alkaloid" content. Comfrey is one of the oldest, most successful, most highly praised wound-healing remedies in folkloric medicine. Our ancestors and present-day herbalists heal countless serious conditions using the whole plant. I have used Comfrey as a reliable healing agent for years and plan to continue using it in the same manner; however, I want to alert the reader to this current reductionist trepidation. It is not harmful for an adult male or female to drink Comfrey leaf tea. For children, occasional use is okay. The precaution I suggest is for pregnant and nursing woman. *Avoid taking Comfrey tea, for it can possibly harm the fetus and nursing infant; and do not use it internally with infants.* External use of Comfrey in salves and poultices is safe and effective for all ages.

Corn Silk – *Zea mays*
Family: Graminaceae
Parts used: Stigma (fine soft threads) from the female flower (ear).
Actions and medical uses: Diuretic, demulcent, tonic.
Systems affected: Genito-urinary, circulatory.
Specific indications: For acute inflammation of the genito-urinary system such as urethritis, cystitis and prostatitis. This herb is especially useful for conditions of purulent (pus forming) decomposition of urine in the bladder. It will cleanse the bladder membranes in cystic catarrh and will manifest antiseptic action when in the presence of morbid deposits. This is one of the most valued of urinary sedatives for treating bladder infections for children. The demulcent action is helpful in treating nocturnal enuresis (bed wetting) especially when this condition is due to weakness or irritation of the renal system. The diuretic action of the silk is due largely to its tonic action on the heart and blood vessels.
Combinations: Combines well with Horsetail and Agrimony for treating bed wetting. For bladder infection, combine with Uva-ursi and Couchgrass.

Combine with Couchgrass, Saw Palmetto and Yarrow for prostatitis or enlarged prostate gland.

Preparations: Eat the fresh (undried) silk like fresh, young corn on the cob. It is sweet and nourishing. *Infusion:* Infusion of the fresh silk is the most active preparation. 1 cup 3 times a day, though not at bedtime when treating bed wetting. *Tincture:* 30 to 50 drops 3 times a day

Note: Use fresh silk or fresh dried green silk from organically grown and unsprayed corn which still smells and tastes like sweet young corn or use the liquid extracts of this fresh stigmata. The dark red-brown Corn Silk sold in most stores is old, oxidized and basically useless.

Couch Grass – *Agropyron repens*
Family: Graminaceae
Parts used: Rhizome.
Actions and medical uses: Diuretic, demulcent, anti-microbial.
Systems affected: Genito-urinary.
Specific indications: Couch Grass is one of our major medicinal grasses. It is a valuable agent used in the treatment of enlarged prostate and/or an infected prostate. Its demulcent action is very soothing when treating the inflammation and irritation of urethritis, cystitis and prostatitis. It is also helpful to soothe the pain of passing kidney stones and gravel. For best results, drink lots of pure water when using diuretics.
Combinations: For all genito-urinary infections, combine with Yarrow, Uva-ursi and Buchu. Combine with Saw Palmetto, Echinacea , Hydrangea and Cornsilk for treating prostate infection and/or enlarged prostate.
Preparations: *Decoction:* 1 cup 3 times a day. *Tincture:* 30 to 50 drops in water 3 times a day.

Cramp Bark – *Viburnum opulus*
Family: Caprifoliaceae
Parts used: Bark.
Actions and medical uses: Anti-spasmodic, sedative, nervine, astringent.
Systems affected: Genito-urinary, skeletal-muscular, nervous.
Specific indications: Cramp Bark is a relaxer of muscular tension and spasm. It has a strong anti-spasmodic effect on the entire skeletal muscle system, on the muscles of the genital-urinary system, both male and female, as well as on the heart muscle for treatment of heart palpitations.
Combinations: For relief of muscular cramps combine with Valerian. For

painful cramping in the genito-urinary organs combine with Chamomile, Ginger and Angelica root. Cramp Bark also mixes well with Wild Yam and Prickly Ash for relief of cramps.

Preparations: *Decoction:* 1 cup 3 times a day. *Tincture:* 30 to 60 drops in water 3 times a day.

Cubeb – *Piper cubeba*
Family: Piperaceae
Parts used: Berry.
Actions and medical uses: Aromatic, diuretic, mild stimulant, carminative.
Systems affected: Genito-urinary, digestive, respiratory.
Specific indications: The actions of these berries have an effect upon the genito-urinary tract as well as upon all the mucous tissues of the body, treating debility with profuse discharges from these tissues. It is used successfully for treating chronic gonorrhea (after the profuse acute discharges have ceased), abscess of the prostate, spermatorrhea, leucorrhea, catarrh of the urinary bladder and chronic inflammation of the bladder. In these conditions, burning in the urethra is an indication for the use of this herb. Very effective for treating dyspepsia which is due to an atonic condition of the stomach. Cubeb berries augment the appetite and improve the digestion. The berries are also used for atonic conditions of respiratory mucous membranes, to treat chronic laryngitis and bronchitis.
Combinations: Combines well with Corn Silk and Bearberry for treating the latter stages of gonorrhea and cystitis.
Precautions: Cubeb berries are often contraindicated in acute active inflammations, but are of great service for treating chronic inflammations.
Preparations: *Infusion:* 1 cup 3 times a day. *Tincture:* 30 to 50 drops in water 3 times a day.
Other uses: Used as a condiment in stews and soups.

Damiana – *Turnera diffusa (aphrodisiaca)*
Family: Turneraceae
Parts used: Leaf and stem.
Actions and medical uses: Tonic, anti-depressant, urinary antiseptic, aperient, mild laxative, aphrodisiac.
Systems affected: Nervous, genito-urinary, digestive.
Specific indications: Tonic for strengthening the nervous and hormonal systems. It also has anti-depressant properties, thus it is excellent for

treating anxiety and/or depression that has a predominant sexual factor. Used to treat impotence, it possibly has a testosterone-like action and may work by strengthening the male system. *Damiana* assists digestion and gives mild laxative action.

Combinations: Combines well with Wild Oat and Scullcap and/or Hops for nervous anxiety conditions, with Wild Oat and Kola for depressed conditions.
Preparations: *Infusion:* 1 cup 3 times a day. *Tincture:* 15 to 40 drops 3 times a day. A Damiana liqueur called Creme de Damiana, sold in Mexico, is reputed to be an aphrodisiac. I have a number of acquaintances who attest to this as fact.

Dandelion – *Taraxacum officinale*
Family: Compositae
Parts used: Root and leaf.
Actions and medical uses: Diuretic, liver tonic, laxative, cholagogue, stomachic, anti-rheumatic.
Systems affected: Digestive, musculo-skeletal, urinary.
Specific indications: A powerful diuretic. It is our best natural source of potassium, making it the safest, most balanced diuretic agent. Also contains a high content of many other easy-to-assimilate minerals and vitamins. Helps reduce blood pressure and aids the action of the heart by safely decreasing water retention due to heart problems. Useful for treating kidney and bladder inflammation and obstructions. Its bitter flavor enhances appetite, digestion and assimilation. It assists the pancreas, being most helpful in both hypoglycemic and diabetic conditions. Dandelion is widely used for inflammation and congestion of the liver, spleen and gall-bladder. It helps these organs clear obstructions and helps the liver to detoxify poisons. Has a toning disease preventive action for the liver as well as a restorative therapy after liver disease such as hepatitis. Dandelion works well as part of a treatment for muscular rheumatism.
Combinations: Combines well with Chamomile for stomach complaints; with Oregon Grape for liver and gall-bladder disease. For treating water retention it combines well with Yarrow and *Couchgrass*. A useful adjunct to most any herbal formula.
Precautions: None. Large amounts can be taken in many forms.
Preparations: *Infusion:* 1/2 cup taken frequently. *Tincture:* 20 to 50 drops 3 times a day.
Other uses: The dried cut root can be lightly roasted, powdered and brewed

as a "dandelion coffee" beverage. If you want to harvest its roots, dig them June to August when they are their bitterest. The blossoms make an excellent wine. The whole blossom can be eaten, having a pleasant mild sweetness, especially if you eat one of its mildly bitter leaves just prior. It is wild, abundantly available and free of charge. Welcome Dandelion into your garden. Pick it, don't poison it.

Devil's Club – *Oplopanax horridus*
(aka Fatsia horrida & Panax horridum)
Family: Araliaceae
Parts used: Bark of the root.
Actions and medical uses: Alterative, tonic, antiarthritic, hypoglycemic, and probably our native Pacific Northwest adaptogen.
Systems affected: Glandular, musculo-skeletal, skin, digestive, respiratory.
Specific indications: Devil's Club is an important plant medicine, ceremonial purifier and protective charm for many Indian peoples in western North America. Its traditional uses are extensive, with few medicinal plants being more widely and consistently used within their native region; the Haida and Tlingit people having the greatest number of medicinal uses for it. The medicinal use of this plant was associated with the observation of bears soothing battle wounds by chewing Devil's Club roots. Bears also ate the berries which were later named "grizzly's fruit." The bark of the root is used to treat an extensive variety of conditions. Rheumatism, arthritis, diabetes, stomach and digestive disorders, tuberculosis, coughs and colds and skin disorders to name a few. Its use for treating arthritis and rheumatism is nearly universal in the native cultures of the Northwest coast. Nancy Turner, ethnobotanist and research associate for the British Columbia Provincial Museum has done extensive research on the native uses of this remarkable plant.

We have here a native plant that is a cornucopia of healing actions. If the Northwestern forests are left with some sort of ecological integrity and this plant is harvested carefully we can continue to learn a great deal from it about preventing and treating diabetes and arthritis and the many other conditions to which it lends its healing virtues. I have received numerous communications from individuals delighted with the results they have experienced by using extracts of this plant as whole or partial substitution for insulin. I have neither seen nor heard any reports of toxic side effects. Respectful inquiry into hundreds of years of local native use and the

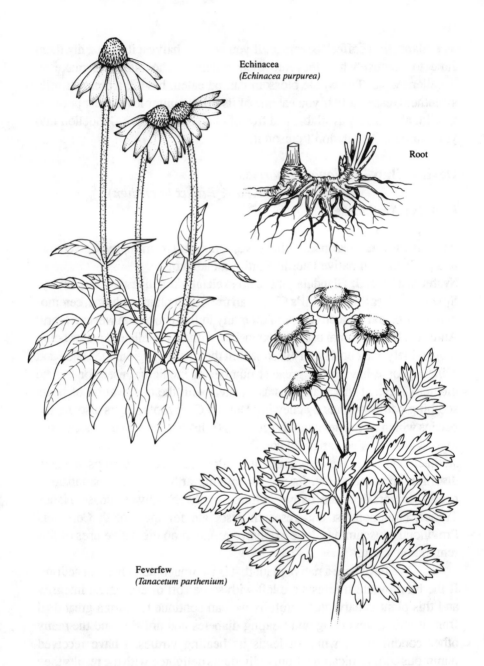

Echinacea
(Echinacea purpurea)

Root

Feverfew
(Tanacetum parthenium)

herbalist's pursuit of further clinical research in the use of *O. horridum* awaits our focus.

Preparations: *Decoction:* 1/2 to 1 cup 3 times a day. *Tincture:* 15 to 30 drops 3 times a day.

Echinacea – *Echinacea spp.*

Family: Compositae

Parts used: Root, seed and juice of the whole plant.

Actions and medical uses: Alterative, lymphatic, anti-bacterial, anti-viral, sialogogue.

Systems affected: Immune, lymphatic, respiratory, reproductive.

Specific indications: Blood and lymphatic purifier, and a most valuable anti-microbial when taken in high doses. Taken internally Echinacea stimulates interferon production enhancing the body's natural defenses by way of the immune system. Echinacea is very useful for treating blood poisoning, boils, carbuncles and abscesses, acute bacterial and viral infection, venomous bites of all sorts as well as allergic reactions to poison oak and poison ivy. Echinacea is an excellent remedy for treating upper respiratory infections such as tonsillitis, bronchitis and laryngitis.

Combinations: Combines well with many plants. Combines with Saw Palmetto for treating prostate infection. Combined in equal parts with Saw Palmetto and used in suppository form for treating inflamed and enlarged prostate. Combines with Burdock root for treating boils and abscesses; with Myrrh resin, Horseradish, Garlic and Golden Seal for tonsillitis and other lymphatic conditions; with Yarrow and Uva-ursi to treat bladder infection.

Precautions: Can, and in most cases probably should, be taken in large amounts; however, it can cause stomach irritation in small children. It will make the mouth tingle and actively salivate.

Preparations: For acute conditions take every hour or two. The actions of this root do not preserve well. Use the fresh root or a tincture of fresh root whenever possible. Dried root must be recently dried. *Decoction:* cupful as a dose. You may want to blend this with Licorice or Fennel for palatability. *Tincture:* 1 teaspoonful as a dose. *Suppository:* Inserted rectally after each bowel movement. *External:* combine with Golden Seal, Calendula and Myrrh as a tincture or salve to treat infected sores and cuts.

Eco-Note: Echinacea has become an immensely popular medicinal. In the wake of this popularity, great strain is being placed on the native Echinacea plant communities. I ask consumers to consciously choose the species

Echinacea purpurea (read the labels on commercial herb products) which is a relatively easy plant to germinate from seed and is therefore cultivated quite successfully by organic growers. This will help the other more vulnerable species, along with wildstands of *E. purpurea*, to survive and thrive in their wild native communities.

Fennel – *Foeniculum vulgare*
Family: Umbelliferae
Parts used: Seed.
Actions and medical uses: Carminative, aromatic, antispasmodic, anti-inflammatory, expectorant, diuretic, anti-microbial.
Systems affected: Digestive, respiratory, urinary.
Specific indications: Fennel's effects have a warming, respiring and loosening nature. Fennel warms and stimulates the digestive organs, especially when they become sluggish. This relieves gas and headaches that are related to improper digestion. An excellent stomach and intestinal remedy for treating flatulence and colic conditions (wonderful for infants and children), while also stimulating healthy appetite and digestion. It also helps children by stimulating milk production in nursing mothers. Fennel frees the respiratory system, rendering a calming anti-spasmodic effect on coughs and bronchitis. It gives a delicious flavor and aromatic lift to herbal blends and cough syrups.
Combinations: Combines extremely well with Catnip for treating childhood fever diseases as well as nervous, respiratory, digestive and intestinal diseases.
Preparations: *Infusion:* grind the Fennel seeds and infuse them. Drink 1 cup 3 times a day. *Tincture:* 25 to 40 drops 3 times a day. *Externally:* apply the infusion as a compress on closed eyelids to treat eye inflammation and eye strain. Fennel essential oil diluted in a fixed oil and rubbed into skin or applied as a compress will ease muscular and rheumatic pains.
Other uses: Chew one or more whole seeds as an after-dinner digestive aid or as an aromatic breath freshener. The young slender leaves are used fresh in salads. Fennel seed is an excellent flavoring agent for blending with most nasty tasting-herbs.

Feverfew – *Tanacetum parthenium*
Family: Compositae
Parts used: Leaf and flower.

Actions and medical uses: Anti-inflammatory, bitter, vasodilator, relaxant.
Systems affected: Digestive, nervous system, musculo-skeletal.
Specific indications: A specific plant for preventing and treating migraine headache, most specifically those migraines that are relieved by the application of warmth to the head. Feverfew also relieves tinnitus and experience of dizziness. Acute rheumatoid arthritic inflammation is frequently relieved by using this plant. An excellent stomach bitter relieving nausea and promoting digestion, reputed to help alleviate melancholy and sadness, enhancing feelings of well being.
Combinations: Combines with Ginkgo and Black Cohosh for treating tinnitus and dizziness.
Precautions: Causes irritation to the mouth in some people .
Preparations: Best to eat 1 fresh leaf 2 to 3 times a day. Feverfew grows prolifically in yards and gardens. *Tincture* (of the fresh plant): take 15 to 30 drops in a little water 3 times a day.
Other uses: Ornamental plant.

Garlic – *Allium sativum*
Family: Liliaceae
Parts used: Bulb.
Actions and medical uses: Universally renowned "panaceaic" home remedy, alterative, tonic, stimulant, diaphoretic, expectorant, hypo-tensive, anti-spasmodic, anti-microbial, nutrient, nervine, cholagogue, carminative and vulnerary.
Systems affected: Respiratory, cardiovascular, immune.
Specific indications: Used for all lung ailments, particularly chronic bronchitis, respiratory catarrh, recurrent colds, influenza, whooping cough and as part of a treatment for bronchitic asthma. Used over a period of time, it is a good treatment for high or low blood pressure and will help reduce blood cholesterol levels. Acting on virus, bacteria and alimentary invaders, Garlic treats infections and rids the body of parasites. Garlic is an effective agent for treating nervous problems such as headache, spasms, cramps and mild seizures. Regular use of Garlic is an excellent nutritional preventative for most respiratory and digestive infectious conditions.
Combinations: Combines well with Coltsfoot and Lobelia for treating bronchitis and asthma; with Echinacea, Wild Indigo and Goldenseal for treating conditions associated with microbial activity. Onion has similar characteristics and is frequently used in combination with or in place

of Garlic.

Precautions: The obvious social breath precautions. When advised to use oil of Garlic in the ear for treating earache, be sure to use an infusion of raw Garlic in a fixed oil; DO NOT use the expressed juice of the Garlic cloves or Garlic essential oil because they will burn.

Preparations: Can be taken in the diet as a raw food (1-3 cloves daily); it is best not to boil or cook Garlic when using it for a medicine. *Syrup:* 1 Tablespoon 3 times a day. *Tincture:* 15 to 40 drops in water 3 times a day.

Ginger – *Zingiber officinale*
Family: Zingiberaceae
Parts used: Fresh or dried root.
Actions and medical uses: Carminative, diaphoretic, rubefacient, diffusive stimulant, anti-spasmodic.
Systems affected: Digestive, circulatory.
Specific indications: Used to stimulate peripheral circulation in cases of poor circulation, chilblains and cramps. Ginger is a very efficient diaphoretic for use in a hot tea to promote sweating in feverish conditions. It is a most effective carminative taken as a tea, tincture or in a capsule for treating stomach and intestinal problems such as stomach cramps, flatulence, dyspepsia, nausea and motion sickness. 1 to 2 #00 capsules full of dried Ginger taken about 1/2 hour prior to exposure has proven to be superior to the common motion-sickness drug Dramamine for suppressing motion induced nausea. Ginger has an effective anti-coagulant action similar to that of aspirin. It is used externally as a compress for treating muscle sprains and inflammation and joint stiffness.

Combinations: Combines well with most all herbs for treating digestive system disorders. Oil infusion of Ginger combines well with oil infusion of Garlic and St. Johnswort for treating earache. Combines well with laxative herbs such as Senna leaves to help prevent gripping. Ginger may be used as a substitute for Cayenne when necessary, but it is a more diffusive stimulant than Cayenne.

Precautions: Don't swallow powdered Ginger unless it is in a liquid preparation or capsule, as it can burn the esophagus.

Preparations: *Infusion of fresh or dried Ginger:* Take one cupful with Lemon and a little honey as needed. *Capsule:* 1 to 2 #00 capsule as needed. *Externally:* Apply a hot tea compress or oil infusion to the affected area, changing the compress as needed to keep the area warm. The skin will become red as the circulation increases. You can also grate fresh Ginger root and place it between hot moist cotton fabric which you apply to the affected area, but apply vegetable oil to the skin first as the ginger can burn sensitive skin. This poultice can work well to bring healing to inflamed or infected lower abdomen and genito-urinary organs.

Other uses: Culinary spice. It is a good food preparation habit to add Ginger to all meat dishes to help the digestive system detoxify the meat.

Ginkgo – *Ginkgo biloba*
Family: Ginkgoaceae
Parts used: Leaf and nut.
Actions and medical uses: Vasodilator, anti-inflammatory, stimulant, antioxidant (free-radical scavenger), anti-clotting.
Systems affected: Cardio-vascular, nervous, brain tissue, genito-urinary, respiratory, whole body cellular level.
Specific indications: Strengthens the cardiac system by increasing arterial tone, reducing inflammation in blood vessel walls and retarding blood cell clumping. Prevents platelet aggregation and blood clotting that can lead to blockage of arteries. Increases blood flow and oxygen circulation throughout the entire body, reversing the effects of insufficient blood circulation. For treatment and prevention of geriatric dementia (cerebral vascular insufficiency), Ginkgo is a protective and therapeutic brain stimulant. It improves brain function such as mental capacity and alertness, memory retention and mental clarity, sociability and mood. Geriatric patients have displayed significant improvement in short term memory loss, vertigo, headache, depression and tinnitus in the ears. Higher than normal doses of this herb can improve concentration and awareness by increasing mental alertness and response time. Ginkgo is an anti-oxidant that traps and neutralizes free-radicals which damage cellular health and accelerate aging; boosts the transmission of signals through deteriorating nerves; inhibits bronchial constriction by reducing inflammation in lung tissue; inhibits water retention in delicate tissues and enhances cellular energy production by beneficially effecting intracellular components. Ginkgo has been shown to be an excellent agent for treating impotence, i.e., arterial erectile dysfunction. It has a direct effect on endothelial cells which enhance blood flow of both penile arteries and veins without any change in systemic blood pressure. Chinese herbal medicine has used Ginkgo nuts as medicine for centuries to treat weaknesses in the genito-urinary system of both male and female persons.

Combinations: Combines well with Hawthorn for a cardio-vascular tonic and with Wild Oat as a nerve tonic. Ginkgo combines well with most other herbs.
Precautions: None when using the ordinary extracts. If a person chooses to use the adulterated "standardized" extracts (standardized percentage content of a particular "active" constituent), he should be aware that European studies have found some side effects inherent in these preparations.
Preparations: *Infusion:* 1 cup 3 times a day. *Tincture:* 1 teaspoon 3 times a day.
Other uses: A beautiful ornamental tree. Ginkgo nuts make a delicious food.

Ginseng – *Panax quinquefolia* (*American ginseng*)

Family: Araliaceae
Parts used: Root.
Actions and medical uses: Alterative, cardiac tonic, liver tonic, stimulant, anti-depressive, aphrodisiac.
Systems affected: Cardiovascular, liver, general effect on whole body helping improve physical and mental performance.
Specific indications: Stimulates the body to overcome weakness and deficiency. Helps normalize blood pressure, particularly low blood pressure, having a strong affinity for the circulatory system. Used to treat blood weakness and anemia. Depressive states; often when associated with debility, exhaustion or sexual inadequacy.
Combinations: Combines well with Saw Palmetto and Damiana for treating glandular weakness.
Precautions: Do not use Ginseng with disease conditions that manifest inflammation, high fever, irritability or burning sensation. Occasionally this herb can produce dizziness or headache.
Preparations: A piece of the root may be chewed. *Decoction:* 1 cup 3 times a day. *Tincture:* 15 to 40 drops 3 times a day.

Golden Seal – *Hydrastis canadensis*

Family: Ranunculaceae
Parts used: Root and rhizome.
Actions and medical uses: Tonic, astringent, oxytocic (stimulant to involuntary muscles), anticatarrhal, antiseptic, bitter, hepatic, stomachic, laxative.
Systems affected: Mucous membranes, musculo-skeletal, digestive, res-

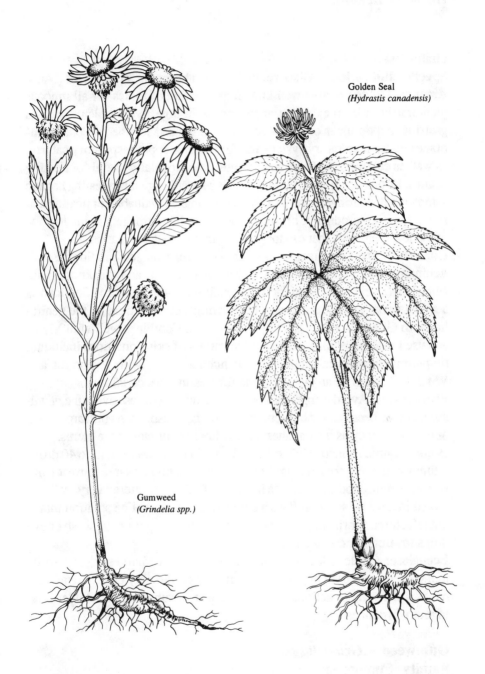

Golden Seal
(Hydrastis canadensis)

Gumweed
(Grindelia spp.)

piratory, skin.

Specific indications: Discovered by the aboriginal cultures of North America, Golden Seal is well known as the king of tonics for all mucous membranes. It is an excellent agent for use in digestive problems such as gastritis, peptic ulcer or inflamed colon. It is used for the mucous membranes of the respiratory system and for treating upper respiratory catarrh, as well as catarrhal deafness and tinnitus. It is especially useful for treating catarrhal sinus conditions. Golden Seal is a specific agent for treating hepatic symptoms. Its astringent and tonic properties make it valuable for treating and strengthening reproductive organs and as an anti-hemorrhaging agent. It is one of the few medicines that can tone and sustain venous circulation.

Combinations: Combines with Chamomile for stomach conditions; with Echinacea and Saw Palmetto for prostate infection and weakness; with Milk Thistle and Dandelion for liver conditions; with Hops and Scullcap as a spinal nerve tonic. Combines with Partridgeberry for treating the genitalia; with Gravel Root for treating the kidneys. Combines well with Myrrh and used externally for treating a wide variety of skin conditions including ringworm, eczema and non-specific itching. Used with Eyebright and Witch Hazel leaf as an eye tonic and for treating eye conditions.

Precautions: Avoid using in prolonged high doses, because over time, it will diminish the beneficial and essential flora of the intestines. Avoid large doses during pregnancy as it stimulates the involuntary muscles of the uterus.

Preparations: *Infusion:* 1/2 to 1 cup 3 times a day. *Tincture:* 15 to 40 drops 3 times a day. *Externally:* Used as infusion, tincture or salve to treat ringworm, eczema, and itching. The infusion of this root, filtered very well and mixed in a saline solution (Use a commercial sterile saline solution that is manufactured for rinsing contact lenses), makes a superior eye wash or eye drops for treating conjunctivitis.

Eco–Note: Golden Seal is being dangerously overharvested due to its immense popularity. Oregon Grape, another remarkably effective medicinal, is a plant whose actions can very adequately substitute for Golden Seal in many instances.

Gumweed – *Grindelia spp.*
Family: Compositae
Parts used: Leaf, bud and flower.
Actions and medical uses: Anti-spasmodic, expectorant, hypotensive.
Systems affected: Respiratory, skin, cardiac.

Specific indications: An excellent antispasmodic and expectorant herb most useful for chronic bronchial cough and bronchial infection. It is effectively used to treat hayfever. Gumweed can be a mild sedative and cardiac relaxant lowering heart pulse and blood pressure. Topical use of the crushed flowers or the tincture as a poultice is used to treat the skin irritation caused by Poison Oak and Poison Ivy and as well for antidoting the poisons of insect bites.

Combinations: Combines very well with Yerba Santa for a relaxing antispasmodic remedy to relieve tight feeling, dry hacking cough. Combine with Lobelia for relief of asthmatic conditions.

Preparations: *Infusion:* 1 cup 3 times a day. *Tincture:* 20 to 50 drops 3 times a day. *Externally:* Crushed leaves and flowers applied as a poultice or the infusion or tincture applied as a compress.

Hawthorn – *Crataegus oxyacantha*

Family: Rosaceae

Parts used: Ripe berry and young (white or pink) blossom.

Actions and medical uses: Cardiovascular tonic, vasodilator, diuretic, astringent, hypotensive sedative.

Systems affected: Cardiovascular, digestive.

Specific indications: The best tonic for the heart and circulatory system. Hawthorn nourishes the heart, assisting it to return to normal activity by either gently stimulating or depressing its activity as needed. Can be used for palpitations of the heart. Used over a period of time, it treats cardiac weakness and/or failure, hypertension, arteriosclerosis and insomnia. Improves digestion.

Combinations: Combines well with Yarrow, Lavender and Motherwort for treating high blood pressure; with Motherwort to specifically treat tachycardia (unduly rapid or arrhythmic heartbeat). Combines well with Ginkgo and Horsechestnut as a vascular tonic.

Preparations: *Infusion:* 1 cup 3 times a day. *Tincture:* 20 to 50 drops 3 times a day. Combined with other appropriate herbs useful as a *syrup* for treating sore throat.

Other uses: Makes excellent jams and syrups. Ornamental tree.

Hops – *Humulus lupulus*

Family: Cannabinaceae

Parts used: Strobile.

Actions and medical uses: Sedative, hypnotic, astringent, bitter.

Systems affected: Nervous, digestive.

Specific indications: First cousin to Cannabis, this herb gives a marked relaxing effect on the central nervous system, easing tension and anxiety of all forms. Treats excessive sexual desire and painful erections associated particularly with gonorrhea. Useful for conditions that manifest restlessness, indigestion and headache. As an astringent and a bitter, it is useful in conditions such as inflammation of the mucous membranes of the digestive system.

Combinations: Combines with Valerian for a hypnotic relaxant to treat insomnia. Combines well with Chamomile for nervous stomach and dyspepsia.

Precautions: Contraindicated in depression.

Preparations: *Infusion:* 1 cup at night to help induce sleep. *Tincture:* 15 to 35 drops 3 times a day.

Ho shou wu – *Polygonum multiflorum*

Family: Polygonaceae

Parts used: Root.

Actions and medical uses: Tonic, alterative, diuretic.

Systems affected: Digestive (liver and pancreas), reproductive.

Specific indications: A rejuvenating tonic herb used to help prevent premature aging. It restores energy, maintaining strength, vitality and fertility in those individuals who are advancing in years. This herb helps normalize the action of the pancreas, kidneys and liver, relieving symptoms of physical deficiency. It is reputed to keep the true color of the hair and benefit the overall body by strengthening the bones, muscles and connective tissues.

Preparations: *Infusion:* 1 cup 3 times a day. *Tincture:* 25 to 40 drops 3 times a day.

Note: This herb is often (erroneously) referred to as Fo-Ti.

Horsechestnut – *Aesculus hippocastanum*

Family: Hippocastanaceae

Parts used: Dried fruit (the nut itself), bark.

Actions and medical uses: The fruit is circulatory tonic and astringent. The bark is tonic, astringent, febrifuge (in this case used for intermittent fever), narcotic and antiseptic.

Specific indications: This plant is specifically used when fluids that are normally free flowing, stagnate. This has occurred in cases of varicose veins and hemorrhoids where the venous blood circulation has become sluggish due to the vessel walls having become slack, atonic and frequently distended in the legs and rectal canal. "The unique actions of Aesculus are on the vessels of the circulatory system . . . increasing the strength and tone of the veins in particular . . . used internally to aid the body in the treatment of problems such as phlebitis, varicosity and haemorrhoids" (D. Hoffmann). Used not so much for active conditions but more for treating congestion and engorgement. "A remedy for congestion and engorgement. Nerve pain in the viscera due to congestion. Soreness of the whole body, with vascular fullness, throbbing and general malaise . . . rectal uneasiness with burning or aching pain" (Felter-Lloyd). This herb has definite potential for use in cases of sluggish, stagnate prostatic terrain.

Combinations used: Combines well with Hawthorn, Yarrow and Prickly Ash for internal use to treat varicosity.

Precautions: Outer husks are toxic. Eating the leaves or green outer husks of the fruit can lead to symptoms of gastroenteritis, reddening of the skin and drowsiness. Do not confuse the nut of this tree with Ohio Buckeye (*Aesculus glabra* and *arguta*), Red Buckeye (*Aesculus pavia*) or California Buckeye (*Aesculus californica*). The actions of these plants are different than Horsechestnut.

Preparation and dosage: *Infusion:* 1/2 cupful 3 times a day of the dried powdered nut. *Tincture:* 10 to 30 drops 3 times a day. *Externally:* used as a lotion for the above conditions and for treating skin ulcers.

Other uses: Shade and aesthetic ornamentation.

Horsetail – *Equisetum arvense*

Family: Equisetaceae

Parts used: Aerial stem and whorl of stringlike branchlets.

Actions and medical uses: Astringent, diuretic, antihemorrhagic, styptic, vulnerary.

Systems affected: Genito-urinary, skin.

Specific indications: Used to treat inflammation or benign enlargement of prostate. Its astringent and diuretic actions make it a valuable herb for treating urinary tract infections, for reducing hemorrhaging, healing wounds, adult incontinence and bed wetting in children. The ancient Horsetail enlivens the kidneys and stimulates the entire excretory process when sluggishness occurs. As a styptic, it aids in coagulation and helps to stop bleeding.

Combinations: Combines well with Hydrangea for treating prostate conditions. Combines with Corn Silk for treating incontinence and bed wetting.

Precautions: Best used in frequent small doses. When large quantities are taken at one time, or if this herb is used continuously over several weeks, it can become an irritant to urinary tract tissue and to the intestinal lining.

Preparations: *Infusion:* 1/2 cup 3 to 4 times a day. *Tincture:* 15 to 25 drops 3 to 4 times a day. *Externally:* In baths it has been used to ease rheumatic pain. Powdered and combined with powdered *Yarrow* in equal parts, formulates a valuable styptic to be applied directly to bleeding wounds.

Other uses: When bundled and dried, it can be used as a scouring pad and as a steel wool substitute.

Irish Moss – *Chondrus crispus*
Family: Gigartinaceae
Parts used: Use the dried thallus of this seaweed.
Actions and medical uses: Nutritive tonic, demulcent, emollient, expectorant.
Systems affected: Respiratory, urinary, digestive, skin, whole body.
Specific indications: A highly nutritive tonic and convalescence supplement. It is well-endowed with iron, iodine, bromine and many other minerals, as well as the vitamins A and B complex. Its mucilaginous, demulcent properties make it valuable primarily for treating bronchitis, pneumonia, stomach inflammation, heartburn and ulcers. It is used in cosmetic care as a skin softener and moisturizer.
Combinations: Combines with Licorice for bronchial inflammation and with Marshmallow for easing stomach inflammation and indigestion.
Preparations: *Infusion:* 1 cup 3 times a day. *Tincture:* 15 to 40 drops 3 times a day.
Other uses: Large quantities are used in the food industry.

Licorice – *Glycyrrhiza glabra*
Family: Leguminosae
Parts used: Root.
Actions and medical uses: Expectorant, alterative, demulcent, anti-inflammatory, adrenal agent, mild laxative.
Systems affected: Respiratory, digestive, endocrine, whole body.

Specific indications: Licorice contains constituents that are similar to the natural steroids of the human body; therefore, its long-term use has a marked effect on the endocrine system, specifically for revitalizing the adrenal glands, with no dangerous side effects. Licorice's expectorant and anti-inflammatory aspects are widely used in throat and upper respiratory conditions such as flu, colds, coughs, catarrh and bronchitis. Good remedy for tickling cough, sore throat and hoarseness. Its demulcent and anti-inflammatory properties effect relief of gastritis, colic and peptic ulcers.

Combinations: Combines with Marshmallow root, Chamomile and Comfrey leaf for peptic ulcer and other gastric problems. Combines well with Coltsfoot, Lobelia and White Horehound for treating bronchitis. Combine with Sage, Ginger or Cayenne for treating colds and flu. For blood cleansing combine it with other alterative herbs such as Red Clover, Echinacea, Dandelion, Burdock or Sarsaparilla. Licorice is often added to herbal formulas to detoxify and alleviate harsh aspects of other plants without interfering with their beneficial actions.

Precautions: The use of Licorice is not recommended for individuals having high blood pressure which is due to water retention. In long term use potassium intake should be increased, so combining Licorice with Dandelion is recommended.

Preparations: *Decoction:* 1 cup 3 times a day. *Tincture:* 15 to 30 drops 3 times a day.

Other uses: Flavoring agent for covering the unpleasant taste of other herbs.

Marshmallow – *Althaea officinalis*

Family: Malvaceae

Parts used: Root and leaf.

Actions and medical uses: Demulcent, diuretic, nutritive tonic, emollient, vulnerary.

Systems affected: Digestive, urinary, respiratory, musculo-skeletal, skin.

Specific indications: Marshmallow supplies an abundance of vegetable mucilage and easily assimilated calcium making it a powerful anti-inflammatory and anti-irritant for the gastrointestinal system. It is used extensively for stomach inflammation, gastric, peptic or duodenal ulcer, also for inflammation of the mouth or pharynx. Triggering reflex mechanisms that travel through the spinal nerves, its demulcent action is valuable for all lung ailments, respiratory catarrh and coughs, and it is effective as a anti-irritant and anti-inflammatory for the joints. Used in combination with other diuretic herbs, Marshmallow is effective for treating kidney stones and gravel. Apply it as a poultice for treating blood poisoning, gangrene, septic wounds, burns and bruises.

Combinations: Combines well with White Horehound and/or Lobelia for coughs; with Comfrey for treating peptic ulcer. Combines with Parsley and Hydrangea as a tea for kidney stones and gravel.

Preparations: *Infusion:* (Prepared as a cold infusion) 1 cup 3 times a day. *Decoction:* Boil the powdered root in milk and drink freely for urinary organ hemorrhaging, diarrhea or dysentery. *Tincture:* 15 to 40 drops 3 times a day. *Externally:* Prepare with St. John's Wort and Calendula as a poultice or salve for soothing and healing skin inflammation and ulcers. The leaves and/or root are used as a fomentation for treating all forms of swelling, pain, abscesses and festering sores. Combine with Red Raspberry leaves as an eyewash to soothe inflamed eyes.

Meadowsweet – *Filipendula ulmaria*
Family: Rosaceae
Parts used: Aerial part.
Actions and medical uses: Antirheumatic, anti-inflammatory, stomachic, antacid, astringent.
Systems affected: Digestive, Musculo-skeletal.
Specific indications: Soothing and protective to the mucous membranes of the digestive system, it counteracts overacidity and the inflammation of the stomach lining due to drug, alcohol and dietary self-abuse. Meadowsweet tones the lining of the small intestines, significantly enhancing the ability of the body to absorb nutrients. It relieves nausea, heartburn, gastritis and peptic ulcer. The use of Meadowsweet is indicated at times when one is suffering with the combined symptoms of upset stomach and headache. It possess a gentle astringent action appropriate for treating diarrhea in children. As a balanced source of salicylates (the active agent in aspirin), it safely reduces fevers and rheumatic pain in joints and muscles due to its anti-inflammatory action.

Combinations: Combines with Marshmallow and Chamomile for treating stomach conditions; with Wild Yam for treating rheumatic pains.

Preparations: *Infusion:* 1 cup 3 times a day, or as needed. *Tincture:* 20 to 40 drops 3 times a day.

Note: The original botanical name of Meadowsweet is *Spiraea ulmaria*. From its genus name, *Spiraea*, came the term aspirin.

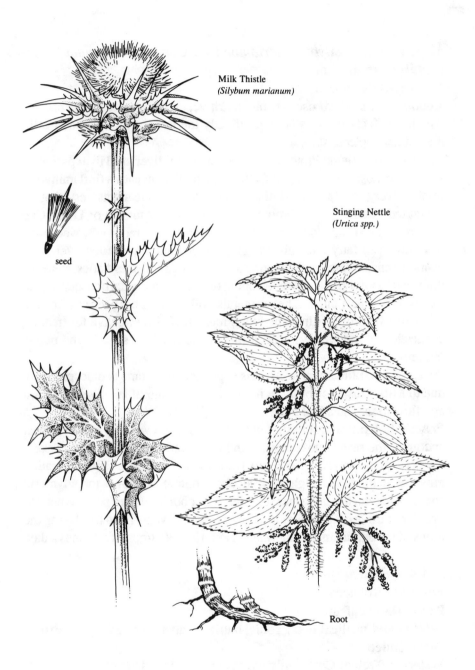

Milk Thistle
(Silybum marianum)

seed

Stinging Nettle
(Urtica spp.)

Root

Milk Thistle – *Silybum marianum (aka Carduus marianum)*
Family: Compositae
Parts used: Ripe seed.
Actions and medical uses: Tonic, nutritive, cholagogue, demulcent.
Systems affected: Digestive (specifically the liver), urinary (specifically the kidney), spleen, skin.
Specific indications: Protects and regenerates the liver in all liver problems such as cirrhosis (hardening of the liver); jaundice; hepatitis (inflammation of the liver); cholangitis (inflammation of the bile ducts resulting in decreased bile flow); mushroom poisoning (from Amanita or Death-Cap mushroom, and immediate medical attention is also required); weakened liver (induced fatty liver disorders). Protects and regenerates liver from damage caused from use of pharmaceutical drugs and anesthetics, steroids, drug or alcohol abuse; or liver poisoning from environmental or occupational toxins such as pesticides or heavy metals. Milk Thistle has been an effective treatment for psoriasis in some individuals. It is also effective for treating congestion of the kidneys, spleen (hypertrophy of the spleen) and pelvic region.
Precautions: Mild laxative effect is experienced in some people, probably due to Milk Thistle's ability to increase bile (a natural laxative) secretion and flow in the intestinal tract.
Preparations: It is best to start with low doses and work up slowly. Roast and grind the seeds into a powder and take as food or in capsules. Take 1 teaspoon of the powdered seed 2 to 3 times a day. *Tincture:* This preparation must be made with a high ethyl alcohol content to extract the silymarin constituent which is not water soluble, so alcohol intolerant persons need to avoid it or drive off the volatile alcohol through evaporation by placing the drops of the extract in boiling water. Take 15 to 30 drops 3 to 4 times a day.

Nettle – *Urtica spp.*
Family: Urticacea
Parts used: Leaf and root.
Actions and medical uses: Tonic, nutritive, alterative, astringent, expectorant, diuretic.
Systems affected: Genito-urinary, respiratory, blood, skin.
Specific indications: Activates metabolism, strengthening and toning the whole body by providing iron, potassium and silicon and aiding the assimilation of these essential minerals; effective for nourishing the blood

and treating anemic conditions. Provides expectorant and antispasmodic actions for the respiratory system giving safe relief for asthma. Strongly affects the excretory processes making it most useful for treatment of a wide variety of skin eruptions and all varieties of adult and infantile eczema, especially nervous eczema. This action is also useful for clearing the toxins that manifest rheumatism and gout. Its astringent action is useful for treating nose bleed or for treating hemorrhaging wherever it occurs in the body. Nettles provide diuretic action for relief of kidney conditions such as chronic cystitis. Nettle root is specific for treating prostate enlargement and inflammation.

Combinations: Combine with Burdock and Dandelion for treating eczema. Combine with Mullein leaf and Comfrey leaf as a nutritive expectorant. Nettle root combines well with *Saw Palmetto* for treating prostate enlargement.

Precautions: Harvest with protective gloves; Nettle sting has the formic acid connection with red ant sting.

Preparations: *Infusion:* 1 cup 3 times a day. *Tincture:* 15 to 50 drops 3 times a day.

Note: Nettles can be blended fresh with a small portion of pure water (in an electric blender); All stinging potential is removed, and according to Ryan Drum, foremost Nettle wildcrafter and connoisseur, this is the best way to take Nettles for food and medicine.

Other uses: Young Nettle leaves are steamed for a delicious pot herb, and its roots make a mineral rich vegetable for those few that know about this. The infusion also makes an effective hair rinse for treating dandruff and to encourage hair growth. Nettle has strong flexible fibers that can be spun and made into cloth.

Oat – *Avena sativa* (cultivated), *A. fatua* (wild)
Family: Gramineae
Parts used: Seed and straw.
Actions and medical uses: Tonic, nervine, antidepressant, nutritive, demulcent, vulnerary.
Systems affected: Nervous, circulatory, skin.
Specific indications: Oat is our best nervous system tonic, as well as an excellent cardiac tonic. It is used primarily for nervous debility and nervous exhaustion manifesting in melancholia and depression.
Combinations: Combines well with all nervine herbs, be they com-

pounded as a relaxant or as a stimulant. Combines with Scullcap for treating depression. Combines with Hawthorn as a heart tonic.

Preparations: *Infusion:* 1 cup 3 times a day. The straw is rich in silica and calcium used to brew a mineral-rich tea for treating skin conditions. *Tincture:* Best made with the fresh green seed harvested while it is still in the milky stage. Take 20 to 50 drops 3 times a day. *External:* Prepare a strong decoction of Oat straw and add it to hot bath for relaxing and treating irritated skin conditions and nervous conditions. Place rolled Oats in a sock and tie off the open end. Put this into your bath water and let it soak; squeeze the soggy bundle and rub the mucilage onto the skin. This will soften the skin and soothe any skin irritation. Grind rolled Oats into a powder and mix with a small amount of cornmeal and powdered Peppermint. Use this blend as a face scrub to cleanse and soften skin, replacing soap.

Other uses: The seed is used to make a nutritious porridge and gruel and as a muscle-strengthening food for domestic animals.

Oregon Grape – *Berberis aquifolium*
Family: Berberidaceae
Parts used: Root and rhizome.
Actions and medical uses: Alterative, cholagogue, hepatic, tonic, laxative.
Systems affected: Digestive, skin, blood, lymphatic, eliminative, genito-urinary.
Specific indications: Has a tonic effect on the liver and gall-bladder similar to that of Golden Seal, and it is an excellent substitute in many instances for the highly overharvested Golden Seal. Oregon Grape has a definite affinity for the genito-urinary tract and is proving to be beneficial for treating male prostate infection. Most useful in treatment of chronic skin conditions such as psoriasis and dry scaly eczema. Its bitter quality has a most beneficial effect on the stomach and gall bladder. It stimulates healthy appetite, promotes digestion and improves assimilation thereby increasing strength and vitality. It is helpful for treating nausea and vomiting, especially when gall bladder related. It is useful in treatments of syphilitic cases and blood diseases that affect the genitals. Being a gentle tonic-laxative, Oregon Grape is a safe and effective plant to use for treating chronic constipation.
Combinations: Combines well with Burdock and Cleavers for skin condition, with Yellow Dock or Cascara Sagrada for improved bowel movement. Combines extremely well with Marshmallow and Saw Palmetto for treating prostate infection.

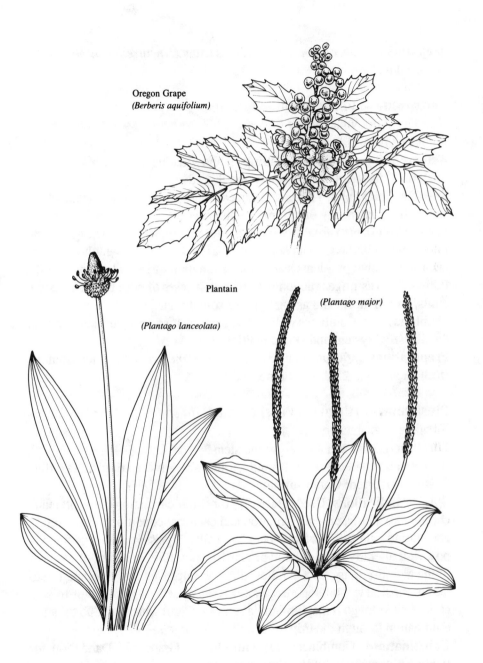

Oregon Grape
(Berberis aquifolium)

Plantain

(Plantago major)

(Plantago lanceolata)

Preparations: *Decoction:* 1 cup 3 times a day. *Tincture:* 15 to 30 drops 3 times a day.

Periwinkle – *Vinca major* and *V. minor*
Family: Apocynaceae
Parts used: Aerial parts.
Actions and medical uses: Astringent and sedative.
Systems affected: Genito-urinary and digestive.
Specific indications: This plant is an excellent all around astringent which can be used internally or externally. Its most common internal use is for treating excess menstrual flow. It is useful as a douch for treating vaginal infection and likewise in a penis soak to assist in couples' health-care. It is use for digestive problems such as inflammation of the colon or diarrhea. Periwinkle's astringent action is also used in cases of nose bleed, bleeding gums, mouth ulcers and as a gargle for sore throat.
Combinations: Combines well with Agrimony for astringent action to treat the digestive system and skin conditions.
Preparations: *Infusion:* 1 cup 3 times a day. *Tincture:* Best made from the fresh plant, 15 to 25 drops 3 times a day.

Pipsissewa – (Prince's Pine) *Chimaphila spp.*
Family: Pyrolaceae
Parts used: Leaf and above-ground stem.
Actions and medical uses: Diuretic, tonic, alterative, astringent, laxative.
Systems affected: Genito-urinary, skin.
Specific indications: Used effectively for chronic irritation of the prostate, chronic prostatitis, chronic irritation and catarrhal condition of the urethra and atonic relaxation of the bladder walls. Pipsissewa has gentle yet powerful alterative and diuretic properties; therefore, irritation of any part of the genito-urinary tract is relieved due to improved nutrition and circulation. Pipsissewa, having also a mild laxative action, gives relief to skin conditions (though it may initially aggravate them) which are due to faulty elimination through the urinary and digestive tracts.
Combinations: Combines well with Oregon Grape and Dandelion for treating kidney, liver and/or skin conditions.
Precautions: Do not boil for this destroys the actions of Pipsissewa.
Preparations: *Infusion:* 1/2 to 1 cup 3 to 4 times a day. *Tincture:* 20 to 40 drops 3 times a day.

Plantain – *Plantago lanceolata (narrow-leaved)*
Plantago major (broad-leaved)
Family: Plantaginaceae
Parts used: Aerial part.
Actions and medical uses: Diuretic, expectorant, demulcent, alterative, astringent, vulnerary.
Systems affected: Digestive, urinary, respiratory, skin.
Specific indications: A gentle expectorant for soothing inflamed and painful membranes caused by bronchitis and coughing. Its diuretic, astringent and alterative actions have a strengthening effect on the genito-urinary tract as well as on the lymphatic system. Very useful for treating blood-poisoning, reducing swelling and promoting healing of highly septic wounds. Fresh juice taken in a cup of warm water is an excellent treatment for treating stomach ulcers. Employing Plantain's astringent action, it is used for treatment of diarrhea, hemorrhoids, gastric ulcers and cystitis where there is bleeding.
Combinations: Combined with Comfrey for treating gastric bleeding or bleeding hemorrhoids. Combines well with Chickweed, Comfrey, Calendula and Goldenseal for a healing, soothing all-purpose salve.
Preparations: Fresh juice taken 1 teaspoon in a cup of warm water before each meal. *Infusion:* 1 cup 3 times a day. *Tincture:* 20 to 40 drops 3 times a day. *Externally:* The fresh juice of bruised or chewed leaves makes an excellent on the spot poultice for treating insect bites and stings especially useful for reducing the swelling and allergic reaction to such wounds. Plantain is very available growing everywhere that bees and insects work and humans tread. Use this poultice on infections, skin wounds and chronic skin conditions. It is often prepared as a salve.

Prickly Ash – *Zanthoxylum Clava-Herculis (aka Z. americanum)*
Family: Rutaceae
Parts used: Bark and berry.
Actions and medical uses: Stimulant, alterative, diaphoretic, tonic.
Systems affected: Digestive, circulatory, lymphatic and skin.
Specific indications: Prickly Ash is a warming, circulatory stimulant that increases the circulation throughout the body; consequently, it is useful for treating cold extremities, rheumatism, arthritis, chilblains, leg cramps, varicose veins, low energy and slow healing wounds. As an alterative it is used for treating skin diseases and for dissipating accumulations in the

joints. Prickly Ash warms the stomach, so it is used for treating sluggish digestion as well as stomach cramps and colic. The bark is used for treating toothache.

Combinations: Having a strong stimulating effect on the circulatory system, lymphatic system and the mucous membranes, it combines well with a number of herbs assisting the treatment of a wide range of specific conditions; e.g., combines well with Horsechestnut for relieving varicosity.

Preparations: *Infusion:* 1/2 cup 3 times a day. *Tincture:* 20 to 30 drops 3 times a day.

Raspberry – *Rubus idaeus*
Family: Rosaceae
Parts used: Leaf and fruit.
Actions and medical uses: Astringent, tonic, antispasmodic.
Systems affected: Genito-urinary tract, digestive, eyes.
Specific indications: One of the most renowned herbal teas for strengthening and toning the female reproductive organs. It renders the same marvelous virtues and nutrients to the male reproductive system. Raspberry is an effective pleasant tea for treating acute stomach problems and for preventing and treating fever diseases such as colds and flu, especially safe and reliable for children. It is a safe and effective astringent for treating diarrhea, and is a safe reliable tonic for the bowels. It makes an effective agent for cleansing and healing canker conditions of the mucous membranes of the mouth throat and stomach. Raspberry infusion makes an excellent anti-inflammatory eye wash and a mouth wash or gargle for treating sore throat, canker on the tongue, mouth ulcers and/or bleeding gums.

Combinations: Combined with Pipsessiwa to treat and strengthen the genito-urinary tract in both male and female. Combine with Sage as a mouth wash or gargle or with Eyebright as tea for an eye wash. Combines well with Catnip, Fennel and Red Clover for children's ailments.

Preparations: *Infusion:* 1 cup 3 times a day. *Tincture:* 15 to 50 drops 3 times a day.

Sage – *Salvia spp.*
Family: Labiaceae
Parts used: Leaf.
Actions and medical uses: Stimulant, astringent, tonic, alterative.
Systems affected: Digestive, nervous, urinary.

Specific indications: Highly regarded as a stimulant tonic in debility of stomach, nervous system and overall digestive weakness. Soothing to the nerves, to quiet nervous excitement and soothe delirium in fevers. Sage decreases secretions, reducing salivation, sweating, excess mucous of the sinuses, throat and lungs. Sage has a beneficial effect on the blood, in biliousness and liver complaints, as well as kidney troubles and internal hemorrhaging. It is a general tonic astringent used in formulas for a wide variety of complaints. It is truly a prudent sage-like herb.

Combinations: Combine the dried or fresh herb with apple cider vinegar and honey and simmer together for 5 minutes to make an excellent gargle and mouthwash.

Precautions: Should not be used internally when sweating is desirable. Should not be used for nursing mothers as it decreases milk secretions, unless this decrease is desired.

Preparations: *Infusion:* Given in small, often-repeated doses, 1/2 to 1 cup 3 to 4 times a day. Cold infusions for treating stomach conditions, warm for treating mouth and throat conditions. *Tincture:* 15 to 25 drops 3 times a day. *Externally:* Fresh leaves rubbed on the teeth will clean them and strengthen the gums.

Other uses: Culinary spice. Ceremonial smudging.

St. John's Wort – *Hypericum perforatum*
Family: Hypericaceae
Parts used: Flowering tops and top leaves.
Actions and medical uses: Anti-inflammatory, astringent, diuretic, vulnerary, sedative analgesic, antiseptic.
Systems affected: Nervous, Musculo-skeletal, urinary, skin.
Specific indications: This plant has a healing, regenerative effect on injured nerves, nervous system functions and all their emotional manifestations. It has sedative effects with specific antidepressant properties. It offers calming and sedative actions in relieving anxiety; is well used as part of a whole treatment for psychological instability. It is reliably used during male and female menopausal stress and excitability, especially if there is resultant depression. As a normalizer, it improves sleep in insomniacs but is also useful for excessive sleepers (hypersomnia). With all wounds, it gives a marked pain relieving effect, and it stimulates the new formation of damaged tissue. Treats neuralgic inflammation and pain. St. John's Wort is remarkably healing to wounds, burns and sunburns. It helps one to control

237

the flow of fluids as in bed-wetting and difficult menstruation. St. John's Wort appears to show anti-retroviral activity giving no serious side effects. It is being empirically researched by AIDS patients. (See resource section AIDS Treatment News). The oil infusion can be taken internally by the teaspoon to treat gastritis, gastric ulcers, and as a retained enema to relieve inflamed conditions of the colon. St. John's Wort is most definitely an herb that blesses humanity in many ways.

Combinations: Excellent anti-inflammatory, vulnerary, analgesic and antiseptic combined with Calendula and Arnica as a compound oil infusion for external use. Combines with Valerian and Calendula as a compound tincture for the nervous system, or with Calendula and Sage as a mouth-wash for gum inflammation and infection. Combines with Feverfew for relief of the severe pain of Tic-douloureux.

Precautions: FDA declared it "unsafe" based on reported toxicity to cattle, not on any reports or studies on human toxicity. Extensive observation by herbal empirical science shows it to be a remarkably safe and effective herb for humans.

Preparations: All forms of preparation are best when made from the fresh undried plant. *Infusion:* 1 cup 3 times a day or as a mouthwash. *Tincture:* 25 to 40 drops 3 times a day. *Externally:* As a fresh plant, deep ruby-red oil infusion. Apply directly to inflamed, injured nerves, bruised areas, any and all skin inflammation and sunburn.

Sarsaparilla – *Smilax officinalis*
Family: Liliaceae
Parts used: Dried root and rhizome.
Actions and medical uses: Alterative, antirheumatic, diuretic, diaphoretic.
Systems affected: Genito-urinary, blood, musculo-skeletal, skin.
Specific indications: Contains constituents that aid testosterone activity in the body. A reliable alterative used to help treat systemic conditions affecting the skin, also for treating gout and rheumatic conditions, especially rheumatoid arthritis. Help relieve the symptoms of menopause.
Combinations: Combines with Saw Palmetto and Echinacea for nourishing and toning the male reproductive organs. Combines well with Burdock, Cleavers and Milk Thistle for treating highly irritated psoriasis or dry scaling eczema. Combines with Sassafras and Dandelion as a blood purifier and tonic.
Preparations: *Decoction:* 1 cup 3 times a day. Drink this strong and hot to

promote sweating for colds and fevers. *Tincture:* 15 to 25 drops 3 times a day.

Sassafras – *Sassafras albidum*
Family: Lauraceae
Parts used: Root bark.
Actions and medical uses: Carminative, alterative, hepatic, diaphoretic, diuretic, antirheumatic, antiseptic, astringent.
Systems affected: Digestive, genito-urinary, musculo-skeletal, skin.
Specific indications: Acts as an alterative, diuretic and stimulating liver tonic to help detoxify the overall system and clear blood disorders; thus it is valuable for treating skin and skeletal conditions such as acne and eczema, gout and rheumatic pains.
Combinations: Combines with Burdock, Yellow Dock and Bearberry for treating acne or eczema. Combines with Sarsaparilla, Burdock, Echinacea and Cleavers for chronic blood disorders and related symptoms.
Precautions: Water extracts when taken in large quantities stimulate the liver and can bring about a strong cleansing reaction. The distilled essential oil of Sassafras is toxic.
Preparations: *Decoction:* 1/4 to 1/2 cup 3 times a day. *Tincture:* 5 to 20 drops 3 times a day. *Externally:* Antiseptic on the skin. Makes a valuable oil infusion for treating head lice and other infestations (do not use this oil internally).

Saw Palmetto – *Serenoa repens*
(aka Serenoa serrulata, Sabal serrulata)
Family: Palmea
Parts used: Berry.
Actions and medical uses: Nutritive, diuretic, urinary antiseptic.
Systems affected: Genito-urinary, nervous, digestive.
Specific indications: Safely and efficiently tones and strengthens the male reproductive system, enhancing the male sex hormones when required. Used specifically in conditions of enlarged, debilitated prostate gland. It is of great value for treating infection of the prostate and associated genito-urinary organs. It increases the tone of the bladder, allowing a better contraction and more complete expulsion of the contents, relieving any straining pain. Nourishes the nervous system and aids assimilation of nutrients. (This herb is discussed in more detail in the chapter titled "Picking the Right Herb," section "About Male Herbs.")

Combinations: Combines exceptionally well with Echinacea, Oregon Grape and Buchu for treating prostate infection and catarrh of the genito-urinary tract. Combined in equal parts with Echinacea and used in suppository form for treating inflamed and enlarged prostate. Combines with Hydrangea and Horsetail for treating enlarged prostate gland and with Damiana and Ginseng for treating general debility associated with un-healthy atonic reproductive system.

Preparations: *Decoction:* 1 cup 3 times a day. *Tincture:* 25 to 50 drops 3 times a day. It helps to mix this tincture in a little water with a 1/4 teaspoon of sour vitamin C crystals for flavor enhancement. *Capsule:* 2 #00 capsules full of powdered berry 3 times a day. Taken it in this form will help get around the flavor of this herb. *Suppository:* Inserted rectally after each bowel movement.

Scullcap – *Scutellaria laterifolia*
Family: Labiaceae
Parts used: Aerial part.
Actions and medical uses: Nerve tonic, sedative, antispasmodic.
Systems affected: Nervous, musculo-skeletal.
Specific indications: High in minerals required for a healthy nervous system, Scullcap is a reliable and safe central nervous system tonic and sedative. It relaxes all states of nervous tension, nourishing and strengthening the nervous system at the same time. Used effectively for treating nervous headache, neuralgia, insomnia and restlessness. Has been useful in cases of seminal weakness. Specifically used to treat conditions of hysteria and/or seizure including petit-mal and grand-mal epilepsy. Useful for assisting people to get through the withdrawal stage of drug and alcohol self-abuse.
Combinations: Combines well with Hops and/or Valerian for treating nervous tension, pre-menstrual tension or seizure. Combined with Chamomile for allaying restlessness and sleeplessness.
Preparations: *Infusion:* 1 cup 3 times a day. *Tincture:* Best to use the fresh undried Scullcap for making a tincture. 15 to 40 drops 3 times a day. Dried or fresh Scullcap herb should never be boiled, and prolonged storage impairs its therapeutic actions.

Siberian Ginseng – *Eleutherococcus senticosus*
Family: Araliaceae

Parts used: Root.
Actions and medical uses: Adaptogen.
Systems affected: Immune, nervous, circulatory, respiratory.
Specific indications: Used as an adaptogen to help a person handle the excessive demands and stress created by his life-style and work conditions (heat, noise, motion, work load increase, exercise and decompression). Increases stamina and mental alertness, thereby countering exhaustion, depression and general debility; this helps improve work performance and increased sense of well being, giving increased resistance to illness. Use of this herb significantly increases resistance to influenza, acute and chronic respiratory infection and hypertension. *Eleuthro* is a circulatory stimulant and a vasodilator. It is used to lower blood pressure, and it also normalizes low blood pressure. It helps reduce cholesterol levels. Effective as an ingredient in compounds formulated to treat impotence. Over time it works to enhance the immune system and obviously assists this system by alleviating the effects of excess stress. Eleuthro positively affects athletic performance, physical endurance, work load capacity and recovery rate after exertion. It is believed to increase longevity, general health, improve appetite and restore memory. The Soviets, Koreans, Japanese and the Chinese are eagerly continuing research on this remarkable plant.
Combinations: Works quite well by itself. Can be used in place of *Panax Ginseng* when *Panax* is too stimulating.
Preparations: A very mild herb, use in large doses. *Infusion:* During times of stress, take 1/2 cup frequently throughout the day. *Tincture:* 25 to 60 drops 3 times a day. *Tablets:* Take up to a gram 3 times a day. Take these doses for up to 60 days to best appreciate results.
Note: Many of the "Siberian Ginseng" products on the herb market are adulterations of *Eleutherococcus senticosus*, many of which do not have the same properties. Make sure of your sources.

Valerian – *Valeriana officinalis*
Family: Valerianaceae
Parts used: Root and rhizome.
Actions and medical uses: Sedative, anodyne, hypnotic, antispasmodic, carminative, hypotensive.
Systems affected: Nervous, digestive.
Specific indications: For conditions presenting nervous excitability. It is probably the most useful relaxing nervine herb, most useful for helping to

reduce high blood pressure. It is most helpful as a pain reliever when the pain is caused by tension, so it is appropriately used in certain kinds of migraine headache and rheumatic pain. Its carminative, mild bitter and antispasmodic properties will aid in the relief of cramping and intestinal colic. This herb is not habit-forming and has nothing whatsoever to do with the allopathic drug Valium.

Combinations: Combines with Scullcap and Wild Oat for tension, anxiety and/or hysteria; with Hops and Camomile for insomnia and with Wild Yam and Cramp Bark for pain and cramping.

Precautions: There are certain rare individuals who react to the use of Valerian by becoming stimulated rather than calmed by its properties.

Preparations: *Infusion:* 1 cup as needed. *Tincture:* 15 to 25 drops 3 times a day or as needed. For best results, this herb should not be boiled.

Wild Lettuce – *Lactuca virosa*

Family: Compositae

Parts used: Leaf.

Actions and medical uses: Sedative, anodyne, hypnotic.

Systems affected: Nervous, respiratory, digestive.

Specific indications: This is the common relative from which our modern hybrid salad lettuce has sprung. It is high in a bitter latex, which at one time was commonly known as "lettuce opium." The older a head of salad lettuce, the more latex it will show and the more bitter flavor it will develop as it matures into a "leaf off the old stalk." Wild Lettuce is an excellent herb for treating an overactive nervous system which develops conditions such as hyperactivity, insomnia, restlessness and irritable excitability, especially in children. It is useful for treating dry irritable coughs. It can relieve colic and other intestinal spasms, and it relieves muscular pain stemming from rheumatic conditions.

Combinations: Combine with Coltsfoot for treating irritable cough, especially with children. Combines with Valerian and Chamomile for treating insomnia and restlessness.

Preparations: *Infusion:* 1 cup 3 times a day. *Tincture:* 15 to 30 drops 3 times a day.

Other uses: Has been used as an anaphrodisiac to mellow out an excessive sexual appetite.

Valerian *(Valeriana officinalis)* Yellow Dock *(Rumex crispus)*

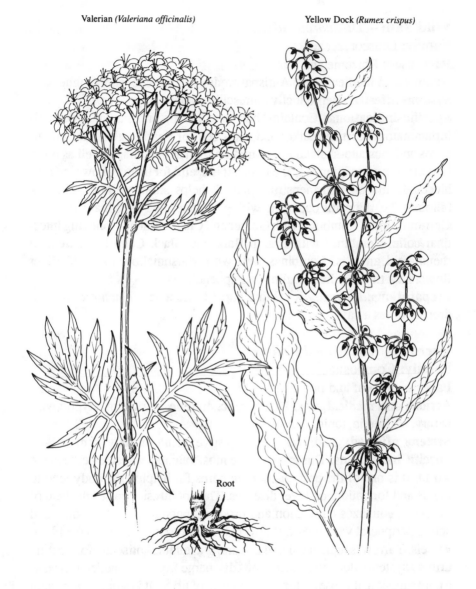

Root

Wild Yam – *Dioscorea villosa*
Family: Dioscoreaceae
Parts used: Rhizome and root.
Actions and medical uses: Antispasmodic, diaphoretic, cholagogue.
Systems affected: Reproductive, musculo-skeletal, digestive.
Specific indications: Contains hormone precursors that provide anti-inflammatory (cortisone-like) actions. Used for treating glandular imbalances and musculo-skeletal inflammation such as arthritis, as well as other inflammation and injuries to the joints. It is useful for treating bowel spasm, hiccough, muscle and menstrual pain. It helps stimulate bile, relieving bilious colic, the pains occurring with gall stones and intestinal gas.
Combinations: Combines with Ginger and Chamomile for relieving intestinal colic. Combines with Cramp Bark and Black Cohosh for treating rheumatoid arthritis. Combines well with Marshmallow root and Elder flowers for treating diverticulitis and appendicitis.
Preparations: *Decoction:* 1/2 to 1 cup 3 times a day. *Tincture:* 15 to 30 drops 3 times a day.

Yarrow – *Achillea millefolium*
Family: Compositae
Parts used: Leaf and flower.
Actions and medical uses: Diaphoretic, diuretic, astringent, styptic, vulnerary, antiseptic, tonic.
Systems affected: Cardiovascular, digestive, genito-urinary, skin.
Specific indications: This is one of the most valuable wayside herbs in the world. It is one of the best diaphoretic herbs for helping the body tend to fevers and for childhood fever diseases. The hot infusion raises the heat of the body, equalizes circulation and produces perspiration. As a tonic and active peripheral vasodilator, it lowers blood pressure and tones the blood vessels. Yarrow is high in volatile oils and is a reliable antiseptic for treating urinary system infections and mucous discharge from the bladder. Given as a cold infusion, it is useful for incontinence of urine. It is a bitter astringent used as an efficient stomach tonic. Taken as a warm tea, it relieves menstrual cramping. Powdered Yarrow used externally is a powerful styptic and wound healer.
Combinations: Combines well with Peppermint, Elder and Ginger as a diaphoretic for treating colds, flu and fever and common childhood fever diseases; when feverish, drink this compound hot. For normalizing blood

pressure, combine with Hawthorn and Garlic. For cramping combine with Crampbark. Combine with powdered Horsetail as an efficient styptic and vulnerary. Combines well with Sage and Chaparrel for use as a penis soak. And with Buchu or Couch Grass it is useful for treating infection of the prostate, bladder and urethra.

Preparations: *Infusion:* 1 cup 3 times a day. Take it as a hot tea hourly for feverish conditions; go to bed, put a hot water bottle to your feet, perspire and fall off to sleep. This is one of our best medicines for treating feverish colds and flu. *Tincture:* 15 to 30 drops 3 times a day. *Externally:* Dry, powder and apply directly to wounds to stop the bleeding, to disinfect and to help the tissue heal.

Other uses: Makes a beautiful cut and dried flower. The dried stalks, stripped of all their leaves, have been used for centuries for keying into the *I Ching* (Chinese Book of Changes).

Yellow Dock – *Rumex crispus*
Family: Polygonaceae
Parts used: Root.
Actions and medical uses: Alterative, cholagogue, laxative, astringent, nutritive.
Systems affected: Digestive, eliminative, blood.
Specific indications: As a blood enhancing alterative high in iron, Yellow Dock works well for treating chronic skin conditions such as psoriasis and eczema. It stimulates digestion and helps improve the function of the liver. It stimulates the action of congested bile flow and is useful for treating jaundice and lymphatic conditions. For constipation, it acts as a firm but not griping laxative by improving the flow of bile and stimulating peristalsis in the intestines.
Combinations: Combines well with Dandelion, Cleavers and Burdock for treating skin by improving blood condition.
Preparations: Use in small doses at first. *Infusion:* 1/2 cup 2 times a day. *Tincture:* 10 to 25 drops 2 to 3 times a day.

Yohimbe – *Pausinystalia yohimba*
Family: Rubiaceae
Parts used: Bark.
Actions and medical uses: Most widely acclaimed herbal aphrodisiac, tonic, stimulant.

Systems affected: Nervous, reproductive, circulatory, respiratory.

Specific indications: Yohimbe has a strong aphrodisiac effect, believed to be due to stimulation of the lower centers in the spinal cord. Some researchers feel this is due rather to the hyperemia (blood engorgement, in this case in the pelvic area) produced. Thought to be of no value when impotence stems from organic nerve trouble, and it is said by some to be harmful when it is used for impotence that is caused by chronic inflammatory disease of the sexual organs or of the prostate (U.S. Dispensatory, 24th ed.). "Its actions appear to go directly to the sexual centers of the spinal cord increasing tonicity. It has long been use by the Aboriginals of Africa in the form of a decoction to increase sexual appetite. Impotence of a functional origin (neurasthenic impotence) appears to be directly affected by its use. It is useful where there is diminished excitability of the sexual centers. In cases where there is a sudden failure of power, producing despondency, foreboding and general mental depression, in young married men, it is satisfactory." (Ellingwood).

Precautions: Much more needs to be learned about the use of this plant. I would advise some initial caution and sensible moderation in experimenting with its actions. It is generally stated that Yohimbe should not be combined with any drugs, including tranquilizers, narcotics, antihistamines or large quantities of alcohol. Please note the above warning of Yohimbe's use in conditions where there are inflamed sexual organs.

Preparations & approximate doses: *Decoction:* Simmer 1 oz. bark in 2 cups water 5 to 10 minutes, strain and add approximately 1000 mg. of ascorbic acid to a cup of the decoction. This helps make the herb's constituents easier to assimilate, avoiding nausea. Take 1 to 2 cups of the decoction 1 hour before desired effects. Stop using this herb after 2 weeks. *Tincture:* Place 1 to 3 teaspoons of the tincture in a small glass, pour boiling water onto it and let it sit until cool to evaporate the alcohol.

Take care of the plants; it's good medicine.

12

And We Wonder Where the Seeds of Male Maturity Fall

One last observation I want to discuss in this book on male-care concerns the subject of old men. Knowledge about old men seems to be similar to common knowledge about prostates. Where are they? Who are they? What are they doing?

I often place myself back into my childhood memories of my grandfather. He was a great big, quiet, living mystery to me. I used to sit next to him on the top stair of his front porch and watch him roll his Prince Albert brand tobacco into a characteristically crooked semi-flat cigarette, light it and stare off deep into who knows where. Frequently, out of the blue, he would whistle portions of an unknown tune or sing some private song quietly to himself. He'd always give me a huge wrap-around hug when I would first see him on my visit to Grandma's and Grandpa's and another one when I left, but in between hugs he left me mostly to be with Grandma. Whenever we went somewhere together (Grandma and Grandpa and me) he would drive his immaculately-kept old Chevrolet about 25 miles an hour, tops; he was in no hurry. You can bet that on long trips he got a lot of "are we there yet?"s out of me. I never knew him. I wished he would spend a whole day with me, but I was too young and too shy to even know that this was what I wanted, so he never did. When I was about 12, I watched him slowly die; he lost all his weight, lost his wits, began to talk to himself incoherently "out of the blue" (but I didn't think much of it, because I was used to listening to his old porch songs anyway).

So, Grandpa Green was the first old man that I missed knowing. Yet even then, I knew inside my little boy's heart that Grandpa knew the many things that old men know. Whatever that wisdom of age is, it was important to me then and it's important to me now, but I didn't know at the time how to ask him to talk to me. Once, many years after Grandpa's death I asked my dad what his father was like and what he thought of his father, but he never answered that letter. So, Grandpa died, and I've not forgotten him. I see him today in other old men, and they unknowingly touch my heart and mind in a deep and private way. I also see these men being ignored, disregarded, ridiculed, or at best, politely tolerated. I'm sure, like my grandfather, they, in some male way, contribute to this isolation, but it seems to me that the male community is ignoring a vital source of insight into the human male spirit that we could easily embrace if we would reach out to our grandelders, and they would reach out to their grandsons. I sincerely hope I can retain trust with the youth who will be living during the years of my old age. It's certainly my intention to be one hell of a grandpa to my daughters' generation's kids, especially to any little boy who might patiently and timidly sit next to me and silently watch me do some silly thing that I always do. I'll try to talk to him, plant some seeds to grow flowers between and around our generations and help him talk to me.

Closing Note

No one knows all that can be contained in the male heart, possibly least of all, we men who caretake the male spirit. We do know that men, too, are sensitive, fragile beings who presently hold the power to evolve or destroy our planetary home. So far, however, amid the current patriarchal power polarity, we don't know if he is either patient enough to perceive and understand the feelings and wisdom of his female side or intelligent enough to make appropriate life-supporting decisions. We do know the collective male spirit needs to be nourished, to be confronted by his species regarding survival and to be re-aligned with the sacred laws of life, balance and Nature's practical plan for perpetual abundance.

Presently, humankind tragically considers itself the highest form of life on the planet when, in fact, it is but a sibling, a *part* of the highest life form — the consummate living planet, Gaia, itself. HOMO SAPIENS JUST HAPPENS TO BE THE FAMILY SPECIES THAT HAS THE INTEL-LECTUAL POWER TO FORGET THIS FACT. *Homo-* is the Latin term for man and *sapiens* is Latin for wise; I hope we have named ourselves accurately. Beholding and experiencing ourselves as a dynamic part of the beauty of this planet Earth, Our first Mother, is our healing. She provides in abundance everything we need. A renewed, simple, nurturing relationship with the herbs reminds our heart and intellect of this connection.

Exploring male wholistic health-care is a journey into the heart of our future. Men are balanced by female, women inspired by male. This includes the male and female parts of one's self. Mightn't we all start sharing and playing again? Must we remain so serious, paranoid and guarded with one another? Doesn't it make good sense to cherish and protect all the diverse species who live with us in our sensual celestial home? Male and female health is simply the reflection of self-empowered, spontaneous, creative, happy beings.

There is a Male Song. The music is our life.

Bibliography

Airola, Paavo. *Stop Hair Loss*. Phoenix, AZ.: Health Plus.

Badgley, Laurence, M.D. *Healing AIDS Naturally*. San Bruno, CA: Human Energy Press, 1986.

Bairacli-Levy, Juliette de. *Herbal Handbook for Farm and Stable*. London: Faber and Faber, 1973.

Biddle, John B., M.D. *Review of Materia Medica*. Philadelphia: Lindsay & Blakiston, 1853.

British Herbal Pharmacopoeia. Scientific Committee. Nr. Keighley, West Yorks, U.K.: British Herbal Medicine Association, 1983.

British Medical Journal. 4–89; 298: 1072

Buri, Deborah. Research paper on alternate views about vaccinations routinely given to children. Vancouver, B.C. Canada, 1980.

Christopher, Dr. John R.. *School of Natural Healing*. BiWorld, Box 412, Springville, UT 84663, 1976.

Cousins, Norman. *Anatomy of an Illness*. New York: Norton & Co., 1979.

Downs, J. & Bleibtreu, H. *Human Variation*. Beverly Hills: Glencoe Press, 1972.

Ellingwood, Finley. *American Materia Medica, Therapeutics and Pharmacognosy*. Portland: Eclectic Medical Publications,1898.

Felter, H.W. *The Eclectic Materia Medica, Pharmacology and Therapeutics*. Portland: Eclectic Medical Publications, 1922.

Felter & Lloyd, J. *King's American Dispensatory,* Vol. I & II. Portland: Eclectic Medical Publications, 1898. Available from Eclectic Institute, 11231 SE Market, Portland, OR 97216.

Franchomme, Pierre. Phytoguide No. 1: *Aromatherapy Advanced Therapy of Infections*. IPF USA, P.O. Box 606, San Rafael, CA 94915.

Gardner, Joy. *The New Healing Yourself*. Freedom, CA: The Crossing

Press, 1989.

Gladstar, Rosemary. *The Science and Art of Herbology*. A correspondence course in fundamental Herbalism. P.O. Box 420, East Barre, VT 05649.

Grieve, M. *The Modern Herbal*, Vol. I & II. New York: Dover, 1971.

Hoffmann, David. *The Holistic Herbal*. Shaftesbury, Dorset, U.K.: Element Books, 1991.

———. *Successful Stress Control*. Rochester, VT.: Inner Traditions, 1987.

Kraus, H. and Raab, W. *Hypokinetic Disease*. Springfield, IL.: Charles C. Thomas, 1961.

Moore, Michael. *Medicinal Plants of the Mountain West*. Santa Fe: Museum of New Mexico Press, 1979.

———. *Medicinal Plants of the Desert and Canyon West*. Santa Fe: Museum of New Mexico Press, 1989.

National Organization of Circumcision Information Resource Center. 731 Sir Francis Drake Blvd., San Anselmo, CA 94960, (415) 454-5669.

Ornstein, Robert & Sobel, David. *The Healing Brain: Medical Discoveries about How the Brain Manages Health*. New York: Simon & Schuster, 1987.

Payer, Lynn. *Medicine in Culture*, as reviewed in *Newsweek* magazine (September, 19, 1988).

Passwater, Richard. *Supernutrition for Healthy Hearts*.

Price, Weston. *Nutrition and Physical Degeneration*. Santa Monica: Price-Pottenger, 1945.

Priest, A.W. and Priest, L.R. *Herbal Medication*. Romford, Essex, U.K.: Fowler & Co., 1982.

Robbins, Stanley L., M.D. *Pathologic Basis of Disease*. Philadelphia: Saunders Co., 1974.

Sawin, Clark T., M.D. *The Hormones: Endocrine Physiology*. Boston: Little, Brown and Co., 1969.

Schnaubelt, Kurt, PhD. *Aromatherapy Course*. P.O. Box 606, San Rafael, CA 94915).

Schauenberg, P. & Paris, F. *Guide to Medicinal Plants*. New Canaan, CT.: Keats Publishing, 1977.

"Sex Over Forty." PHE Inc., P.O. Box 1600, Chapel Hill, N.C., 27515.

Shook, Edward. *Advanced Treatise on Herbology*. Mokelumne Hill, CA: Health Research, Trinity Center Press.

Steinberg, Franz. *The Immobilized Patient*. New York: Plenum Medical Co., 1980.

Thomas, Lewis. *The Lives of Cells*. New York: Bantam, 1974.

Tierra, Michael. *Planetary Herbology*. Santa Fe: Lotus Press, 1988.

———. *The Way of Herbs*. New York: Simon & Schuster, 1980.

U.S. Dispensatory, 24th ed., Philadelphia: Lippincott Co., 1947.

Vogel, A., N.D. *The Nature Doctor*. Teufen, Switzerland: Bioforce-Verlag, 1960.

Weiss, Rudolf Fritz, M.D. *Herbal Medicine*. Beaconsfield, U.K.: Beaconsfield Publishers Ltd., 1988.

Herbal & Other Resources

Herb books

Christopher, Dr. John R. *School of Natural Healing*, (BiWorld,1976)

Ellingwood, Finley. *American Materia Medica, Therapeutics and Pharmacognosy*, 1898

Felter, H.W. *The Eclectic Materia Medica, Pharmacology and Therapeutics*, 1922

Foster, Steven. *Herbal Bounty, The Gentle Art of Herb Culture*, Gibbs M. Smith/Peregrine Smith Books, Salt Lake City, UT, 1984

——— and Duke, James A., *Eastern/ Central Medicinal Plants*, A Peterson Field Guide, Houghton Mifflin, 1990.

Gardner, Joy. *The New Healing Yourself*, Crossing Press, Box 1048, Freedom CA 95019

Gladstar, Rosemary, *Sage Healing Ways* (A series of herbal pamphlets), P.O. Box 420, East Barre, VT 05649

Green, James. *The Herbal Medicine-Maker's Handbook*, Simpler's Botanical Co., Box 39, Forestville, CA 95436

Grieve, Mrs. M. *The Modern Herbal*, Volumes I and II, Dover Publications, 1971

Hobbs, Christopher. *Echinacea! The Immune Herb*, Botanica Press, Box 742, Capitola, CA 95010

——— . *Medicinal Mushrooms*, Botanica Press, Box 742, Capitola, CA 95010

Hoffmann, David. *The Herbal Handbook*, Inner Traditions, Vermont, 1988

——— . *The Holistic Herbal*, Element Books, 1983

——— . *Successful Stress Control*, Inner Traditions, Vermont, 1987

Kenner, Daniel & Requena, Yves. *Botanical Medicine Paradigms*, Paradigm

Publications, 1990.

Keville, Kathi. *Country Herbs*. Publication date 1991.

———. *Illustrated Encyclopedia of Herbs*. Publication date 1991.

Levy, Juliette de Bairacli. *Herbal Handbook for Farm & Stable*, Faber & Faber, London, 1973.

———. *Nature's Children*, Warner Paperback, N.Y., 1972.

Moore, Michael. *Medicinal Plants of the Mountain West*, Museum of New Mexico Press, 1979.

———. *Medicinal Plants of the Desert and Canyon West*, Museum of New Mexico Press, 1989.

Parvati, Jeannine. *Hygieia, A Woman's Herbal,* Freestone Books, Bookpeople, Berkeley CA, 1978.

Robbins, Tom. *Jitterbug Perfume*, Bantam Books, N.Y., 1984. An olfactory classic.

Thie, Krista. *A Plant Lover's Guide to Wildcrafting,* Longevity Herb Press, 1549 W. Jewett Blvd., White Lalmon WA, 98672, 1989.

Thomson, William. *Medicines from the Earth,* McGraw-Hill, 1978.

Tierra, Michael. *The Way of Herbs*, Orenda/Unity Press, 1980.

———. *Planetary Herbology*, Lotus Press, 1988.

Tisserand, Robert. *Aromatherapy to Heal and Tend the Body*, Lotus Press, 1988.

Valnet, Jean, M.D. *The Practice of Aromatherapy*, Destiny Books, 1980

Vogel, A. *The Nature Doctor*, Bioforce-Verlag, Teufen Switzerland, 1960

Weed, Susun. *Healing Wise,* Ash Tree Publishing, Woodstock, New York, 1989.

Weiss, Rudolf Fritz. *Herbal Medicine*, Beaconsfield Publishers Ltd., Beaconsfield, England.

Other Books

Airola, Paavlo., Ph.D. *Hypoglycemia: A Better Approach*, Health Plus, Arizona, 1977.

Airola, Paavlo., Ph.D. *How to Get Well*, Health Plus, 1974

Baker, Jeanine Parvati and Baker, Frederick. *Conscious Conception: Elemental Journey Through the Labyrinth of Sexuality*, North Atlantic Books, Berkeley, California, 1983.

Brauer, Alan and Donna. *ESO, Extended Sexual Orgasm,* Warner Books, N.Y., 1983.

Brooks, Svevo, *The Art of Good Living*, Houghton Mifflin, Boston, 1990.

Chia, Mantak. *Taoist Secrets of Love; Cultivating Male Sexual Energy*, Aurora Press, N.Y.

Chia, Mantak & Chia, Maneewan. *Healing Love Through the Tao; Cultivating Female Sexual Energy*, Healing Tao Books, Huntington, 1986

Cousins, Norman, *Anatomy of an Illness: As Perceived by the Patient*, Norton & Co., N.Y., 1979.

Dossey, Larry, M.D. *Space, Time & Medicine*, Shambhala, Colorado, 1982.

Graedon, Joe. *The People's Pharmacy*, Avon Books, N.Y., 1976.

Griggs, Barbara.*Green Pharmacy*, Norman & Hobhouse, 1981.

Grossinger, Richard. *Planet Medicine*, Shambhala, Colorado, 1982 .

Herer, Jack. *The Emperor Wears No Clothes*, HEMP Publishing, 5632 Van Nuys Blvd., Van Nuys, CA 91401, 1990. And supplementary video, "Hemp for Victory" 1942 USDA, WW 2, Reefer Madness 1936.

Kaptchuk, Ted, O.M.D. *The Web That Has No Weaver*, Congdon & Weed, N.Y., 1983.

Koehler, Nan, *Artemis Speaks: Vaginal Birth After Cesarean Section Stories & Natural Childbirth Information*, Self-published by author, 13140 Frati Ln. Sebastopol, CA 95472, 1989.

Lovelock, James E. *Gaia, A New Look at Life on Earth*, Oxford U. Press, 1979.

Merck Manual 15th Ed., Merck & Co., New Jersey.

McDougall, John A., M.D., *A Challenging Second Opinion*, New Century, N.J., 1985.

McDougall, John A., M.D., *The McDougall Plan*, New Century, N.J., 1983.

Mindell, Earl, *Vitamin Bible*, Rawson, WAde Publ., N.Y., 1980.

Passwater, Richard, Ph. D., *Super-Nutrition for Healthy Hearts*, Jove Books, N.Y., 1975.

Pei, Mario, *The Story of Language*, Lippincott Co. New York, 1965.

Robbins, Tom. *Skinny Legs and All*, Bantam Books. New York, 1990. To help drop the final veil on the bottom line of the Desert Shield.

Tompkins & Bird, *The Secret Life of Plants*, Harper & Row, N.Y., 1972.

Wood, Bill, *Marty the Marathon Bear*, Rallysport Video Productions, Box 29809, L.A., CA 90020.

Tools

Medicine Cards, Jamie Sams & David Carson, Bear & Co., P.O. Drawer 2860, Santa Fe, NM 87504. An esthetic key into the intelligent wisdom of animals that teaches respect, compassion and pathways to personal power and peaceful coexistance.

OH cards, Eos Enterprises, Inc., Box 3655, Vancouver, B.C., Canada, V6B 3Y8. For creating a safe atmosphere to explore ones personal issues through both the left and right brain.

Videos

Herbal Preparations and Natural Therapies, By Debra Nuzzi, Morningstar Publications, 997 Dixon Rd., Boulder, CO 80302.

"Hemp for Victory" 1942 USDA, WW 2, Reefer Madness 1936. 5632 Van Nuys Blvd., Van Nuys, CA91401. Regardless of your politics, you gotta see this one.

Schools

California School of Herbal Studies

The author, James Green and his wife, Mindy Green are directors and teachers at this school. P.O. Box 39, Forestville CA 95436, (707) 887-7457.

Herbal Healing Journey

C/O Self-Heal Herbal Centre, 1106 Blanshard St., Victoria, B.C., Canada V8W 2H6. Offers a 9 week course of study.

Southwest School of Botanical Medicine

701 1/2 East Broadway, Silver City, NM 88061.

The Australasian College of Herbal Studies

P.O. Box 4451, Aucklund, New Zealand.

Correspondence Courses

Aromatherapy Course, basic aromatherapy course with emphasis on chemistry. Dr. Kurt Schnaubelt, P.O. Box 606, San Rafael, CA 94915.

Dominican Herbal College

7527 Kingsway, Burnaby, British Columbia, V3N 3C1, Canada.

East West Course in Herbology, a course in Eastern & Western sciences of herbalism by Michael Tierra, P.O. Box 712, Santa Cruz, CA 95061

Herbal Studies Course, offers a basic and advanced course.

by Jeanne Rose, 219 Carl Street, San Francisco, CA 94117.

The Science and Art of Herbology, a complete course in fundamental, practical herbalism by Rosemary Gladstar, P.O. Box 420, East Barre, VT 05649.

The School of Herbal Medicine, American branch of the National Institute of Medical Herbalists, Box 168, Squamish, WA 98392.

Therapeutic Herbalism, an introduction to European & American phytotherapy by David Hoffmann, 9304 Springhill, Sebastopol, CA 9547.

Publications

American Herb Association, Quarterly Newsletter
P.O. Box 353, Rescue, CA 95672
An exceptionally well rounded forum for all professional herbalists and student herbalists.

HerbalGram
P.O. Box 201660, Austin, TX 78720, (512) 331-8868
The journal of the American Botanical Council and the Herb Research Foundations.

Medical Herbalism
P.O. Box 33080, Portland OR 97233
A clinical newsletter for the herbal practitioner.

Mother Jones
P.O. Box 58249, Boulder, CO 80321-8249
About "People, Politics and Other Passions"
Agree with it or not; it's a reader supported mag.

The Animal's Voice Magazine
P.O. Box 16955, N. Hollywood, CA 91615-9931
"A powerful voice that must be listened to." A nationally acclaimed animal rights magazine.

Wildfire
P.O. Box 9167, Spokane, WA 99209, (509) 326-6561
Multi-topic publication from the Bear Tribe non-profit educational organization.

Wildflower
Canadian Wildflower Society, 75 Ternhill Crescent, North York, Ontario, Canada, M3C 2E4
Dedicated to the study, conservation & cultivation of this continent's native plants.

Wildlife Conservation
New York Zoological Park, Bronx, New York 10460
Beautifully photographed presentation of Earth's remaining wildlife.

Places one can buy high quality herbs and herbal extracts
Abundant Life Seed Foundation
P. O. Box 772, Port Townsend, WA 98368
Blessed Herbs
Route 5, Box 1042, Ava, Missouri 65608 • (417) 683-5721
Frontier Cooperative Herbs
Box 299, Norway, IO 52318 • 1-800-669-3275
Herb Pharm
Box 116, Williams, OR 97544 • (503) 846-7178
Herbalist & Alchemist
Box 458, Bloomsbury, NJ 08804-0458 • (201) 479-6679
Island Herbs — Ryan Drum
Waldron Island, WA 98297
Mountain Butterfly Herbs
Box 1365, Hamilton, Montana 59840 • (406) 363-6683
Oak Valley Herb Farm
14648 Pear Tree Lane, Nevada City, CA 95959
Pacific Botanicals
4350 Fish Hatchery Road, Grants Pass, OR 97527 • (503) 479-7777
Rainbow Light
207 McPherson St., Santa Cruz, CA 95060
Simplers Botanical Co.
Box 39, Forestville, CA 95436 • (707) 887-2012
Trinity Herbs
Box 199, Bodega, CA 94922 • (707) 874-3418.
Trout Lake
Rt. 1, Box 355, Trout Lake WA 98650
Turtle Island Herbs
Salina Star Route, Boulder, CO 80302 • (303) 442-2215
Walter H. McDaniel
Box 15, Waycross, Georgia 31502 • (912) 287-0188 or 285-2057
Wildflowers on Hawthorne
3202 S.E. Hawthorne Blvd., Portland OR 97214 • (503) 230 9485

Other Resources
AIDS Treatment News
P.O. Box 411256, San Francisco, CA 94141. (415) 255-0588
Reports on experimental and complementary treatments. Collects information from health practitioners, and persons with AID or ARC. Reports on combinations that have worked for long-term survivors. Seeks to increase the options available. Examines ethical and public-policy issues around AIDS treatment research and access.

Co-op America
2100 M Street, N.W., #310, Washington, DC 20063
A co-operative listing and catalog of socially responsible small businesses.

Earth Care Paper, Inc. (Write for 'Recycled Paper' Catalog)
Box 3335, Madison, WI 53704.

Impotents Anonymous
Box 1257, Maryville, TN 37802
Send for free pamphlet titled, "Answers to the Most Often Asked Questions About Impotence."

National Organization of Circumcision Information Resource Center
P.O. Box 2512, San Anselmo, CA 94960, (415) 488-9883

People for the Ethical Treatment of Animals (PETA)
Box 42516, Washington, DC 20015

Rocky Mountain Herbalist Coalition
412 Boulder Street, Gold Hill, Boulder, CO 80302, (303) 442-2215
An organization of Herbalists setting standards for ethics in herbalism.

ROMP (Recovery of Male Impotence)
2711 Lahser, Suite #208, Southfield, MI 48038 • 1-800-Tel-ROMP
A self-help support group with 27 chapters nationwide.

Seventh Generation
Colchester, VT 05446-1672, 1-800-456-1177
Products for a Healthy Planet. Send for catalog.

The National Anti-Vivisection Society
53 West Jackson Blvd, Suite 1550, Chicago, Ill. 60604-3795, (312) 427-6065.

The Nature Conservancy
1815 North Lynn Street, Arlington, Virginia 22209

Working Assets Visa Card
230 California St., San Francisco, CA 94111, (800) 522-7759.

For each credit card purchase Working Assets makes a donation to socially responsible, non-profit organizations working for either the Environment, Human Rights, Peace and/or Hunger. Each individual card user can direct to which catagory(s) his or her percentage of the donations go.

World Wildlife Fund

1250 24th St., NW, Washington, DC 20037

Glossary

actions — The specific nutritional and therapeutic energies of a plant.

acute — manifesting symptoms of some severity and coming quickly to a crisis. Sharp, painful.

aerial — The parts of a plant that grow above the ground.

alimentary canal — the tubular food-carrying passage extending from the mouth to the anus.

allopathy — The theory or system of medical practice which combats disease by the use of remedies producing effects different from those produced by the disease being treated.

antioxidant — A substance that prevents oxidation.

anus — Posterior opening of the alimentary canal.

apiarian — Relating to bees and beekeeping.

Apollo — Twin brother of Artemis. Physician. Greek God of healing.

apoplexy — Sudden coma, paralysis and sometimes death from sudden hemorrhage into or upon the brain.

Artemis — Twin sister of Apollo. Herbalist and midwife. Greek Goddess of healing.

astrology — Human beings' first science. A dynamic mythology for modern mankind.

atonic — Lack of tone or vital energy. Weakness of an organ or system.

avitaminosis — Any condition resulting from a deficiency of vitamins.

Ayuvedic — An East Indian science of health-care.

Bach Flower Essences — The powerfully subtle essences of wildflower blossoms drawn out by the sun and retained in water. The system of using these essences to heal a patient through the personality was developed by an

English physician, Dr. Edward Bach, over forty years ago.

bile — A very bitter, greenish-yellow fluid secreted by the liver, stored in the gall-bladder and poured into the small intestine as required. Bile aids the digestion of fats and helps prevent putrification in the intestines.

biliary — Pertaining to bile.

binomial — A species (plant or animal) name consisting of two terms.

Calvin, John — French theologian, (1509–64), patriarch of Calvinism.

cardiovascular — pertaining to the heart and blood vessels.

Chi (Qi) — A term used in Chinese medical thinking to represent the unifying energy of all things. It is best perceived as function rather than substance. Everything is composed of and defined by its Chi. Chi protects and warms the body, is the source of all movement in the body and is the source of harmony in the body.

chronic — Continuing for a long time. Having long had a condition or habit.

C.O. — A conscientious objector. Conscious objection to participating in war.

companion species — Every species native to the planet Earth. Planetary siblings. Family. Relatives.

compost — a fertilizing mixture composed of peat, leaf mold, manure, food scraps, and other organic and inorganic waste mingled and decomposed. Recycled scraps transiting back to fertile soil.

conjunctivitis — Inflammation of the white of the eye.

cutaneous — Pertaining to the skin.

cystitis — inflammation of the urinary blader.

dermal — pertaining to the true skin.

diastolic — Pertaining to the rhythmic period of relaxation of a heart chamber during which it fills with blood.

digestive system — Pertaining to the stomach and intestines.

duodenum — The first part of the small intestine leading from the stomach.

empirical — Depending upon experience or observation alone.

endocrine glands — Glands whose secretions pass directly into the blood or lymph.

estrogen — Predominently female hormone. A substance possessing the biological activity of estrus producing hormones. It stimulates the production of an egg. It too stimulates aggression.

estrus — Sexual desire. The mating period of animals especially the female.

fecund — Full with creative potential and passion.

fixed oil — An oil that does not easily vaporize such as common vegetable food oils.

flatulence — The presence of gas in the stomach and intestinal canal, also the spontaneous release of that gas into society.

free radical — highly active fractions of molecules generally harmful to the body.

free radical scavenger — A substance that removes or inactivates a free radical.

Gaia — The living planet, Earth, including all her inhabitants and the atmosphere they create communally.

gastro-intestinal — Pertaining to the stomach and intestines.

genito-urinary — pertaining to the genitalia and the urinary organs or functions.

geriatric dementia — loss of the intellectual faculties, reasoning, memory and will in old age.

gerontology — The study of the phenomenon of old age.

glycerine — The sweet fraction of oil. A clear, colorless, emollient, syrupy liquid of sweet taste, miscible with alcohol and water obtained by hydrolysis of fats.

glycerite — An herbal extract prepared with glycerine as the principle solvent.

hemorrhage — an escape of blood from the vessels either through intact blood vessel walls or through ruptured walls.

herb — Any plant ally.

herpes simplex — An acute inflammation of the skin and vesicular eruptions occurring on the borders of the lips or oral mucous membrane.

herpes zoster (shingles) — An acute infection of the central nervous system characterized by a vesicular eruption and neuralgic pain distributed in relation to the course of a cutaneous nerve.

homeopathy — A system of healing advocated by Hahnemann, whose motto was *Similia similibus curantur*: likes cure likes. Hahnemann taught that drugs should be tested upon normal human beings; that the symptoms caused by drugs given to a healthy person (proving) would cure those same symptoms when given to a person suffering from an illness.

homologous — having the same relative position, proportion, value or structure.

hydrolysis — Reaction with water.

immune enhancer — An agent that assists or strengthens the immune system.

incontinence — Unable to restrain natural evacuations. Bed wetting.

infusion — An herbal extraction using water as the principle solvent.

in vitro — In glass; in a test tube, beaker, petri dish, etc.

in vivo — In a living organism, as a human, animal or plant.

lipid — Fat substances.

magic-bullet medicine — a term used for the illusion that a particular medicine will automatically and magically eliminate a disease.

marc — The residue remaing after extraction of the active principles from an herb or after extraction of juice from fruit.

medulla — The deep or inner tissue of an organ or gland.

menstruum — A solvent.

miscible — Capable of mixing or dissolving.

M.N.I.M.H. — Member of the British National Institute of Medical Herbalists

mucilage — A solution of gum in water. Gelatinous substances found in plants.

musculo-skeletal — Pertaining to the muscles, skeleton and skeletal connective tissue.

mutagen — An agent that causes biological mutation.

naturopathy — A system of medicine which emphasizes assisting nature. It sometimes includes the use of certain medicines such as herbs, vitamins, and nutrition and of certain physical means such as manipulation and hydrotherapy.

neurology — The science dealing with the nervous system.

nutrient — A nutritious substance.

nutritious — Nourishing; promoting growth and repair.
orchitis — Inflammation of the testis.
oxidation — Reacts with oxygen.

palliate — To cloak or hide. To ease without curing.
parasympathetic nervous system — That part of the autonomic (involuntary) nervous system that tends to regulate and respond to the internal enviroment of the body.
part, a — Relative unit of measure used to prepare a given formula.
parturition — Giving birth.
pathology — The condition, as of an organ or fluid, produced by a disease.
peripheral — Away from the central nervous system. In higher animals and some lower there is formed a central nervous system with peripheral connections. Also those blood vessels that are away from the central (heart and major blood vessel) circulatory system.
pheremone — (Gr. *pherin-* to bear along, *hormon-* an excitement) A term used to designate the scent secreted into the environment at the right time and place to the related sex of one's own species.
Physician's Desk Reference — Physician's standard reference guide listing indications, counter-indications and side effects of allopathic drugs.
phytomedical — Plant medicine.
phytotherapy — The therapeutic use of plants.
plant gum — Plant exudates. They are soluble in water, thus forming a mucilaginous liquid or jelly-like adhesive mass.
platelets — cellular elements in blood that are active in the blood clotting process.
precursor — A forerunner, one that precedes.
progesterone — A predominantly female steroid sex hormone, which stimulates the preparation of the uterus lining for implantation of a fertile egg. Once pregenant the female body produces large quantities of this hormone.
pulmonary — Pertaining to the lungs.

recycling — Environmental doctor of the present and future.
reductionist — One who practices reductionism.
reductionism — The theory or system of research which focuses on the individual, separated pieces and parts of a whole.

renal system — Pertaining to the kidneys.

respiratory — Pertaining to the lungs and air passages.

ritual — a conscious, though often unconscious, observance or practice of rites which reflect deep meaning to the performer.

salient — prominent, noticeable, conspicuous, outstanding.

saponin — Any of a group of glucosides characterized by the property of producing a soapy lather.

scrotum — The external pouch containing the testicles.

secondary action (of an herb) — actions attributed to an herb which enhance its primary action and system affinity.

smudge — A thick smoke used in ceremonies to cleanse and protect an area.

somatic — Pertaining to or affecting the physical body as distinguished from the mind.

specieism — Assumption of the inherent superiority of a certain species, and consequent discrimination against other species; also any doctrine, occupation or program of species domination, abuse, exploitation and discrimination based on such an assumption.

spermatogenesis — Development of mature sperm.

standardized extract — An extract that has been prepared in accordance with a particular set of arbitrary standards.

Stonehenge — The elder computer built by the ancients to compute future astronomical and astrological events.

strobile — A multiple fruit whose seeds are enclosed by prominent scales.

sympathetic nervous system — That part of the autonomic nervous system that tends primarily to the body's reaction and response to its external environment.

synergism — Cooperative action of distinct components such that the total effect is greater than the sum of the individual effects taken independently.

system — Combination of parts into a whole, as the nervous system, digestive system.

systemic — Working through systems. Throughout the whole body.

system affinity — The affinity (dynamic bio-medical relationship or attractive force) that the actions of an herb have for a particular body system.

systolic — pertaining to the contraction phase of the heart beat (cardiac cycle).

tachycardia — Excessive rapidity of the heart's acton.

T'ai-chi — Also known as T'ai-chi ch'uan, the way to good health. A marshal art of balance, grace, stretching, exercise and self-defense.

tannin — Any group of astringent plant principles characterized by their ability to precipitate collagen.

tinnitus — A subjective ringing, roaring or hissing sound in the ears.

testicles — Male genital glands.

testosterone — Male sex hormone. Androgenic compound derived mainly from the testes. It too stimulates aggression.

thallus — A simple type of plant structure without root, stem and leaf.

tincture — An herbal extract prepared with ethyl alcohol as the principle solvent.

tissue — An aggregation of similar cells and their intercellular substances.

uremia — Retention in the blood of urinary constituents, due to the kidneys failure to excrete them.

venous — Pertaining to the veins.

vertigo — A sensation of a lack of equilibrium. Dizziness.

volatile — Readily evaporates.

volatile oil — a readily vaporizable oil distinguished from a fixed oil which does not vaporize easily.

whole-plant — Plant preparations and extracts that contain most all of the original plant constituents aside from the indigestable cellulose and woody fiber.

Yang — The practicle experience of energy on the sunny side of a hill; hot, firm, light, dry, also external, aggressive, creative and so forth.

Yin — The practicle experience of energy on the shady side of a hill; cold, yielding, dark, moist, also internal, passive, receptive and so forth.

Index

A Challenging Second Opinion 255
A Plant Lover's Guide to Wildcrafting 254
Abcesses 215
Acids: fatty 184
Acne 179–180, 201
Adaptogen 89, 150, 213, 241
Adaptogenic herbs 133, 141
Adenoids 207
Adrenal glands 35, 147, 174, 227
Adrenal hormones 90–92
Adrenal system 141
Adrenaline 95
Aduki beans 185
Advanced Treatise on Herbology 251
Aerobic activities 89, 144
Agarose diffusion 24
Agave 15
Agrimony – Agrimonia eupatoria 47, 73,
    76, 77, 100, 188, 193, 198, 209
AIDS 117, 161, 164, 166, 238
Airola, Paavlo 138, 146, 148, 174, 183, 250,
    254, 255
Alcohol 89, 92, 99, 105, 113, 228
Aldomet 136
Alfalfa 68, 129, 188
Allopathic medicine 4, 6, 13, 20, 31, 106,
    156, 168-70
Almond butter 150; oil 89
Aloe vera 186
Alterative 66, 69, 88, 100, 141, 151, 180,
    194, 200, 201, 205, 206, 213, 215,
    217, 220, 224, 227, 230, 232, 234,
    235, 236, 238, 239, 245
Aluminum: cooking utensils 145
Alzhemier's disease 145
American Alliance for Health, Physical Educa-
    tion, Recreation and Dance 48
American Dietitian's Association 172
American Ginseng 69, 81, 220
American Herb Association, Quarterly
    Newsletter 257
American Materia Medica, Therapeutics and
    Pharmacology 79, 253, 250
Amino acids 20, 148, 177
Amphetamines 136
Anaerobic bacteria 171
Analgesic 69, 204, 237
Anand, Margo 115, 255
Anatomy of an Illness As Perceived by the
    Patient 85, 250, 255
Anderson-Geller, Cascade 121
Androgens 102, 136
Anemia 220, 231
Anemopsis 74
Angelica – Angelica archangelica 68, 71,
    73, 188, 194, 200, 205, 211
Anger 29
Animals: and herbal research 23–26
Animal's Voice Magazine 257
Anise 70, 71
Anodyne 69, 203, 241, 242

Anomalies and Curiosities of Medicine 36
Antacid 69, 228
Anthelmintic 69
Antiemetic 70
Antiarthritic 213
Antibacterial 148, 149, 171, 215
Antibilious 69
Antibiotics 171, 205
Anticatarrhal 69, 88, 204
Anticlotting 219
Antidepressant 41, 43,
    66, 96, 141, 211, 220, 231
Antifungal 202
Antihistamines 137
Antiinflammatory 68, 70, 75–76, 96,
    113, 124, 130, 182, 195-196, 202, 204,
    206, 216, 217, 219, 228, 237
Antilithic 70
Antimicrobial 66, 70, 88, 107, 108,
    113, 121, 123, 148, 170-171, 180, 182
    205, 210, 216, 217
Antimicrobial action 170–171
Antioxidant 123, 219
Antirheumatic 194, 212, 228, 238
Antiseptic 66, 96, 194, 198, 202-205,
Antispasmodic 77, 88, 89, 96, 130, 194-
    195, 200, 203- 204, 208, 210, 216-217,
    218, 222, 236, 240-241, 244
Antispetic 198, 202, 203, 205, 211, 220, 237
Antiviral 123, 124, 127, 148, 149, 215
Anus 107
Aperient 73, 211
Aphrodisiac 70, 133, 141, 147, 152, 196,
    201, 211, 220, 245
Apollo 7
Appendicitis 77, 193, 244
Appetite 211, 216, 241
Apple cider vinegar 89, 92, 186, 237
Apricots 174
ARC/AIDS 161
Arnica – Arnica spp. 70, 75, 76, 182, 188,
    195, 202, 238
Aromatherapy 98, 112–113, 127, 141–142,
    168–172
Aromatherapy Course 170, 251, 257
Aromatherapy to Heal and Tend the Body 254
Aromatherapy: Advanced Therapy of
    Infections 171, 250
Aromatic 71, 211, 216
Art of Good Living, The 255
Art of Sexual Ecstacy: The Path of Sacred
    Sexuality 114, 255
Artemis 7
Artemis Speaks: Vaginal Birth After Cesarean
    Section 255
Arterial walls 94
Arteries 90, 137, 177
Arteriosclerosis 90–94, 223
Arthritis 51, 74, 145, 147, 166, 203, 205
    213, 217, 235, 238, 244
Artichoke 71, 76, 138, 185, 188

Asclepius 7
Ashwagandha – *Withania somnifera* 68, 69
  126, 139, 188, 196
Asparagus 175, 185
Aspartame 178
Aspartic acid 147
Aspirin 228
Asthma 96, 217, 223, 231
Astragalus – *Astragalus spp.* 69, 97, 108, 109
  151, 153, 167, 188, 197
Astringent 66, 71, 76, 88, 100, 107,
  123, 193, 196, 197-198, 202-203, 206,
  207 210, 220, 223, 224, 225, 228, 230, 234,
  236, 237, 239, 244, 245
Atheroma 92
Atherosclerosis 92
Athlete's foot 207
Australian College of Herbal Studies 257
Avitaminosis 194
Avocados 176
Avoirdupois 58
Ayurvedic 185, 196

Back 197
Bacteria 172
Badgley, Laurence 250
Baker, Frederick 135, 255
Baker, Jeanine Parvati 255
Baker, Rico 28
Baldness 128, 183
Balm 70, 188
Balmony 69
Baptisia 180
Barberry 69, 71
Barley 138
Basil 93, 167, 188
Baths 98
Bay leaves 153
Bayberry – *Myrica cerifera* 73, 74, 76,
  100, 188, 197
Beans 127, 176
Bearberry (Uva-ursi) – *Arctostaphylos uva-*
  ursi 68, 75, 76, 188, 198-199, 211
Bed-wetting 198, 209, 238
Bee pollen 134, 147, 148, 150; wax 145
Beer 43, 107
Beet greens 47
Beet root 73
Bergamot 127
Bernard, Claude 156
Beta-carotene 174
Biddle, John B. 250
Bile 71, 73; ducts 230
Bites 182
Bitter 42, 43–47, 66, 71, 76, 77, 88, 90, 99,
  137, 138, 141, 178, 201, 217, 220, 224, 242
Black Cohosh – *Cimicifuga racemosa* 41-42
  74, 95, 180, 188, 199, 200, 205, 217, 244
Black Haw 67, 130
Black Haw tincture 126
Black Pepper 70, 74
Black Walnut hulls 70
Blackberry 73, 188

Bladder 79, 102, 104, 108, 110, 115, 195
  198, 204, 205, 207, 209, 211, 212, 234,
  239, 244; stones 70; infection 215
Bladderwrack 147, 148, 188
Bleeding 202, 234
Bleibtreu, Hermann 165, 250
Blessed Thistle 47, 188
Blood 194, 197, 219, 223; anemia 220;
  bleeding 74; cells 15; circulation 74,
  85, 141, 219, 225; cleansers 69; clotting
  219; flow 85; hemoglobin 15;
  plasma 15; poisoning 215, 228; pressure
  69, 73, 88, 89, 94, 136, 177, 212, 217,
  220, 223, 242, 245; purifier 215; sugar
  43, 69, 137-138, 195; tonic 78; toxicity 69;
  vessels 75, 184, 209, 219, 225
Blue Chamomile 113, 182
Blue Cohosh 40, 75, 188
Blue Flag 180, 188
Blueberry 138
Bogbean 76, 188
Boils 215
Bone tissue 48
Boneset 72, 73, 188
Botanical Medicine Paradigms 254
Bowel function 43
Bowels 197, 204, 207, 244
Brahmi Oil 185
Brain 144, 177
Brauer, Alan 111, 135, 255
Brauer, Donna 111, 135, 255
Breathlessness 96
Brewer's yeast 175
Brith Milah 118
British Herbal Pharmacopoeia 250
British Medical Journal 116, 250
Broccoli 138, 175, 177
Bromine 226
Bronchial catarrh 195; disorders 147
Bronchitis 195, 207, 211, 215, 217, 226,
  227, 235
Brooks, Svevo 255
Bruises 181, 193, 196, 202, 207, 228
Buchu – *Agathosma betulina* 70, 108, 137
  188, 198, 200, 210, 240, 245
Buckwheat 176
Burdock – *Arctium lappa* 68, 69, 76, 126,
  138, 141, 180, 188, 201, 215, 227, 231, 232
  238, 245
Buri, Deborah 250
Burns 182, 202, 228
Butter 89, 92

Cabbage 101
Cadmium 176
Caffeine 90, 105, 113, 153
Calcium 127, 146, 177, 184, 227
Calculus: in bladder 198; in kidney 198
Calendula (Marigold) – *Calendula officinalis*
  68, 70, 73, 75, 124, 167, 180, 182,
  188, 196 202, 205, 207, 215, 235, 238;
  flower tincture 126

California Buckeye 225
California Poppy – *Eschscholzia californica* 188, 203
California School of Herbal Studies 1, 58, 77, 170
California Spikenard 174, 188
Cancer 123, 166; penis 123; prostate 175
Candida infections 121
Canker sores 236
Carbuncles 215
Cardiovascular system 89, 138, 217, 219-220, 244
Carminative 71, 88, 100, 194, 203-204, 211, 216, 217, 218, 239, 241
Carob 127, 150
Carotenoids 174
Carrot 15, 138, 174
Carrot Seed 181
Carvacrol 171
Cascara Sagrada 73, 188, 232
Castration 102
Catapres 136
Catarrh 217, 222, 227; of bladder 198; of kidneys 198; of urinary bladder 211
Catecholamines 85
Catnip 69, 73, 121, 129, 188, 216, 236
Cauliflower 138
Cayenne – *Capsicum spp.* 70, 73, 74, 88, 127, 147, 188, 198, 203, 218, 227
Celery 138, 185
Celery seed 188
Centaury – *Centaurium umbellatum* 47, 69, 188
Central nervous system 144
Cereals 177
Cervix 123
Chamomile – *Matricaria chamomilla* 47, 70, 71, 73, 75-76, 100-101, 126, 180, 188, 203-204, 211-212, 224, 227, 228, 240, 242, 244; German 204; Roman 204
Chaparral – *Larrea mexicana* 70, 105, 122, 123, 188, 205, 245
Chaste Tree – *Vitex agnus* 38, 41–42, 189, 206
Cheese 127
Chemotherapy 4, 147
Cherries 175
Chi (Qi) 78
Chia, Maneewan 135, 255
Chia, Mantak 111, 135, 255
Chiccory 47, 189
Chickweed 72, 75, 189, 235
Chilblains 218, 235
Childhood fever 216
Chinese Ginseng 69
Chives 89
Chocolate 43, 127
Cholagogue 71, 88, 89, 193, 202, 212, 217, 230, 232, 244, 245
Cholangitis 230
Cholesterol 148, 177, 217, 241; serum 89
Christopher, John R. 100, 205, 250, 253
Cichorium endiva 45

Cinnamon – *Cinnamomum zeylanicum* 71, 152, 153, 189, 193
Circulatory system 42, 66, 75, 94, 96, 197, 203, 205, 209, 218, 231, 235, 241, 246
Circumcision 115–118
Cirrhosis 230
Citrus bergamia 122, 127
Citrus Peel 71
Clary Sage 98
Cleavers - *Galium aparine* 68, 69, 70, 73, 108, 180, 189, 201, 206, 232, 238, 245; tincture 126
Clitoris 36, 117
Clostridium 171
Clove 70, 152
Cocaine 136
Cocoa butter 56
Coconut 127
Coffee – *coffea arabica* 43, 73, 89, 127, 189
Cold pack 107, 130
Colds 147, 203, 213, 217, 227, 236
Colic 96, 195, 216, 227, 242, 244
Collards 175
Colon 77, 234
Coltsfoot 68, 72, 73, 74, 75, 189, 195, 217, 227, 242
Comfrey – *Symphytum officinale* 14, 72, 74-75, 108, 120– 121, 152, 189, 202, 208, 227-228, 231, 235; Comfrey root 100
Compress 57
Conscious Conception: Elemental Journey Through the Labyrinth of Sexuality 255
Constipation 147, 232, 245
Copper 176
Coriander – *Coriandrum sativum* 151, 189
Corn Silk – *Zea mays* 70, 72, 75, 108, 129, 189, 198, 201, 209-210, 211, 226
Cornstarch Soak 121
Couch Grass – *Agropyron repens* 72, 75, 108, 185, 189, 198, 201, 208-210, 212, 245
Cough 72, 195, 213, 217, 223, 227, 235, 242
Cousins, Norman 85, 155, 255, 250
Cramp Bark – *Viburnum opulus* 40, 67, 73, 88, 95, 106, 130, 189, 195, 200, 203, 210, 242, 244-245
Cramps 71, 96, 203, 204, 210, 217, 218, 242, 244; genito-urinary 195; leg 235 menstrual 195
Cranberry 138
Cranesbill 189
Cress 47
Cryptorchism: hidden testis 128
Cubeb – *Piper cubeba* 189, 211
Curry 127
Cuts 74, 182, 215
Cystitis 109, 121, 193, 198, 209, 210, 235

Dairy products 92, 174, 180
Damiana – *Turnera diffusa* 40–42, 58, 66-68, 70, 73, 96, 109, 133, 141, 151-152, 189, 202, 211, 220, 240
Dandelion – *Taraxacum officinale* 68-73,

89, 108, 138, 175, 178, 189, 212–213,
222, 227, 231, 234, 238, 245; greens 47;
leaf 47; root 73
de Bairacli-Levy, Juliette 38
Death-Cap mushroom 230
Decoction 53, 108
Demulcent 70, 71, 75, 100, 107, 121, 123,
129, 198, 207, 209, 210, 226, 227, 230, 231
Depression 89, 203, 219
Devil's Club – Oplopanax horridus 69, 138,
189, 213
DHT 79
Diabetes 43, 51, 89, 137–138, 195, 212, 213
Diaphoretic 66, 72, 88, 194, 197, 201,
217, 218, 235, 238, 239, 244
Diarrhea 71, 158, 193, 197, 228, 234, 235,
236
Diet 86, 89, 92, 111, 142, 144, 172–177,
180, 184; cholesterol 86; fruit 86; low
fiber 99; seeds 86; sugar 86;
vegetables 86
Digestion 42, 46, 69, 71, 96, 121, 141, 147,
178, 193, 195, 211, 217, 222, 223
Digestive juices 66, 201
Digestive system 42, 75, 201-205, 207,
211-213, 216-218, 224, 226-228, 230,
232, 234, 237, 239, 242, 244-245
Dihydrotestosterone (DHT) 79, 104
Dill 70, 71, 189
Diptheria 157
Disease: resistance 148
Diuretic 66, 72, 88, 180, 193-194, 197-198,
200, 201, 202, 205-206, 209-212, 216,
223, 224, 225, 227, 230, 234, 237, 238,
239, 244
Diverticulitis 77, 244
Dizziness 217
Dominican Herbal College 257
Dong Quai 68, 78, 130, 189, 195
Dossey, Larry 255
Downs, James 165, 250
Draize test 24
Drum, Ryan 51
Duke, James A. 253
Dulse 173, 184
Dysentery 197
Dyspepsia 195, 211, 224
Dysuria 104

East West Course in Herbology 257
Eastern/Central Medicinal Plants 253
Echinacea – Echinacea angustifolia 58, 66–
67, 70, 73, 74, 97, 100, 101, 105, 108, 109,
121, 137, 167, 180, 189, 201, 205, 207,
210, 214, 217, 222, 227, 238, 240
Echinacea! The Immune Herb 253
Eclectic Materia Medica, Pharmacology and
Therapeutics, The 253, 250
Eclectic physicians 78
Eczema 201, 222, 232, 239; infant 231
Egg yolks 177
Eggs 92, 127
Ejaculation 102, 106, 114, 132, 136, 142;

premature 106
Elder 72, 73, 189, 244; blossom 73;
flowers 244
Elecampane 72, 74, 189, 200, 205, 207
Eleuthro 241
Eliminative system 205
Ellingwood, Finley 79, 253, 250
Emetic 72
Emmenagogue 194, 195, 200, 202
Emollient 70, 72, 226, 227
Emperor Wears No Clothes, The 255
Endive –Cichorium endiva 45, 47
Endocrine 102, 227; gland 69, 128, 177;
system 35
Endorphins 85
Enema 112
Engstrand, Lars 183
Epididymis 130, 131, 132
Epilepsy 240
Epimedium 139
Eraldin 25
Erection 115, 135
ESO, Extended Sexual Orgasm 111, 135, 255
Essential oils 171–172, 181, 204; antimicro
bial action of 170–171
Estrogen 35, 41, 102, 136, 143, 144, 206
Ethyl alcohol 54
Eucalyptus 70, 127, 189; Eucalyptus
globulus 127, 189; Eucalyptus
polybractea 113
Everclear 54
Everywoman's Book 146, 255
Exercise 47–51, 85–86, 92, 105, 142, 143,
154
Expectorant 68, 72, 88, 205, 207, 216, 217,
222, 226, 227, 230
Eyebright 69, 189, 222, 236
Eyes 236

False Unicorn 189
Fatigue 88
Fats 146; saturated 89; unsaturated 89
Fatty acids 176, 184
FDA See Food and Drug Administration
Febrifuge 73, 224
Felter, H.W. 250, 253
Fennel – Foeniculum vulgare 67, 69, 70, 71,
75, 96, 109, 121, 129, 152, 189, 193, 215,
216, 236
Fenugreek 138, 189
Fever 72, 73, 195, 228, 237; childhood 216, 244
Feverfew – Tanacetum parthenium 74, 189,
214, 216, 238
Flatulence 195, 204, 216
Flavonoids 149
Flaxseed 112, 189; oil 176
Flu 203, 217, 227, 236, 241
Folk Medicine 17–18, 209
Fomentation 57
Food and Drug Administration (FDA) 17–18,
133, 238
Foods: Longevity 145–148
Foot bath 203

Foreskin 115, 118; inflammation of 119–123
Foster, Steven 253
Franchomme, Pierre 171, 250
Frankincense 181
Free radicals 177, 205, 219
Fringe Tree 137, 189
Fruits 86, 89, 107
Fry, William F. 85

Gaia, A New Look at Life on Earth 168, 255
Gall stones 244
Gall-bladder 43, 70, 71, 212, 232
Gandhi, Mohandas 27
Gangrene 228
Gardner, Joy 121, 253, 250
Gardnerella 121
Garlic – Allium sativum 68, 69, 70, 73, 88,
   92–93, 137, 138, 139, 167, 175, 180, 189,
   215, 217, 245; oil 218
Gas 71, 88, 96, 204, 216, 244
Gastric ulcers 43, 207, 235
Gastritis 227, 228
Gastroenteritis 225
Gelatin 57
General Adaptation Syndrome 94
Genital Herpes 124–127; warts 123–124
Genitalia 222
Genito-urinary system 66, 102, 107, 193,
   198, 201, 205, 206, 209, 210, 211, 219,
   225, 232, 234, 236, 238, 244; tonics 107
Gentian – Gentiana spp. 47, 70, 71, 74, 76,
   137, 141, 189
Geranium 98, 127, 182
Gerard, John 206
Geriatric dementia 219
Germs 156–157
Ginger – Zingiber officinale 58, 70, 71, 72,
   74, 75, 88, 127, 150, 151, 152, 153, 190,
   211, 219, 227, 244; root 147
Ginkgo – Ginkgo biloba 65, 74, 87, 88,
   93–94, 94, 96, 137, 139, 140, 141, 144,
   145, 190, 217, 219, 223
Ginseng 15, 68, 70, 97, 133, 140, 141, 150,
   151, 152, 153, 174, 190, 240; American
   69, 220; Chinese 69; Panax ginseng
   77–78; Siberian 69
Gladstar, Rosemary 150, 253, 251
Glans penis 36, 115, 118, 119
Glycerine 57
Glycerite 55
Goat's Rue 138, 190
Golden Rod 70, 75, 76, 190
Golden Seal – Hydrastis canadensis 47, 68,
   69, 70, 71, 73, 76, 100, 101, 120–121, 141,
   190, 202, 204, 205, 215, 217, 221, 232, 235
Gonadotropic hormone 134
Gonadotropin: chronic 128
Gonads 129, 177
Gonorrhea 195, 198, 211
Gotu Kola 145, 148, 185, 190
Gould, G. 36
Gout 231, 238, 239
Graedon, Joe 255

Gravel Root 70, 190, 222
Green, James 253
Green, Mindy 170
Green Pharmacy 255
Grieve, M. 253, 251
Grieves, M. 63
Griggs, Barbara 255
Grossinger, Richard 255
Guarana 153, 190
Guide to Medicinal Plants 251
Gum 67
Gums 234, 236
Gumweed – Grindelia spp. 72, 77, 96, 190,
   200, 205, 221, 222; tincture 126

Hair 175, 183–186; care 184–186; color
   224; loss 183, 201
Hawthorn – Crataegus oxyacantha 42, 68,
   87, 93–94, 96, 140, 141, 144, 145, 190, 220,
   223, 225, 232, 245; berries 73, 75, 86,
   88, 109, 137; blossoms 86; flowers 73;
   leaves 86
Hayfever 223
Headache 203, 216, 219, 240, 242; migraine 217
Healing AIDS Naturally 254
Healing Brain: Medical Discoveries about
   How the Brain Manages Health, The 167, 251
Healing Love Through the Tao: Cultivating
   Female Sexual Energy 135, 255
Healing Wise 254
Health Protection Branch of Canada 17–18
Heart 42, 144, 147; arrhythmic heartbeat
   223; attack 203; damage 175; disease
   51, 177; muscle 210; obesity 85;
   palpitations 88, 210, 223; pulse
   223; rate 48, 95; stroke 203
Heartburn 226, 228
Hemoglobin 146
Hemolysis 15
Hemophilus 121
Hemorrhaging 73, 197, 203, 207, 222, 225,
   231, 237
Hemorrhoids 205, 225, 235
Hemostatic 73
Hepatic 73, 88, 96, 201, 220, 232, 239
Hepatitis 212, 230
Herb Preparation: concentrate (very strong
   tea) 53; decoction (strong tea) 53;
   glycerite 55; infusions (tea) 53;
   liniment 54; materials 52; oil
   infusion 55; syrup 53; tincture 54
Herbal: Use of 62–67
Herbal Bounty, The Gentle Art of Herb
   Culture 253
Herbal Formulas & Recipes 150, 150–151
Herbal Gram 257
Herbal Handbook for Farm & Stable 38,
   250, 254
Herbal Handbook, The 253
Herbal Handbook: A Formulary 253
Herbal Healing Journey (School) 256
Herbal Medication 251
Herbal Medicine 254, 252

Herbal Medicine-Maker's Handbook, The
   58, 253
Herbal Preparations and Natural Therapies 256
Herbal Studies Course 257
Herbalism   9; and mainstream medicine
   19–20; and plants 8;
Herbalists   9, 21; Simpler, 52
Herer, Jack 255
Herpes 124, 164
Hidden Testis: cryptorchism 128
Hill, Amie 98
Hill, Ray 149
Hittleman, Richard L. 86, 255
Hiziki 107, 173
Ho shou wu – *Polygonum multiflorum* 68,
   141, 145, 148, 151, 185, 190, 224
Hobbs, Christopher 206, 253
Hoffmann, David 76–77, 101, 225, 253, 251
Holistic Herbal, The 76, 254, 251
Honey 145, 237; raw 93
Honey Bee 145
Hops – *Humulus lupulus* 45, 47, 71, 73, 76,
   79, 88, 96, 100, 190, 204, 212, 222, 223,
   240, 242
Horehound 73, 190, 207
Hormonal imbalances   43; building
   assistance 41
Hormones: Endocrine Physiology, The 251
Horsechestnut – *Aesculus hippocastanum* 14-
   15, 17, 62, 64, 68, 71, 75, 76, 137, 190,
   223, 224, 236
Horseradish 74, 109, 138, 167, 190, 215
Horsetail – *Equisetum arvense* 72, 74, 76,
   108, 186, 190, 198, 209, 225, 240, 245
Hot packs 107
How to Get Well 255
Human papilloma virus (HPV) 123, 164
Human Variation 165, 250
Hydrangea– *Hydrangea arborescens,*
   canadensis 70, 108, 109, 190, 210, 226,
   228, 240
Hydrastis 190, 221
Hygieia, A Woman's Herbal 254
Hygiene 154, 165
Hyperacidity 69
Hyperactivity 242
Hyperemia: Blood engorgement 246
Hypertension 88–90, 175, 223, 241
Hypnotic 73, 203, 224, 241, 242
Hypoglycemia 43, 138, 212-213
Hypoglycemia: A Better Approach 138, 254
Hypogonadism 140
Hypokinetic Disease 49, 251
Hypopituitarism 140
Hypotensive 73, 96, 217, 222, 223, 241
Hypothyroidism 140
Hyssop – *Hyssopus officinalis* 68, 70, 72, 190
Hysteria 240

Illustrated Encyclopedia of Herbs 254
Immobilized Patient, The 48, 251
Immune system 51, 66, 70, 96, 105, 108,
   109, 121, 133, 149, 151, 154, 164, 172,
   174, 175, 197, 215, 217, 241
Impotence 51, 69, 70, 88, 89, 134, 138,
   139, 148, 241
Incontinence 193, 244
Indigestion 43, 88, 193, 203
Infections 46, 69, 72, 217; bladder 215;
   bacterial 215; bronchial 223;
   prostate 222; respiratory 215;
   vaginal 121; viral 215; yeast/
   candida 121
Infertility 140–141
Inflammation 46, 711
Infusion 53, 108
Insect bites 223
Insomnia 147, 196, 204, 223, 237, 240, 242
Insulin 89, 137; substitute 213
International Foundation for Ethical
   Research 25
Intestines 99; small 228
Iodine 184, 226
Ipecac 72
Irish Moss – *Chondrus crispus* 147, 190, 226
Iron 184, 226, 245
Ismelin 136

Jaundice 69, 230
Jerusalem Artichoke 138
Jing 114, 185
Jitterbug Perfume 254
Joints 48–49, 74, 196, 201, 205, 218, 228
Jokl, Ernst 143
Juniper 180

Kale 175
Kaptchuk, Ted 255
Kegel, Arnold 110
Kegel exercises 109–111, 139
Kelp 89, 107, 173, 184
Kenner, Daniel 254
Keville, Kathi 104
Kidneys 20, 71, 102, 108, 147, 185, 198,
   201 204, 205, 207, 212, 222, 224, 230,
   237; stones 70, 210, 228
King's American Dispensatory 250
Knees 196
Koch, Robert 25, 156–157
Koehler, Nan 255
Kola 190, 212
Kombu 173
Kraus, H. 49, 251

L-lysine tablets 127
Labia 36, 117
Lady's Mantle 75, 190
Lard 89
Laryngitis 193, 211, 215
Larynx 128
Laughter 83–84
Lavandula vera 122, 182
Lavender 71, 95, 96, 112, 122, 172, 181,
   182, 190, 223
Laxative 66, 71, 73, 89, 96, 211, 212, 218,
   220, 227, 230, 232, 234, 245

LD-50 24; test 24
Lecithin 177
Lemon 98, 124
Lemon Balm 86, 96
Lettuce 175
Leucorrhea 198, 211
Licorice – *Glycyrrhiza glabra* 15, 42, 69, 70, 72, 75, 97, 133, 141, 151, 152, 153, 190, 205, 215, 227, 227; root 147; tea 126
Limbic system 168
Linden 93–94, 190; blossoms 75, 96
Liniment 195, 205; preparation 54
Linoleic acid 107
Liver 20, 43, 46, 71, 73, 95, 124, 133, 141, 147, 180, 205, 212, 222, 224, 232, 234, 237, 239
Lives of Cells, The 158, 252
Lloyd, J. 250
Lobelia – *Lobelia inflata* 72, 73, 96, 190, 200, 217, 223, 227, 228
Longevity 143–149, 241; foods 145–148
Lovage 185
Lovelock, James E. 168, 255
Lungs 197, 205, 207, 217, 219, 227
Lymph 197; nodes 207
Lymphatic 66, 73, 100, 215; actions 180; glands 158; system 206, 215, 232, 235
Lysine foods 127

Ma Huang 190
Magnesium 176, 184
Male: reproductive system 66; contraception 142–143; pattern baldness 183; problems: prostate 101–114
Mammary glands 79
Marc 54
Margarine 89, 176
Marijuana 136
Marjoram 98
Marshmallow – *Althaea officinalis* 53, 72, 75, 96, 108, 153, 190, 198, 201, 202, 204, 207, 227, 228, 232, 244; root 100, 105, 121, 123, 136
Marty the Marathon Bear 48, 256
Massage 97, 141, 185; oils 205
Masturbation 117–118
McDougall, John A. 86, 255
McDougall Plan, The 255
McQuade-Crawford, Amanda 42, 77, 152, 254
Medical Herbalism 257
Meadowsweet – *Filipendula ulmaria* 69, 70, 75, 100, 101, 190, 207, 228
Meat 89, 92, 127
Medicinal Mushrooms 253
Medicinal Plants of the Desert and Canyon West 254, 251
Medicinal Plants of the Mountain West 254, 251
Medicine & Culture 162
Medicine Cards 256
Medicines from the Earth 254
Meditation 97

Melilot 190
Memory 144, 219, 241
Meningitis 157
Menopause 206, 237, 238
Men's Health 50
Menstrual cramps 195; cycle 142, 244
Merck Manual 138, 255
Migraine headache 43, 217
Milk 127, 176
Milk Thistle – *Silybum marianum* 124, 190, 205, 222, 229, 230, 238
Milk Thistle 230
Mindell, Earl 174, 255
Mineral supplements 173–177
Minerals 20, 146, 194, 212, 226, 240
Miso 107, 127
Modern Herbal, The 253, 251
Monilia: yeast/candida infections 121
Moore, Michael 254, 251
Motherwort 68, 88, 96, 191, 223
Mother Jones 257
Mouth: inflammation 227; ulcers 77, 234, 236; wash 236
Moxa 129
Mucilage 227
Mucilaginous 101, 107, 112
Mucous membranes 100, 198, 211, 222, 228
Mucus 69, 72
Mugwort 40, 42, 47, 71, 76, 77, 88, 138, 141, 191
Muir, Caroline 114, 256
Muir, Charles 114, 256
Mulberry 138, 191
Mullein 69, 72, 73, 74, 191, 200, 202, 231
Mumps 130, 195
Muscle: atrophy 51; pains 242; sore 196
Musculo-skeletal system 75, 203, 204, 207, 210, 213, 217, 228, 237, 238, 244
Mushrooms 175, 176; poisoning 230
Mustard 74, 109, 176
Mustard seed 74
Myrrh 70, 97, 182, 191, 202, 204, 205, 215, 222

Narcotic 225
Nasal catarrh 204
National Anti-Vivisection Society 25
National Organization of Circumcision Information 119, 251
Nature Doctor, The 254, 252
Nature's Children 254
Nausea 217, 228, 246
Nerve: pain 196; tonic 66
Nervine 73, 88, 89, 100, 113, 121, 129, 130, 210, 217, 231
Nervous system 42, 66, 73, 75, 79, 90, 95, 126, 127, 141, 144, 148, 154, 164, 197, 203, 204, 210, 211, 217, 219, 224, 231, 237, 241, 242, 246
Nettle 68, 69, 138, 152, 177, 180, 186, 191
Neuralgia 240
Neurasthenia 196
New Healing Yourself, The 121, 253, 250

Newsweek 162, 251
Nicotine 89, 99, 113, 136
Nori 107, 173
Nutmeg 153
Nutrient 66, 194, 217
Nutrition 251
Nutritional yeasts 127
Nutritive 129, 207, 230, 239, 245
Nuts 86, 127, 176, 177

Oak Bark 76, 123, 191
Oat – Avena sativa 41, 68, 73, 138, 191
Obesity 89
Oil Infusion: preparation 55
Oils 89, 92; almond 89; Bergamot
  122; canola 89; flaxseed 176; garlic
  218; Lavender 122; lemon 98;
  massage 205; palm 89; palm
  kernel 89; peanut 89; rose 141;
  Rosemary 186; safflower 89, 176;
  sesame seed 89, 176, 185; skin
  205; sunflower 89; sunflower seed
  176; Tea Tree 122; Thuja 124;
  vegetable 92, 176; volatile 70-71, 244;
  wheat germ 89
Olfactory nerve cells 169
Olive Leaf 138, 191
Olive oil 138, 181
Onion 69, 73, 88, 138, 177, 217
Opium Poppy 203
Orange 191
Orange Peel 152, 153
Orchitis 130, 195, 206
Oregon Grape 68, 69, 70, 71, 105, 109, 191,
  201, 205, 212, 222, 233, 234, 240
Ornstein, Robert 168, 251
Osha 72, 191
Osteoporosis 49, 51
Ovaries 35, 79
Oysters 175

Palm kernel oil 89
Palm oil 89
Panax ginseng 77-78, 241
Panax quinquefolius 81
Pancreas 71, 137, 174, 212, 224
Pancreatic juices 178; secretions 43
Pantothenic acid 148
Papaya 175
Parasites 172, 217
Parasympathetic blocking agents 136
Paris, F. 251
Parsley 93, 176, 185, 191, 228
Partridgeberry 71, 191, 222
Parvati, Jeannine 135, 254
Pasque Flower 191
Passion Flower 69, 74, 88, 96, 191
Passwater, Richard 174, 177, 256, 251
Pasteur, Louis 24-25, 156-157
Pasteurella pestis bacteria 164
Pathologic Basis of Disease 251
Payer, Lynn 162-163, 251
Peaches 175

Peanut butter 127, 150
Peanut oil 89
Peanuts 127
Pectoral 74
Pei, Mario 10, 20, 256
Pelargonium Asperum 127
Penis 36, 109, 115-126, 128; cancer
  123; health-care 120-121; inflamma
  tion 119-123; soaks 121-122
Pennyroyal 40, 191
People's Pharmacy, The 255
Peppermint 70, 71, 72, 73, 75, 96, 191, 244
Peptic ulcers 194, 202, 227
Perineum 113
Peristalsis 71
Peristaltic muscles 205
Periwinkle 123, 191
Pesto 93
Pharmacology 13
Pharynx inflammation 227
Phimosis 120
Phlebitis 196, 225
Phosphorus 177, 184
Physicians' Desk Reference 15
Phytomedical research 169-170
Phytosteroids 174
Phytosterols 92
Phytotherapists 109
Phytotherapy 169, 169-170, 172
Pineal glands 177
Pipsissewa 71, 108, 191, 236
Pituitary glands 140, 177, 206
Placenta 128
Planet Medicine 255
Planetary Herbology 254, 252
Plant: gum 67; mucilage 67
Plantain 72, 74, 75, 89, 101, 182, 191, 233
Plants: and the human body 20-22;
Plaque 177
Play 83-84
Pleurisy 195
PMS 43
Pneumococcus 159
Pneumonia 226
Poison Ivy 223
Poison Oak 77, 223
Polarity reversal 144
Polio 157
Pollen 145, 146
Pomegranate seeds 143
Poppy seeds 107
Potassium 89, 184, 212, 230
Potato 15
Poultices 57, 182, 195, 209, 219
Practice of Aromatherapy, The 254
Pregnancy 175, 195
Prepuce 115, 118
Price, Weston 251
Prickly Ash 74, 152, 191, 211, 225, 235
Priest, A.W. 251
Priest, L.R. 251
Progesterone 41, 206
Pronatec International 178

Propolis 145, 148–149
Propolis — The Natural Antibiotic 149
Prostate 35, 41, 66, 101–114, 128, 148, 176, 198, 210, 211, 222, 234, 239, 245; benign enlargement 104, 225; enlargement 231; gland 58, 177; malignant enlargement 111–112, 175; tonic 151
Prostatic fluid 102; urethra 105
Prostatitis 175, 195, 210, 234
Prostitis 105–109
Protein 194
Prune plums 175
Psoriasis 201, 230, 232, 245
Puberty 128
Pubococcygeal muscle 109
Pumpkin 175, 191
Pumpkin seeds 107, 150, 175
Punctures 182
Pyelitis 198

Qi 78

Raab, W. 49, 251
Radiation therapy 4
Raisins 127, 176
Rashes 182
Raspberry 38–40, 68, 76, 152, 191, 236
Raw honey 53
Recipes: Herbal 150
Rectum 207
Red Clover 69, 96, 191, 202, 227, 236
Red pepper 175
Red Raspberry 38–42, 141, 228
Red Sage 77
Red-to-Orange Chakra Express 152
Rejuvenation Secrets From Around The World—That Work 146
Relaxant 73, 217
Reproductive organs 126; atrophy 174
Reproductive system 41, 42, 66, 75–76, 77, 107, 200, 215, 224, 244, 246
Requena, Yves 254
Respiration 48
Respiratory system 71, 72, 74, 75–76, 197, 200, 203, 205, 207, 211, 213, 215, 216, 217, 219, 223, 226, 227, 235, 241, 242, 246
Restorative tonic 150
Review of Materia Medica 250
Rheumatic inflammation 200
Rheumatism 74, 196, 205, 212, 213, 228, 231, 235, 238, 242
Rhubarb root 73
Ringworm 222
Robbins, Stanley L. 102, 251
Robbins, Tom 254, 256
Rose oil 141, 172
Rosemary 70, 76, 98, 145, 191; oil 186
Rosewood 98
Royal Jelly 145, 148
Rubefacient 70, 74, 203, 218
Rue 69

Saccharin 178

Sachs, T. Elder 8, 29, 84, 99, 132, 142
Safflower oil 89, 176
Sage 70, 76, 122, 186, 191, 227, 236, 245
Sage Healing Ways 253
St. John's Wort 124, 192, 207, 237, 228
Saliva 74, 149
Salivary glands 74, 130
Salt 92, 184
Salve 205, 209; preparation 56
Sandalwood 98, 182
Saponins 15, 67, 133
Sarsaparilla 15, 68, 70, 105, 133, 138, 140, 141, 147, 150, 152, 153, 174, 180, 191, 201, 202, 227
Sarsparilla 141
Sassafras 42, 151, 153, 191, 238
Saw Palmetto 40–42, 58, 66–67, 68, 70, 78–80, 81, 105, 107, 108, 109, 126, 129, 133, 140, 141, 148, 150, 151, 152, 191, 200, 210, 215, 220, 222, 231, 232, 238, 239
Sawin, Clark T. 251
Scalds 182
Schauenberg, P. 251
Schizandra 69
Schnaubelt, Kurt 170, 251
School of Natural Healing 100, 253, 250
Science and Art of Herbology, The 251
Sclera 92
Scrapes 182
Scrotum 36, 107, 128, 130, 206
Scullcap 40–42, 42, 68, 69, 74, 79, 90, 95, 106, 124, 126, 140, 180, 192, 212, 222, 232, 242
Sea salt 93
Seafoods 184
Seaweed 184
Sebaceous glands 120
Secret Life of Plants 256
Sedative 74, 88, 96, 196, 200, 203, 210, 223, 224, 234, 237, 240, 241, 242
Seeds 86, 107, 177
Seizures 217, 240
Selenium 177
Selye, Hans 94
Semen 102, 132, 175, 177
Seminal fluid 28, 132, 176
Seminal vesicles 128
Septic wounds 235
Serenoa serrulata 78, 191
Sesame oil 176, 185
Sesame seeds 107, 150; butter 150; oil 89
Setchenov, I.M. 156
Sex glands 147
Sexual intercourse 121
Sexual organ dysfunctions 43
Sexual vitality 151
Sharlip, Ira 106
Sheperd's Purse 73, 192
Shingles 75
Shook, Edward 251
Sialogogue 74, 215

Siberian Ginseng   69, 74, 88, 97, 105, 107, 108, 133, 137, 138, 140, 141, 148, 150, 151, 167, 192, 197
Silica   184
Silicon   230
Simple   52
Simpler   52
Sinus   69
Skin   72, 74, 75, 127, 170, 175, 178–181, 193, 196, 197, 201, 202, 204, 213, 222, 232, 239; diseases   207; disorders   213; eruptions   69, 207; mature   181; normal to dry   181; normal to oily   181; oils   205; perspiration   71; sun damaged   181; ulcers   202
Skinny Legs and All   256
Skullcap   145
Slant board   185
Sleep   73, 237
Slippery Elm   53, 69, 72, 75, 100, 120–121 192, 194
Smegma   120
Smith, Ed   143
Smoking   89, 135, 175
Sobel, David   168, 251
Sodium   89
Sore throat   149, 193, 197, 234, 236
Sores   215
Sorrel   192
Southernwood   192
Southwest School of Botanical Studies   256
Soya beans   15, 175, 177
Space, Time & Medicine   255
Sperm   28, 34, 114, 127–130, 132, 140, 177
Spermatogenisis   128
Spermatorrhea   211
Spermatozoa   28
Spike Lavender   180
Spinach   138, 175
Spinal nerves   71
Spirulina algae   150, 174
Spleen   174, 212, 230
Sprains   74, 196, 207, 218
Stamina   147, 241
Staphylococci bacilli   157
Staphylococcus   148, 159
Star Anise   151, 153, 192
Starches   86
Steinberg, Franz   48–49, 251
Sterility   35, 130
Steroids   227, 230
Stimulant   74, 194, 197, 203, 211, 217, 218, 219, 220, 235, 236, 245
Stinging Nettle   69, 74, 92, 186, 229
Stings   182
Stomach   71, 72, 99, 100, 195, 207, 211, 212, 222, 228, 236; acids   178; disorders   213; pain   203; ulcers   235
Stones   70, 198, 207
Stop Hair Loss   250
Story of Language, The   10, 256
Strawberry   152, 192
Streptococcus   148, 159

Stress   51, 74, 94–98, 96, 105, 106, 126, 133, 137, 140, 144, 154, 184, 241
Styptic   74, 202, 225, 244
Sucanat®   178
Successful Stress Control   101, 254, 251
Sugar   46, 113, 127, 178
Suma   69, 97, 107, 109, 137, 138, 140, 141, 192, 197
Sunflower seeds   107, 138, 175
Super-Nutrition for Healthy Hearts   256
Supernutrition for Healthy Hearts   177, 251
Suppository: Preparation   56
Syrup: Preparation   53
System tonics   141
Szent-Gyorgi, Albert   20

Tagamet   136
Tai Chi   50–51, 97
Tannins   67
Tantra the Art of Conscious Loving   114, 256
Tantra Yoga   114
Taoist Secrets of Love: Cultivating Male Sexual Energy   111, 135, 255
Tea   101, 129; Licorice   126; White Sage   126
Tea Tree   122, 124, 127, 172, 192
Tension   224, 240
Terpenoid compounds   171
Testicles   35, 122, 127–130, 177, 195, 206
Testicular Self-Examination   130–131
Testis   140
Testosterone   34–35, 79, 104, 127–130, 133, 136, 144, 174, 175, 183
Tetanus   171
Thalidomide   25
Therapeutic Herbalism   257
Thie, Krista   254
Thomas, Lewis   158, 252
Thomson, William   254
Thuja   192; oil   124
Thyme   69, 70, 152, 167, 192
Thymol   171
Thyroid gland   140
Tierra, Michael   254, 252
Tincture   101, 107, 121, 129; Preparation   53–54
Tinnitus   217, 219
Tisserand, Robert   254
Tissues   211
Tobacco   92, 135
Tomato   16, 175, 177
Tonic   68, 78, 123, 151, 193, 194, 196 197, 206, 209, 211, 212, 213, 217, 220, 223, 224, 226, 227, 230, 231, 232, 234, 235, 236,
Tonsils   207; tonsillitis   215
Toxins   71
Trace elements   194
Traditional Chinese Medicine   46, 106, 114
Tranquilizers   25
Travel sickness   204
Trichomonas   121
Tsitsin, Nicolai   146

Tuberculosis 213
Tumeric 192
Tumors 207
Turmeric 69
Turner, Nancy 213

Ulcers 99–101, 136, 202, 207, 226; duodenal 99, 202, 207, 227; gastric 99, 207, 235; mouth 77; mouth 234, 236; peptic 194, 202, 227; skin 202; stomach 235
Upton, Roy 106
Urethra 102, 115, 195, 211, 234, 245
Urethritis 121, 198, 209, 210
Urinary antiseptic 66
Urinary system 75–76, 108, 197, 200, 204, 206, 207, 212, 216, 226, 230, 235, 237
Urinary tract infection 105, 106, 117
Urine 20, 72, 79, 102, 104–106, 107, 108, 132, 209
Usnea 167, 192
Uterus 123
Uva Ursi 70, 72, 108, 137, 192, 201, 207

Vagina 36, 123
Valerian 69, 73, 74, 79, 88, 96, 100, 106, 152, 180, 192, 204, 224, 238, 240, 242, 243
Valnet, Jean 254
Varicose veins 225, 235
Vas deferens 128, 131
Vasodilator 70, 74, 88, 217, 219, 223, 241, 244
Vegetables 86, 89, 107, 174, 176, 177; leafy 127
Venereal disease 105; warts 121
Vertigo 219
Vervain 68, 89, 96, 192
Vinegar 123
Virchow, Robert 163
Vitamin A 15, 174, 184; B 142, 184; B₁₂ 146; C 108, 124; D 184; E 107, 124, 174, 177, 184; F 107, 184; supplements 173–177
Vitamin Bible 255
Vitex 38
Vitex! The Female Herb 206
Vogel, A. 252, 254
Volatile oils 244
Vomiting 70, 72
Vulnerary 70, 74, 88, 96, 193, 195, 196, 204, 225, 231, 237, 244
Vulva 123

Watermellon seed 108
Way of Herbs, The 252, 254
Web That Has No Weaver, The 255
Weed, Susun 254
Weiss, Rudolf Fritz 206, 254, 252
Wheat 176
Wheat germ 176; oil 89, 176
White Horehound 72, 76, 227, 228
Whooping cough 217

Wild Cherry 192; bark 96
Wildfire 258
Wildflower 258
Wildlife Conservation 258
Wild Indigo 192, 217
Wild Lettuce 47, 73, 96, 192
Wild Oat 42, 90, 91, 96, 124, 140, 147, 148, 192, 212, 220, 242
Wild Yam 15, 68, 70, 71, 73, 77 96, 133 138, 141, 151, 152, 174, 192, 205, 211, 228, 242
Willow 75
Willow Bark 192
Winston, David 126
Witch Hazel 14, 71, 76, 96, 192, 196, 202, 222
Wood, Bill 48, 256
Worms 69
Wormwood 47, 69, 70, 74, 192
Wounds: septic 228

Yam 175
Yarrow 40, 42, 47, 58, 66–67, 68, 69, 70, 72, 73, 74, 75, 76, 87, 88, 93–94, 108, 109, 122, 123, 137, 141, 167, 185, 192, 198, 200, 210, 212, 215, 223, 225, 244
Yeast 172
Yeast infections 121
Yellow Dock 68, 73, 152, 180, 192, 201, 232, 243
Yerba Manza 167, 192
Yerba Maté 192
Yerba Santa 70, 74, 200, 205, 223
Yin Yang Huo 139
Ylang Ylang 98
Yoga 97, 255
Yoga 86
Yohimbe 70, 133, 139, 152, 192
Yucca 133, 192

Zinc 107, 124, 175–176, 177